Phytochemicals Targeting Tumor Microenvironment in Gastrointestinal Cancers

Ganji Purnachandra Nagaraju
Editor

Phytochemicals Targeting Tumor Microenvironment in Gastrointestinal Cancers

Springer

Editor
Ganji Purnachandra Nagaraju
Winship Cancer Institute
Department of Hematology
and Medical Oncology
Emory University
Atlanta, GA, USA

ISBN 978-3-030-48404-0 ISBN 978-3-030-48405-7 (eBook)
https://doi.org/10.1007/978-3-030-48405-7

This Springer imprint is published by the registered company Springer Nature Switzerland AG
The registered company address is: Gewerbestrasse 11, 6330 Cham, Switzerland

Preface

Recent studies from global cancer statistics have revealed that gastrointestinal (GI) cancers include esophagus, gastric, pancreas, colorectal, liver, and gallbladder cancers. These cancers collectively depict public health issues in the USA and around the globe. According to the American Cancer Society (ACS), GI cancers are reported to have the highest incidence rate and are the second leading cause of cancer-related mortality. Colorectal cancer (CRC) exhibits increased incidence rate in high-income countries, whereas other cancers like gastric, liver, and esophageal most frequently occur in low-income countries. GI cancers are among the five most common cancers detected in both males and females. The most common risk factor associated with GI cancer is diet. It is clearly elucidated from previous studies that GI cancer incidence is highly correlated with food intake. Other common factors include *Helicobacter pylori*, gastric ulcers like gastroesophageal reflux disease, smoking, and alcohol. Conventional therapies including surgery followed by chemo- and radiotherapies are usually the only therapeutic strategies, which can be effective, but the patient survival rate is only 5 years. Even though advanced research techniques treat patients for a certain period of time, the issue of recurrence and metastasis still persist. This could be due to the resistance that is developed by tumor cells and dysregulated signaling pathways. The tumor microenvironment is an extracellular matrix that includes collagens, glycoproteins, dendritic cells, tumor-associated macrophages, and mast cells. Moreover, the tumor microenvironment regulates the behavior of cancer stem cells (CSC) via modulating immune surveillance and cell-to-cell signaling. Thus, it has gained attention as it is required to induce initiation, progression, and metastasis. Phytochemicals are now a focus for researchers due to their antioxidative property to treat cancer cells. Therefore, including fresh fruits and vegetables rich in antioxidants can control the growth of tumor. This book illustrates various dysregulated signaling pathways and the role of phytochemicals. This also includes novel nanotechniques used to enhance the therapeutic efficacy of drugs in use.

Our book mainly focuses on CRC, gastric, hepatic, and pancreatic cancers. These cancers are the most prevalent cancers that are detected worldwide. Besides the genetic and environmental alterations, gut microbiota plays a profound role in causing GI cancer. The human body has significant microorganisms among which gut microbiota and *H. pylori* play a chief role in the advancement of GI cancer, especially CRC. The gut microbiota shows its impact on epithelial cells and drives cancer progression. This chapter outlines the process to control the growth of gut microbiota in order to avoid the risk of GI cancer. Moreover, tumor resistance and recurrence are the main reasons for poor prognosis of these cancers. Cancer stem cells (CSCs) were suggested to play a crucial role in recurrence as well as developing resistance to traditional therapies. The extracellular matrix continuously maintains cross talk between the cancer cell and tumor microenvironment to maintain the stemness of CSCs. The authors focus on the biology of CSCs in the tumor microenvironment. They are widely detected in various cancers and are suggested as an important therapeutic target. Additionally, the CSCs of GI cancers express unique surface markers including CD24, CD44, CD133, CD26, CD166, and CD90. They play an important role in the self-renewal of tumor cells and activate Wnt, Hedgehog, and Notch signaling pathways. Therefore, targeting these specific CSC markers could offer new therapeutic approach to eradicate GI malignancies.

Diet and nutrition are the two primary factors to uphold good health. Diet can show both positive and negative effects equally. These are the principal determinants for causing chronic diseases like cancer. They are also studied as antioxidant determinants to prevent cancer. Thus, diet can be studied as a blend of mutagenic, carcinogenic, and protective agents. The relationship of GI cancers with diet has been widely studied in various epidemiological research data. High intake of fruits and vegetables probably reduces the risk of GI cancer occurrence. Using these natural agents and their derivatives for the therapy of human chronic diseases like cancer is known as naturotherapy. This form of therapy includes use of plant derivatives, supplements, herbs, and nutrients. These therapies are completely free of chemical exposure and may or may not include marginal processing. Our book focuses on various herbal medicines and has highlighted preclinical evaluations against GI cancers. Phytochemicals, on the other side, are nonnutritive bioactive secondary compounds abundantly extracted from fruits, vegetables, and grains. Consumption of these phytochemicals keeps chronic disorders like neurodegenerative and cardiovascular diseases away. Moreover, they are also studied as chemopreventive agents against cancers like GI cancer. They were determined to alter various signaling pathways like PI3K/Akt and NF-κB. Authors of this book describe various phytochemicals including resveratrol, genistein, curcumin, and EGCG. Curcumin and its relation with gut microbiota are highlighted in the book to direct its association to decreased GI cancer progression and its role in inhibiting CRC. Additionally, garlic and its natural constituents are found to possess medicinal benefits. These constituents are sulfur compounds and are found to inhibit GI cancer angiogenesis. They downregulate the expression of VEGF and NO signaling.

Furthermore, phytochemicals are used in combinational therapies to potentiate the therapeutic efficacy of various inhibitors like checkpoint inhibitors that are used against GI cancers. They induce cell cycle arrest and block cell cycle to mediate apoptosis of tumor cells. With the advancement of nanotechnology in the field of research, drug efficiency has increased tremendously. This chapter focuses on the combination of nanoparticles and phytochemicals. The phytochemical usage is limited in the medical field due to their poor bioavailability and low stability. Researchers are now combining nanoparticles and phytochemicals, which can improve the bioavailability, solubility, and half-life and increase the stability of phytochemicals.

Our book summarizes the contemporary advances performed so far for managing GI therapy. The biology and molecular mechanisms explained would enable researchers to concentrate on markers. A clear understanding regarding the development of resistance and metastasis would support in drug designing and therapeutic strategies for improving the drug delivery mechanisms. It is our pleasure to present the novel advances with updated clinical information to the research community. This will encourage novel thoughts and ideas for innovative therapeutic to benefit GI patients.

Atlanta, GA, USA Ganji Purnachandra Nagaraju

Contents

About the Editor

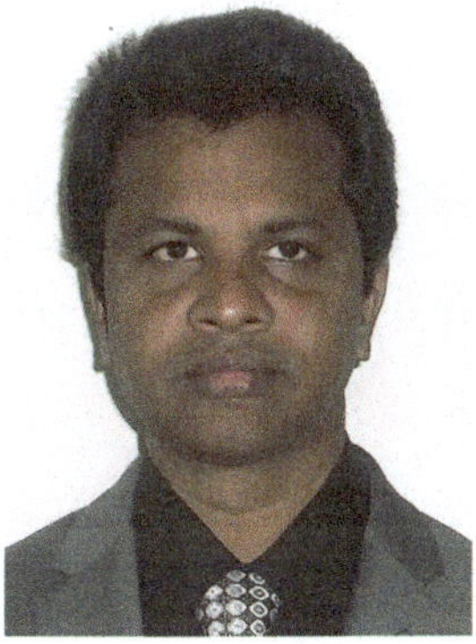

Ganji Purnachandra Nagaraju is a faculty member in the Department of Hematology and Medical Oncology at Emory University School of Medicine. Dr. Nagaraju obtained his MSc and PhD, both in Biotechnology, from Sri Venkateswara University in Tirupati, Andhra Pradesh, India. Dr. Nagaraju received his DSc from Berhampur University in Berhampur, Odisha, India. Dr. Nagaraju's research focuses on translational projects related to gastrointestinal malignancies. He has published over 100 research papers in highly reputed international journals and has presented more than 50 abstracts at various national and international conferences. Dr. Nagaraju is author and editor of several published books including (1) *Role of Tyrosine Kinases in Gastrointestinal Malignancies*, (2) *Role of Transcription Factors in Gastrointestinal Malignancies*, (3) *Breaking Tolerance to Pancreatic Cancer Unresponsiveness to Chemotherapy*, (4) *Theranostic Approach for Pancreatic Cancer*, and (5) *Exploring Pancreatic Metabolism and Malignancy*. He serves as editorial board member of several internationally recognized academic journals. Dr. Nagaraju is an associate member of the Discovery and Developmental Therapeutics Research Program at Winship Cancer Institute. Dr. Nagaraju has received several international awards including FAACC. He also holds memberships with the Association of Scientists of Indian Origin in America (ASIOA), the Society for Integrative and Comparative Biology (SICB), the Science Advisory Board, the RNA Society, the American Association for Clinical Chemistry (AACC), and the American Association of Cancer Research (AACR).

Chapter 1
Role of Specific Phytochemicals Against Gastrointestinal Malignancies

Dariya Begum, Neha Merchant, and Ganji Purnachandra Nagaraju

Abstract The estimation from the American Cancer Society recorded cancer with the highest incidence and mortality rate every year. The most common cancer as estimated from the global cancer statistics is the gastrointestinal cancers with a major mortality rate. The common conventional therapies including chemo- and radiation therapies can improve prognosis of the patient only up to 5% due to adverse toxic side effect and multidrug resistance (MDR) developed by the patient against therapeutic drugs. The onset of these digestive system-related cancers is due to the Western lifestyle and food habits. The epidemiological studies evidenced that use of phytochemicals has significant health benefits. They are bestowed with their antioxidant and anticarcinogenic properties that control multiple signalling pathways involved in tumor progression like PI3k/Akt/MAPK and sensitize the tumor-suppressor gene like p53 to the chemo-drugs. This chapter presents cancers of the upper gastrointestinal tract (esophagus and gastric) and a part of lower intestine (colon and rectum) with specific phytochemicals inhibiting the tumor. It also focus on the molecular mechanism involved in promoting cancer and role of the phytochemicals in regulating these signalling pathways. It also include derivative forms of phytochemicals and their enhancement efficacy when used in combinational therapies. We further focus on novel nano-formulated phytochemicals used against cancer therapy. Thus, our chapter summarizes the use of phytochemicals that strengthen as a therapeutic candidate against gastrointestinal malignancies.

Keywords Gastrointestinal cancers · Phytochemicals · CRC · Esophageal cancer · Gastric cancer · Chemo-drugs

---

D. Begum
Department of Biosciences and Biotechnology, Banasthali University, Banasthali, India

N. Merchant · G. P. Nagaraju (✉)
Dept. of Hematology and Medical Oncology, Winship Cancer Institute, Emory University, Atlanta, GA, USA
e-mail: pganji@emory.edu

G. P. Nagaraju (ed.), *Phytochemicals Targeting Tumor Microenvironment in Gastrointestinal Cancers*, https://doi.org/10.1007/978-3-030-48405-7_1

Abbreviations

5-FU	5-Fluorouracil
ABCB	ATP-binding cassette subfamily B member
ACF	Aberrant crypt foci
AMPK	5′-AMP-activated protein kinase
APC	Adenomatous polyposis coli
Chk1	Checkpoint kinase 1
COX-2	Cyclooxygenase-2
CRC	Colorectal cancer
CSC	Cancer stem cells
DCA	Deoxycholic acid
EC	Esophageal cancer
EGCG	Epigallocatechin-3-gallate
EGFR	Epidermal growth factor receptor
EMT	Epithelial mesenchymal transition
GC	Gastric cancer
HER2	Human epidermal growth factor
IL-8	Interleukin-8
iNOS	Inducible nitric oxide synthase
JAK	Janus kinase
MDR	Multidrug resistance
MMP	Matrix metalloproteinases
mTOR	Mammalian target of rapamycin
NF-κB	Nuclear factor kappa B
NRF2	Nuclear factor erythroid 2-related factor 2
PARP	Poly (ADP-ribose) polymerase
PEG	Polyethylene glycol
P-gp	P-glycoprotein
PLGA	Poly (lactic-co-glycolic acid)
ROS	Reactive oxygen species
STAT3	Signal transducer and activator of transcription 3
TNF-α	Tumor necrosis factor-alpha
VEGF	Vascular endothelial growth factor

1 Introduction

The American Cancer Society estimated 1,762,450 new cancer cases with 606,880 deaths recorded for the year 2019 [1]. The current results from the global cancer statistics, 2018, estimated that the most common cause for the mortality was gastrointestinal cancers worldwide that mainly include colorectal (CRC), gastric, and liver cancers [2]. The incidence for this disease varies in terms of both geography and population showing social and environmental variations [3]. For instance, the highest incidence rate diagnosed is for CRC in high-income countries and esophageal, gastric, and liver cancers in low-income countries [2, 4]. The tumor initiates in the small intestine commonly and causes symptoms only after the tumor is stabilized at a certain location and attains a certain size. The risk factors including usage of opium, biomass, *H. pylori*, smoking, and alcoholism with an incidence rate increased exponentially in respect to the individual' s age and lifestyle. Diagnosing and screening GI malignancy at its higher risk followed by surgical resection and conventional therapies are considered as the golden standards for GI malignancy therapy. The novel adjuvant chemo- and radiation therapies may increase the overall survival rate of patients but are with serious symptoms. The widely used drugs are cisplatin, methotrexate, doxorubicin, taxanes, and many molecular targeting agents [5]; however they are with serious unwanted adverse side effects including cardiac toxicity, hair loss, lesions in the gastrointestinal tract, bone marrow suppression, and neurological dysfunction [5–7]. Additionally, development of resistance against the drugs used is a serious hurdle and results in poor prognosis of patients. In this regard, new anticancer drugs with more efficacy, less side effects, and less toxicity to healthy cells are necessary and are continued.

Earlier, the natural compounds extracted from herbal medicinal plants were traditionally used for the therapy of various diseases like cancers. Phytochemicals are the heterogenous, bioactive compounds extracted from medicinal herbs and are naturally obtained from fruits and vegetables that include compounds like quercetin, resveratrol, isoflavones, curcumin, and epigallocatechin gallate [8]. They are found to show chemopreventive properties. Cancer chemoprevention includes the use of varied forms of natural and biological agents that inhibit the tumor growth via participating in various signalling pathways that are involved in tumor suppressing, apoptosis, and cell proliferation [8–12]. Moreover, they are found to possess antioxidant, anticarcinogenic, and anti-inflammatory characteristics [8]. Thus, as evidenced from the earlier research works on chemoprevention, the higher the consumption of fruits and vegetables the lower the occurrence of gastrointestinal malignancies. This chapter focuses on the therapeutic role of various phytochemicals used for the prevention of gastrointestinal cancer.

Gastrointestinal malignancies include a group of cancers that affect the digestive system. The tumors included are esophagus, gallbladder, hepatic, gastric, pancreatic, and colorectal cancer.

2 Esophageal Cancer

Esophageal cancer [EC] is the eighth most serious gastrointestinal cancer worldwide and sixth leading cause for mortality [13]. As estimated from the American Cancer Society for the year 2020, the new EC cases diagnosed were 18,440 and deaths recorded were 16,170. It is a common disease detected mostly in male than in female. It exists as two common forms, adenocarcinoma and squamous cell carcinoma; it is revealed from their etiological and epidemiological studies that the main cause of EC is the severity in gastroesophageal reflux disease, Barrett's esophagus, human papilloma virus infection, alcohol, and smoking. Jenkins et al. [14] reported that the patients with reflux disease are highly prone to EC since deoxycholic acid (DCA) which is a secondary bile acid is carcinogenic and causes the nonlinear response for the activation of NF-κB. The molecular alteration in EC includes changes in the genes like APC, telomerase, p12, and p53 as well as signalling pathway including Wnt, Hedgehog, and Notch.

Many chemo-drugs like 5-fluorouracil (FU), mitomycin, cisplatin, and gemcitabine are used for the treatment of EC but the tumor cells have developed resistance against these drugs. Therefore, combinational therapies in chemo- and radiotherapies have emerged. The combinational therapy of 5-FU and cisplatin was regarded as a standard combo for the therapy of EC with the survival rate improved to 9.2 months [15, 16]. Wagner et al. reported that the addition of anthracycline to the 5-FU and cisplatin as a third agent showed an improvement in the survival period [17]. With the development of neoadjuvant chemoradiotherapy the combo forms of oxaliplatin-capecitabine (OxCap), paclitaxel-carboplatin (CarPac), and irinotecan-5-FU showed promising results in EC therapy. The multitargeted therapies including tyrosine kinase inhibitors (erlotinib and gefitinib) targeting EGFR [18, 19], COX-2 inhibitors, monoclonal antibodies for EGFR, and FOLFIRI (leucovorin/5-FU/irinotecan) with cetuximab and matuzumab [20] are few therapies reported from phase I/II clinical trials against EC. However EC is widely considered as pathogenic worldwide; therefore, the conventional chemotherapy is made more effective via combining it with novel molecular targeted drugs and neoadjuvant therapies. However, the usage of these multiple drugs is associated with multidrug resistance (MDR) in tumor cells and are highly toxic to the healthy cells. The serious side effects include gastrointestinal lesion, pigmentation in skin, hair loss, cardiac toxicity, and neurologic dysfunction. Moreover, the current interventions are with poor prognosis; therefore this reflects the search for better anticancer agents without side effects and better efficacy. Researchers, are now finding interest on using naturally available phytochemicals like resveratrol for cancer therapy. The phytochemicals extracted from herbs and medicinal plants are used since ancient time for the therapy. These phytochemicals are found to possess anti-cancerous, antioxidant, and anti-inflammatory properties. Earlier studies also revealed that these phytochemicals behave like chemopreventive agents against cancer cells. They induce apoptosis and inhibit proliferation and metastasis. Furthermore, they are used as an adjunct to chemo-drug as they sensitize the resistant EC cells to chemo-drugs and are non-toxic to the healthy cells compared to them. Thus, these novel therapeutic approach can be considered as advantageous for EC therapy in the future. The status of the phytochemicals in clinical trials is illustrated in Table 1.1. In this chapter we focus on few phytochemical compounds used widely for the therapy of EC.

Table 1.1 Clinical trial status of phytochemicals performed against gastrointestinal cancers

Phytochemical	ClinicalTrials. gov Identifier	Status	Condition	Cancer	Phase
Green tea (EGCG)	NCT00233935	Completed	Barrett's esophagus	Esophageal cancer	Phase I
Curcumin	NCT02782949	Recruiting	Chronic atrophic gastritis	Gastric cancer	Phase II
Resveratrol	NCT00433576	Completed	Adenocarcinoma of colon and rectum/ stage I, II, III of colon and rectal cancer	CRC	Phase I
Resveratrol Drug: SRT501	NCT00920803	Completed	Neoplasms, CRC	CRC	Phase I
Curcumin C3 tablet	NCT01333917	Completed	CRC	CRC	Phase I
Curcumin	NCT00027495	Completed	CRC	CRC	Phase I
Genistein	NCT01985763	Completed	CRC	CRC	Phase I Phase II

Source: https://clinicaltrials.gov/

2.1 *Isothiocyanates*

Isothiocyanates are naturally available phytochemicals in various cruciferous vegetables like cauliflower, cabbage, turnips, and sprouts [21]. They occur as glucosinolates that are later converted into isothiocyanates in the presence of myrosinase enzyme through hydrolysis. They are otherwise released from these vegetables while chewing or by the action of microflora present in the intestine of humans. They are found to possess chemopreventive properties and its active metabolites include phenethyl isothiocyanate (PEITC), sulforaphane (SFN), allyl isothiocyanates (AITC), and benzyl isothiocyanate (BITC) that actively showed chemopreventive properties. For instance, PEITC effectively inhibits EC in rats induced with tobacco-induced carcinogen (N-nitrosobenzylmethylamine) [22–24]. Additionally, PEITC is also found to inhibit cytochrome P450 enzyme in EC [25–27]. A P450 enzyme is a phase I enzyme that plays a crucial role in carcinogen and xenobiotic absorption that is later converted into electrophilic metabolites, which eventually disturb the genomic stability, causing damage to DNA. PEITC inhibits DNA methylation and inhibits O^6-methylguanine formation in the DNA of esophagus [24]. Stoner et al. [28] determined that various compounds including isothiocyanates from berries inhibit the growth of tumor in esophagus. They suppress the metabolic activation of carcinogens that are responsible for converting the lesion into cancer, via inhibiting iNOS, VEGF, COX-2, and c-Jun expression. Similarly, SFN was found to downregulate the expression of p63-iRHOM2, where p63 targets iRHOM2. iRHOM2 is the gene encoded by RHBDF2 which is an inherited dominant-mutated form that forms a genetical base for the occurrence of palmoplantar keratoderma associated with dermal diseases and EC. The antioxidant property of SFN thus reduces survival, inflammation, and ROS production [29]. The 4-methylthio-3-butenyl isothiocyanate was found to induce cleavage of caspase-3, caspase-9, PARP, and reduced expression of Bcl-2 and thus promotes the mitochondrial associated apoptotic pathway in EC cell lines. Additionally, it was also found to induce cell cycle arrest at G2/M phase by upregulating the expression of Chk1 and Akt proteins with the downregulation of p27 expression [30]. Thus, the metabolites of isothiocyanates are associated to treat dermal diseases and neoplasia. However, future research should include still more molecular targets for isothiocyanates for the therapy of EC.

2.2 *Resveratrol*

Resveratrol is a phytoalexin and stilbene based comprising of two phenolic rings interconnected by styrene double bond that produces 3,4′,5-trihydroxy-stilbene. It exists in both cis and trans forms, where trans form is the widely studied form. It is found in various plants like grapes, berries, and peanuts. Additionally, it is also produced during fungal infection, exposure to UV radiations, and injury [31]. It has extensive properties including antioxidant, anti-inflammatory, and anticarcinogenic [32]. As an antibacterial agent it inhibits the growth of multiple strains of *H. pylori* and increases the production of ROS and IL-8 [33–36]. It is found to induce cytotoxicity in various cancers including ECs by inhibition initiation and progression of tumor cell growth, cell division, and metastasis [37–40]. For instance, Tang et al. [41] for the first time determined that resveratrol inhibits cell growth of esophageal squamous cell carcinoma in a dose- and time-dependent manner. It induces cell cycle arrest at sub-G1 phase resulting in apoptosis not in AMPK/mTOR-dependent pathway but by the inhibition of pharmacological and genetical autophagy cells that enhances the pro-apoptotic effects of resveratrol in cancer cells. The data from Swedish nationwide population recruited cases from esophageal adenocarcinoma, esophageal squamous cell carcinoma, and gastroesophageal junctional adenocarcinoma wherein a survey analysis was performed. The data from the population-based control study revealed that a high combination of food intake that is rich in resveratrol, lignans, and quercetin as represented from the intake of red wine, tea, tomato, lettuce, and vegetables could prevent the occurrence and development of the esophagus-related cancers [42]. The natural demethylated analogue of resveratrol, pterostilbene, was also found to fight against esophageal cancers [43]. Feng et al. [44] determined that pterostilbene acts as a potent anticancer pharmaceutical agent in a dose- and time-dependent manner against EC cells. It enhanced the apoptotic index with the increase in caspase-2 and ROS levels. Furthermore, decrease in intracellular GSH levels with reduced tumor cell adhesions and migration is detected. Additionally, pterostilbene upregulated the expression of endoplasmic reticulum stress-related molecules including p-PERK, CHOP, GRP78, and p-elF2α [45–47]. This resulted in upregulation of pro-apoptotic proteins and downregulation of Bcl-2 expression. Further, this also promoted translocation of cytochrome c from mitochondria to cytosol and activating caspase-9 and caspase-12 expression. On the other hand, ERS signalling when downregulated is responsible for developing resistance as detected by using CHOP siRNA that desensitizes the tumor cells. However, its upregulation sensitizes esophageal cells to pterostilbene. Thus, resveratrol can be used as a pharmaceutical anticancer agent for the therapy of cancers like EC.

2.3 EGCG

It was reported that consumption of decaffeinated green and black tea reduces the occurrence of EC. This is due to the presence of chief constituent polyphenol, whereas epigallocatechin-3-gallate (EGCG) is the abundantly present constituent in the tea polyphenols. The antitumor efficacy of EGCG is detected in multiple cancer cell lines, animal models, and their related clinical studies [48–50]. As an anticarcinogenic agent, EGCG mediates various signalling pathways regulating MAPK, AP-1, EGFR, and DNA methyltransferase activity. It also induces cell cycle arrest at G0/G1 phase, inducing apoptosis. In EC, EGCG was found to inhibit the phosphorylation of ERK, COX-2, and c-Jun in vitro and in vivo [51]. This suggests that EGCG reduces the expression of pro-inflammatory mediators along with c-Jun and ERK in EC. Similarly, Liu et al. [52] determined the molecular mechanism of EGCG involved in inhibiting the growth of EC; they found that EGCG inhibits the EC growth in a time- and dose-dependent manner in vitro and in vivo. Moreover, the tumor cells showed cell cycle arrest at G1 phase and with induced apoptosis supported by the production of ROS. It significantly reduced the expression of VEGF and upregulated the expression of cleaved caspase-3. Later, Liu et al. [53] determined a specific mechanism of EGCG in inducing apoptosis and inhibiting EC. The mitochondrial transmembrane potentiality is an essential effector in the apoptotic intrinsic pathway that plays a crucial role in reducing apoptosis in tumor cells. EGCG downregulates the mitochondrial membrane potential and induces the expression of caspase-3 subsequently inducing apoptosis. The telomerase on the other hand produces short DNA repeats and ensures the genomic stability during cell division. However, its activity is always essential for the growth of tumor cells. Thus, from their work EGCG was also found to modulate the activity of telomerase to inhibit tumor growth. Genetically, it was previously found that the dysregulation of p16 gene that is caused due to methylation at its promoter site induces vigorous cell proliferation and tumorigenesis that subsequently causes ECs [54]. In general, p16 protein induces cell cycle arrest at G1 phase and inhibits tumor progression in various cancers [55]. It was determined by Meng et al. [56] that EGCG reverses the methylation status of p16 to induce cell cycle arrest. However, their work did not give evidence if EGCG is the inhibitor of DNA methyltransferase enzyme. Therefore, further investigation about the efficacy of EGCG in this regard is warranted. The ascorbic acid, an effective antioxidant, was found to enhance the activity of both EGCG and theaflavin-3-3′-digallate in human lung adenocarcinoma and EC. It was determined that ascorbic acid induces apoptosis by the activation of caspase-3 and caspase-9. Additionally, it was also found to induce activation of MAPK and its subfamilies including ERK and SAPKs [57]. Furthermore, EGCG also reverses the MDR in cancer cells. Thus, EGCG is also used in combinational therapy that potentiates the efficacy of drug. For instance, EGCG potentiates the efficacy of adriamycin in EC cells when compared with the drug alone. It reverses the resistance towards drug by downregulating the expression of ABCG2 protein, whose overexpression increases the efflux of drug and induces resistance. Moreover, it was also found to induce apoptosis by inhibiting the expression of Bcl-2 and upregulating the expression of caspase-3 and Bax proteins [58]. Recently, EGCG is also used as a promising therapeutic option for the therapy of serious toxic side effects including acute radiation-induced esophagitis caused due to the radio- and chemoradiotherapy in EC patients. Patients from Shandong Cancer Hospital and Institute in China were taken to conduct a phase II study for the validation of safety and efficacy of EGCG used after the chemoradiotherapy in EC patients. They were monitored for dysphagia, esophagitis-related pain, and radiation therapy oncology group. The tumor response rate estimated was about 86.3% and overall survival rates of the patients for the subsequent 3 years were 74.5%, 58%, and 40.5%. Thus, the oral administration of EGCG might be feasible for the ARIE-suffering EC patients who received radiation therapy [59]. However, further evaluation for the randomized study is essential. Thus, future clinical applications are still vital for the use of EGCG in the therapy of EC.

2.4 Curcumin

Curcuma longa, traditionally called as turmeric, is widely used for flavoring in foods. The yellow color of *Curcuma longa* is due to the bioactive polyphenol curcuminoids [60–63]. The three main curcuminoids extracted are demethoxycurcumin, curcumin, and bisdemethoxycurcumin. The therapeutic activities of curcumin are known since ancient times and it is widely used against various diseases including arthritis, diabetes, inflammation, and skin diseases. Besides this, it is widely studied as an efficient chemotherapeutic and chemopreventive agent against various cancers like ECs [64–66]. Curcumin is found to regulate various signalling pathways that evidence its therapeutic potentiality for the therapy of many diseases including cancer [67, 68]. Zang et al. [69] gave evidence that curcumin inhibits the EC cell growth by downregulating the expression of glycolytic enzyme, which is essential for the tumor cells that respond during metabolic stress. Moreover, in general AMPK signalling pathway is activated during metabolic stress in order to conserve energy and improve glucose uptake [70]. However, in tumorigenesis it acts as a metabolic checkpoint and is highly activated under energy stress and high AMP/ATP ratio, thus inhibiting cell proliferation [71, 72]. Here, they demonstrated that curcumin downregulated the expression of glycolytic enzymes via activating AMPK signalling pathway and inhibiting Warburg effect as well. In another work Li et al. [73] studied the molecular mechanism of curcumin against EC proliferation inhibition. They determined that curcumin increases PTEN signalling pathways, upregulates the expression of GSK3β and caspase-3, and inhibits the expression of PI3K/AKT signalling pathway. Thus, curcumin promotes apoptosis and inhibits proliferation of EC cells. As evidenced that EC is also characterized due to the pro-inflammatory pathway activity, Chemnitzer et al. [74] performed in vitro cell culture cell lines including normal squamous cells, dysplasia, Barrett' s metaplasia, and esophageal adenocarcinoma to investigate the progression of tumor of Barrett' s sequence from the usual squamous epithelial cells to esophageal adenocarcinoma. They determined that TNF-α expression mediated the expression of IL-8 in a time-, dose-, and stage-dependent manner. Moreover, TNF-α expression also induced the expression of mesenchymal markers including vimentin and slug with decrease in the expression of E-cadherin that significantly resulted in malignant behavior of esophageal adenocarcinoma. Additionally, TNF-α was also found to activate PI3K/AKT and NF-κB pathway inducing tumor growth and metastasis. The anti-inflammatory compound curcumin efficiently represses the proliferation of tumor cells and induces apoptosis in the esophageal adenocarcinoma cancer cell lines. STAT3 signalling pathway is also found to promote various cancers. It is activated by the action of cytokines including TNF-α, IL-6, and IL-10 that bind to their respective receptors and activate JAK which sequentially phosphorylate STAT eventually causing inflammation and carcinogenesis. In EC, STAT3 plays a crucial role in developing progression as it is discovered as a DNA-binding protein and controls its downstream targets including Bcl-xL, Bcl-2, CDKN1A, c-MYC, and cyclins D1/D2 that are responsible for cell growth and survival. Curcumin was found to inhibit JAK2 and further block phosphorylation of STAT3, which results in promoting apoptosis and inhibiting progression and can be an effective target for therapy to prevent cancer [75]. Later, Wang et al. [76] synthesized curcumin analogues including 2-pyridyl cyclohexanone and determined the molecular mech anism played by it in the EC cell lines. They showed that the curcumin analogue inhibits the activation of STAT3 and its binding activity on DNA for the expression of Bcl-2 genes to inhibit progression and survival of EC cells. Moreover, the bioavailability of the drug is always a hurdle for the therapy. Curcumin is hydrophobic in nature and is with poor bioavailability [77]. When compared, its metabolite tetrahydrocurcumin was found to show better bioavailability than curcumin and has effective antitumor properties. Additionally, when used in combination with 5-FU, the tumor cell proliferation was inhibited efficiently when compared with 5-FU alone [78]. Recently prepared Theracurmin® is the preparation of curcumin that possesses 30% of curcumin in it [79]. The bioavailability of curcumin in Theracurmin® is remarkably improved that showed better antitumor effects when compared with curcumin. Moreover, Theracurmin® induced ROS production along with the activation of NRF2-NMRAL2P-NQO1 pathway that improved the cytotoxicity of curcumin, whereas the NQO1 inhibitor enhanced the antitumor efficacy of Theracurmin®. Thus, it can be used in combinational therapy and combination of

Theracurmin® and NQO1 inhibitor effectively suppressed EC cell progression [80]. The development of nanotechnology is now encouraged to overcome the limitations faced due to the low bioavailability of the drug. Hosseini et al. [81] used SinaCurcumin®, a nano-micelle, to determine its efficacy against the EC cells. It was compared with paclitaxel and carboplatin as reference drugs. They determined that the novel nano-micelle showed efficient cytotoxicity with reduced IC_{50} concentration and downregulated the expression of cyclin D1 which resulted in inhibiting the proliferation of EC cells. Among the use of nanomedicine, use of magnetic nanoparticle is widely emerged to enhance the drug delivery and bioavailability. Martin et al. [82] prepared curcumin loaded into polymeric micelles together with gold nanorods encapsulated together as PLGA-*b*-PEG copolymer in vitro and in vivo to evaluate the drug delivery and systemic permeability against Berrett's esophageal cells and EC cells. The synthesized novel nano-system showed effectiveness in delivery of drug and in eradicating premalignancy of esophageal adenocarcinoma. Thus, these studies indicate that curcumin serves as a promising anticancer drug. Moreover, the formulations of curcumin should be thoroughly tested for clinical trials that would form the path for novel therapeutic options in improving the drug delivery and bioavailability to treat EC cells.

3 Gastric Cancer

Gastric cancer (GC) is recorded as the deadly cancer worldwide especially in older men. As estimated by the GLOBOCAN 2018, GC is the fifth most common and third most deadly cancer with death rate recorded as 783,000 [83]. The high incidence and mortality rate are due to the dietary habits and infection of *Helicobacter pylori*. The major risk factors are inherited mutations in certain genes (including GSTM1 or CDH1 gene, APC gene), gastric ulcers, gastroesophageal reflux diseases, smoking, alcohol, chemical exposure, and obesity [83]. It is asymptomatic, and can be diagnosed only in their advanced stages that show variation geographically. The GC can be differentiated into two types in respect to their anatomical location-gastric cardia cancer joining esophagus to the stomach and non-cardia cancer also called distal stomach cancer that arises from the lower part of stomach. The pathogenesis involved in the occurrence of GC is unclear and there are multiple factors involved in altering the molecular mechanism including genetical and environmental characteristics. The *H. pylori* is a serious environmental factor determined and is classified as a class I carcinogen for the occurrence of cancer. Moreover, the dysregulated pathways including Hippo, Notch, and Wnt/β-catenin with the upregulation of EGF and NF-κB resulted in the progression of GC.

5-FU is considered as the best adjuvant with better prognosis for GC therapy but showed toxicity in the patient's body. Ustaalioglu et al. [84] compared adjuvant 5-FU chemotherapy taken together with leucovorin (LV) and cisplatin with capecitabine combined with radiotherapy; the patient however developed high toxicity in the body. In the targeted therapies, 5-FU and cisplatin are together used to target HER-2-positive metastatic adenocarcinoma and recommended only under overexpression of HER2 [85]. Oxaliplatin is a platinum analogue and non-nephrotoxic, used in combination with capecitabine as XELOX in chemotherapy against miR-17-92 which is associated with advanced GC [86]. It is also used against targeted therapies against HER-2. Trastuzumab is a monoclonal antibody used in combination with XELOX and is efficient in treating GC as proved in their phase II clinical trials [87]. The efficacy and safety of oxaliplatin taken as SOX(with S-1), combined with Endostar (recombinant human endostatin YH-16), are investigated by Xu et al. against the advanced GC; however trails for the safety and efficacy are still needed [88]. Gemcitabine is another chemo-drug used in combination with other chemo-drugs. Gemcitabine is used along with cisplatin; Lange et al. reported that this combination is effective in patients with advanced GC and showed manageable toxicity that was even confirmed from the phase II trials [89]. Wang also reported that gemcitabine inhibits the cell cycle phases, cell proliferation, and cell apoptosis taken together with 5-FU [90]. MDR is however considered as the major hurdle, where the GC cells get in-sensitized to multi-chemo-drugs. The use of phytochemicals would reduce the cytotoxicity of the healthy cells, prevent serious adverse reactions, and sensitize cancer cells to therapy. The clinical trials for determining the efficacy of phytochemicals against gastric cancer are illustrated in Table 1.1.

3.1 Curcumin

The mechanism and potential therapeutic efficiency of curcumin are investigated in various cancers like GC cell lines in vitro and in vivo. It is even suggested that curcumin inhibits the infection caused by *H. pylori* in mice reducing the growth of tumor [91]. Curcumin was found to inhibit the expression of NF-κB and VEGF signalling pathways along with the ability to form tube driven via HUVECs in GC mesenchymal stem cells that showed a direct involvement of both the proteins in angiogenesis [92]. MicroRNA-21 (miR-21) is onco-miRNA and is upregulated in GC cells. It targets various genes responsible for tumorigenesis of cancer cells including PTEN/PI3K/Akt pathways. Curcumin was found to inhibit these molecular pathways, whereas PD98059, a potent inhibitor of MAPK, enhances apoptotic efficacy of curcumin when used against GC cell lines [93]. Liu et al. [94] investigated the molecular mechanism played by curcumin to inhibit proliferation, migration, invasion and induce apoptosis. They determined that the GC cell growth and migration were significantly decreased by curcumin in a dose- and time-dependent manner. It was found that curcumin upregulates the expression of E-cadherin and Bax increasing the activity of caspase-3, -8, -9 and downregulates the expression of N-cadherin, Bcl-2, Snail1, β-catenin, and Wnt3, thus inducing apoptosis and inhibiting EMT pathway. Thus, this might offer potential therapeutic strategy for the therapy of cancer. Curcumin, as a part of its anticancer properties, upregulates the expression of tumor-suppressor proteins p53 and p21. Additionally, it was also evidenced that it downregulates the expression of PI3K, p-mTOR, and p-Akt. Thus curcumin induces apoptosis and autophagy as well as inhibits proliferation in GC cells [95]. The mitochondria also play a crucial role in cellular bioenergetics that consists of mitochondrial respiration (OXPHOS) and glycolysis for the survival and death of cells. The mitochondrial associated apoptosis is related with the disruption of mitochondrial homeostasis that is carried by the mitochondrial DNA and its encoded 13 proteins. In case of tumor cells the program switches off from the OXPHOS to glycolysis to reach the demand for higher energies by the tumor cells called as Warburg effect. Moreover, POLG is a DNA polymerase enzyme that participates in the replication of mitochondrial DNA and repairing DNA which is found overexpressed in GC cells. Wang et al. [96] suggested that curcumin inhibits cellular bioenergetics as well as POLG that was accompanied by the decrease in mitochondrial DNA. This resulted in the control of GC cell proliferation through the regulation of mitochondrial respiration and aerobic glycolysis. The late-stage diagnosis of GC always resulted in poor prognosis and therapeutic outcome, which is attributed to the dissemination of circulating tumor cells (CTCs) in the bloodstreams that resulted in the distal tumor like liver metastasis [97–99]. The CTCs are found to possess the receptor CXCR4 for the stromal cell-derived factor-1 that is highly expressed in various cancers. It was also suggested that the signalling pathway of CXCR4 plays a crucial role in tumor progression, angiogenesis, and metastasis. Gu et al. [100] evidenced anti-CTC property of curcumin and showed that it reduces the expression of CXCR4 in the extracted primary GC cells in vitro and in vivo through the inhibition of CXCR4 signalling that significantly reduced circulating CTCs and metastasis. The researchers have now started investigating on the derivatives of curcumin as they increase the bioavailability when compared. As such, CL-6 is a curcumin derivative that showed effective inhibition in proliferation, migration, invasion and induced apoptosis. It was evaluated that it increased the levels of Bax and reduced the expression of Bcl-2 with an increase in Bax/Bcl-2 ratio. Additionally, it was determined that CL-6 derivative was found to activate Hippo-YAP signalling pathway, with the increase in phosphorylated YAP protein and LATS expression [101]. Similarly, another analogue CH-5 induces apoptosis and decreases cell viability through the downregulation of MMP-2 expression that plays a key role in migration and metastasis [102]. Curcuminoid WZ35 potentiates the therapeutic efficacy of cisplatin by inhibiting the expression of TrxR1 that is overexpressed and associated with tumor progression in GC. The inhibition resulted in production of ROS and activation of p38 and JNK signalling pathway that significantly induced apoptosis and suppressed tumor growth [103]. Recent advancement in research developed curcumin-encapsulated chitosan nanoparticles along with photodynamic therapy against overexpressed EGFR cells. The photodynamic therapy involves the combinations of photosensitizers and produces ROS to harm the tumor cells. The results showed low IC_{50} value and increased production of ROS [104]. Taken together, curcumin and its derivatives can be a promising therapeutic strategy; however still more nano-formulations should be worked on to improve the bioavailability of curcumin.

3.2 Resveratrol

Resveratrol, a non-flavonoid polyphenol, has pharmacological properties including antioxidative, antitumor, and anti-mutation characteristics. *H. pylori* that induces oxidative stress and plays a crucial role in developing inflammation is a major risk factor for the cause of GC. Resveratrol was proposed to inhibit *H. pylori*-induced inflammation and its underlying mechanisms. It was further determined that this phytochemical downregulates the *H. pylori*-induced transcription and protein expression of IL-8 and iNOS as evidenced from their decreased levels of lipid peroxide and myeloperoxidase activity with improved histological infiltration in the gastric mucosa. Additionally, resveratrol also inhibits the phosphorylation of IkBα and inhibits NF-κB with the activation of Nrf2 pathway [105]. It inhibits cell cycle progression and induces cell cycle arrest at G0/G1 and apoptosis via suppressing the activity of kinase C. Moreover, cyclin D1 is repeatedly regulated by phosphor-glycogen synthase kinase 3B (p-GSK3B), a protein regulated by PI3K/Akt signalling pathway that plays a crucial role in the progression of tumor. PTEN, a tumor suppressor, downregulates the expression of PI3K/Akt to inhibit tumor. When exposed to resveratrol, cell proliferation was decreased with the increase in apoptosis. The PTEN phosphorylation is decreased significantly, resulting in negatively controlling PI3K/Akt signalling pathways by resveratrol. This further targeted the dephosphorylation of GSK3β and cyclin D1 degradation and thus promoted cell cycle arrest and apoptosis [106]. Furthermore, cyclin D1 and c-myc are considered as the target in Wnt/β-catenin signalling pathway. The β-catenin is tumorigenic and is important for promoting cell adhesions. The presence of β-catenin in nucleus will reduce the adherence of cells [107] . Moreover, the overexpression of cyclin D1, β catenin, and c-myc is always associated with tumor progression via activation of Wnt signalling pathway. It was found that resveratrol inhibits the expression of these three cyclin D1, β-catenin, and c-myc at the mRNA and protein levels. Thus resveratrol inhibits proliferation in GC cells via inhibiting the Wnt signalling pathway [108]. IL-6, a multifunctional cytokine, is oncogenic and protects the cells from apoptosis and promotes Akt and NF-κB signalling pathways. Yang et al. [109] found that IL-6 serum level increased in the GC lines and it increases the activation of Ras-MAPK pathway promoting invasion. They also suggested that resveratrol blocks IL-6 to inhibit invasion via blocking these pathways. Metastasis-associated lung adenocarcinoma transcript 1 (MALAT1) is potentially taken as a biomarker for GC and is found to undergo EMT in various cancer types. This could induce migration and invasion as demonstrated from the comparison done with the knockdown MALAT1 mice. Resveratrol was found to decrease the expression of MALAT1 in a time- and dose-dependent manner mediated by EMT in GC cells [110]. Additionally, resveratrol was also found to inhibit metastasis by inhibiting hedgehog signalling pathways [111]. Furthermore, it was also found to induce apoptosis through the activation of mitochondrial pathway. The PARP cleavage with the increase in the expression of caspase-3 was found with the downregulation of pro-caspase-9 and release of cytochrome c into the cytosol from mitochondria when exposed to resveratrol. Additionally, Bax/Bcl-2 ratio was found increased in the treated GC cells [112]. Wu et al. [113] investigated the effect of resveratrol on the progression and apoptosis of GC cells. They found that as mentioned earlier resveratrol upregulates the expression of Bax, cleaves caspase-3 and caspase-8, and downregulates the expression of Bcl-2 in a dose-dependent manner. Additionally, it also inhibits the activation of NF-κB (p65) and significantly induces apoptosis. Supplementing with other phytochemicals, resveratrol was combined together with curcumin to inhibit progression more efficiently that significantly upregulated the expression of p53 and modulated p53 posttranslational modification in GC [114]. Resveratrol was also found to reverse the resistance against various drugs including doxorubicin. The combinational treatment of resveratrol and doxorubicin modulated PTEN/Akt pathways and achieved EMT reversion, where only with doxorubicin GC cells showed EMT with Akt activation via the activation of PTEN [115]. In general the MDR is associated with the overexpression of ATP-binding cassette subfamily B member 1 (ABCB) that encodes P-gp and contributes to the efflux of drugs out of the cells [116–121]. In addition to this there are other typical mechanisms involved whose overexpression in annexin A1 (ANXA1) and thioredoxin (TXN) proteins also involved in developing MDR via reverse binding of Ca2+ ion and phospholipids present in the plasma membrane [122]. Mieszala et al. [123] experimented on the gastric cell lines that are resistant against daunorubicin and mitoxantrone compared with their controls. They determined the cellular levels of P-gp, TXN, and ANXA1 after treatment with the combination of these chemo-drugs with resveratrol and only with the chemo-drugs. Resveratrol showed a significant influence on the expression of the MDR proteins at their mRNA and protein level. Despite many positive features of resveratrol, the hydrophobicity nature of resveratrol makes it unsuitable for in vivo administration. The present nanotechnology is now highly encouraged to encapsulate resveratrol and enhance its stability. Hu et al. [124] combined resveratrol along with anti-miR21 loaded into mesoporous silica nanoparticles that is conjugated with hyaluronic acid. miR-21 is oncogenic that induces MDR and is found upregulated in various cancers like GC. They performed TUNEL staining and determined that the percentage of TUNEL-positive cells is significantly high with increased apoptotic cells in the designed nanoparticle when compared to the free resveratrol. This represents that combinational inhibitors along with resveratrol with a triggered nanocarrier would be a promising therapeutic strategy for GC therapy. Future clinical trials are still essential for determining the efficacy of the so developed formulations.

3.3 Genistein

Genistein is an isoflavone present in soybeans; it is antioxidant and is focused for its anti-cancerous properties against various cancers like GC [125–127]. The previous studies evidenced its efficiency in altering the genes that are involved in regulating cell cycle [128, 129]. It suppresses the activation of Akt signalling pathways that play a crucial role in cell proliferation and survival. It also induces the expression of tumor-suppressor genes by the activation of PTEN pathway [130–133]. It was later suggested by Liu et al. [134] that genistein induces cell cycle arrest at G2/M phase via decrease in the expression of phosphor-Wee1 (Ser642) and increase in the expression of phosphor-cdc2 (Thr15) through the inactivation of Akt. Isoflavone (genistein) and lignans (enterolactone) are the two main classes of phytoestrogens. Moreover, phytoestrogen has the property to mimic and modulate the action of endogenous estrogens binding to their receptors [135, 136]. Moreover, phytoestrogens are also found to inhibit the *H. pylori*-induced GC progression by deactivating Akt and NF-κB pathway, thus reducing the risk for the cause of cancer [137]. Similarly, the gene-environment interactions demonstrated that FAS and MAP3K1 genes interact with enterolactone; these genes play a key role in activating Akt/NF-κB pathway. This reduces the risk for GC cause [138]. Prostaglandin endoperoxide synthase 2 is a human gene that encodes COX-2 and have binding sites for NF-κB at its promoter region. Therefore, NF-κB upregulation is always associated with the expression of COX-2 [139]. As discussed, genistein was found to inhibit the activation of NF-κB; however the effect of genistein on COX-2 is unknown. Li et al. [140] determined that genistein inactivates NF-κB signalling pathway in a dose- and time-dependent manner that even resulted in decreased levels of COX-2 expression in GC. Thus, the suppression of COX-2 would be an efficient step of genistein in showing the antiproliferative effect mediated via NF-κB. The hedgehog signalling pathway along with its activator Gli1 is oncogenic and induces cancer stemness. This pathway results in the upregulation of CD44, surface markers for cancer stem cells. Genistein was found to inhibit the expression of Gli1 gene via deactivating hedgehog signalling pathway, with the reduction of Gli1 and CD44 mRNA and protein level [141]. Additionally, ornithine decarboxylase (ODC) poly amine pathway that elevates polyamine is associated with GC that controls chronic inflammation and determines *H. pylori* infection and innate immunity of the host with DNA damage. Cho et al. [142] initially determined genes that encode ODC pathway including ODC1, OAZ2, NQO1, NOS2A, and AMD1 responsible for the risk of GC. They have taken 76 GC cases within the Korean Multi-center Cancer Cohort and a total of 30 single-nucleotide polymorphs; these 5 genes were determined. Their pooled analysis showed NQO1 rs1800566 to be the most significant for the cause of GC; the other AMC1 rs1279599, OAZ2 rs7403751, and AMD1 rs7768897 showed significant interaction with genistein and altered the development of GC; and reduced polyamine synthesis was determined. Cancer cachexia is a metabolic syndrome, associated with underlying illness and loss of fat mass and musculature [143, 144]. Isoflavone treatment of the cachexia induced GC cell line, attenuated cachexia, and improved the survival reducing proliferation of tumor cells, whereas discontinuation of isoflavone resulted in weight loss and tumor growth. It was determined that isoflavone in the sequence AglyMax>daidzein>genistein showed inhibitory effect against GC cells [145]. Furthermore, genistein is also suggested to reverse the resistance properties against 5-FU and cisplatin. It inhibits the expression of ABCG2 and ERK1/2 activity reducing the chemoresistance and GC stem cell-like properties [146]. Among other resistance-developed protein, kinesin superfamily (KIF) protein is found to induce mitotic spindle formation and chromosome partitioning [147]. Furthermore, the high levels of KIF20A were associated with the progression in GC and correlated with the poor prognosis of patients. Genistein was found to inhibit the expression of KIF20A as well as enhance antitumor property of 5-FU and cisplatin [148]. The analogue of genistein, 7-difluoromethoxyl-5,4′-di-n-octyl genistein, is more efficient than genistein. The novel synthetic analogue inhibits the cancer cell stemness in GC reversing EMT. The inhibition of self-renewal and migration was accompanied with the downregulation of FoxM1 expression and EMT-related protein (Twist1). FoxM1 is associated with cell cycle progression and its progression resulted in poor progression. Additionally, genistein was also found to inhibit the expression of CSC markers CD133, ALDH1, and CD44 along with the expression of N-cadherin and upregulation of E-cadherin [149]. With the advancements in the nanotechnology and improvising of the combinational therapy to make the therapeutic strategies more efficient and effective genistein is combined with curcumin encapsulated with nanostructure lipid carriers against inhibition of prostate cancer cells. The stability of both the phytochemicals is enhanced and they are with no adverse reactions [150]. However, there are as such no nano-formulations designed for the therapy of GC. Therefore, further investigations are still essential to improvise the therapeutic strategies using these conventional agents for the therapy of human malignancies.

4 Colorectal Cancer

Colorectal cancer (CRC) is the third most common cancer diagnosed in both men and women in the USA. As estimated from the American Cancer Society, for the year 2020, the newly diagnosed cases for colon cancer are 104,610 and for rectal cancer are 43,340. The expected deaths during 2020 would be 53,200. The risk factors associated with the occurrence of CRC are modifiable factors that include physical inactiveness, obesity, smoking, taking alcohol, and consuming food rich in red meat, whereas the non-modifiable factors include intestinal bowel disease and being elderly. Despite these factors, the foodborne mutagens cause mutations and epigenetic alterations. Moreover, the chronic inflammation caused by the bacteria *H. pylori* are associated with 20% of CRC occurrence [151]. CRC is a multifactorial disease initiated as tubulovillous (premalignant neoplasm) and later progressed into invasive adenocarcinoma. The anatomical polyps developed in the lining of epithelium are detected as dysplastic aberrant crypt foci (ACF) that are hyperplastic polyps and benign in nature. These however further induce mutation in the tumor-suppressor genes including adenomatous polyposis coli (APC) gene that becomes oncogenic causing dysfunction in KRAS gene leading to proliferation and survival of tumor cells. Additionally, Wnt signalling pathway is the primary cause for CRC that has β-catenin as its key regulator. The Wnt signalling pathway functions by suppressing the destruction complex that constitutes β-catenin along with APC, axin, and glycogen synthase kinase-3β. This results in the accumulation of β-catenin and as it is prevented from degrading it gets further translocated into nucleus and binds with T-cell factor/lymphoid enhancer factor family molecules promoting the expression of c-myc and cyclin-D1 involved in cell proliferation. The Wnt signalling is potentiated in another way via the risk factor obesity. This promote the overactivation of PI3K/Akt and MAPK signalling pathway inducing their downstream proteins including mTOR. The activating mutations in KRAS resulted in 30–50% of CRC occurrence that drives tumorigenesis [152]. Moreover, BRAF and KRAS signalling pathways are associated with tumorigenesis, whose 90% of activating mutation causes CRC is due to the alteration in the nucleotide 1799 of exon 15 [153]. Thus, both KRAS and BRAF can be taken as targets for the therapy of cancer.

The adjuvant therapies include use of various drugs like 5-FU are often given along with folinic acid, capecitabine (Xeloda®), irinotecan (Campto®), oxaliplatin (Eloxatin®), trifluridine and tipiracil (Lonsurf®); additionally there are drugs used as combinational drugs including FOLFOX (folinic acid, 5-FU, and oxaliplatin), FOLFIRI (folinic acid, 5-FU, and irinotecan), and CAPOX (capecitabine and oxaliplatin). Earlier 5-FU and folinic acid were recommended to be given intravenously after surgery for 6 months and at present capecitabine and oxaliplatin are recommended for stage III after surgery by National Institute for Health and Clinical Excellence [154]. Capecitabine is given as a precursor for improvising the cytotoxic moiety of 5-FU and the platinum-based oxaliplatin is another drug used along with 5-FU that prevents DNA replication [154]. Use of these chemo-drugs taken individually or in combination is effective to some extent and these are with serious adverse reactions and toxicity. For instance, celecoxib, a COX-2 inhibitor found effective for preventing FAP, however it develop serious cardiovascular adverse side effects [155]. Additionally, the use of chemo-drugs develops MDR in cells. miR-106a-5p, a typical oncogene, is found overexpressed in various cancers like CRC. The CRC cell lines are found to develop resistance against 5-FU. Additionally, it also downregulates the expression of TGFβR2 [156]. Similarly, there are other ABC transporter proteins that also develop resistance and promote drug efflux [157]. Thus, phytochemicals have the capacity to reduce toxicity and are antitumor in nature that sensitize the tumor cells during the therapy. Moreover, having a healthy diet filled with vegetables and fruits keeps intestinal related cancers like CRC away, as they are the source for phytochemicals [158–161]. The current clinical trials performed for CRC therapy with the phytochemicals are illustrated in Table 1.1.

4.1 Resveratrol

The phytoalexin compound is anti-cancerous; as evidenced from various in vitro studies it is an efficient anti-CRC that inhibits initiation and proliferation of tumor. For instance, the inflammatory response is reduced by resveratrol via reducing NO levels along with the inhibition of IkB complex phosphorylation and NF-κB activation [162]. When compared with 5-aminosalicylic acid, resveratrol taken 20 times lower concentration is efficient in significantly decreasing the production of NO and expression of PGE2, iNOS, and COX-2. Similarly, Gong et al. [163] also showed that resveratrol inhibits the progression of CRC through the inhibition of COX-2. It is also found to promote AMPK signalling pathway with the inhibition of MAPK and PI3K/Akt signalling pathways [164]. Li et al. [165] demonstrated that resveratrol inhibits Akt and its signalling downstream targets together with STAT3 that had Akt as an upstream regulator of STAT3. Their computational docking results gave evidences that resveratrol docks with Akt1 and Akt2 at their ATP-binding pockets; moreover silencing of Akt 1/2 induced cell cycle arrest at G1 phase and promoted apoptosis. Thus, resveratrol shows its anti-cancerous effect through the suppression of Akt/STAT3 signalling pathways. Bone morphogenetic proteins (BMPs) are a subgroup of TGF-β superfamily involved in the development of embryo, growth, differentiation, and apoptosis. However, the aberrantly acting BMPs sometimes behave as promoter as well as inhibitor in various cancers. In CRC, BMP7 is associated with the anticancer activity, where resveratrol upregulates it to suppress the phosphorylation of PTEN to inactivate PI3K/Akt signalling pathway [166]. Lao et al. [167] also showed that resveratrol promotes the expression of PTEN, p53, and caspase-3 to promote inhibition and induce apoptosis. As evidenced from previous reports the upregulated PTEN always targets Akt signalling pathway to inactivate it. The epigenetic modification of p53 causes posttranslational modifications leading to its inactivation. SET7/9 domain on the other side has lysine methyltransferase that transfers methyl group to the target site of lysine residue of proteins like p53. Resveratrol was found to upregulate the expression of this SET7/9 in the treated CRC cell lines leading to the methylation of p53 at its K372 residue. This resulted in improving the stability of p53 and inducing apoptosis with the upregulation of PARP cleavage and caspase-3 [168]. mMiR-200c plays an essential role as a tumor suppressor, inhibiting EMT. Moreover, resveratrol was found to upregulate the expression of miR-200c in CRC-treated cells, resulting in inducing of apoptosis and inhibiting of invasion and migration via switching of EMT to MET [169]. The resveratrol analogue is now found to be efficient enough against the tumor growth of CRC. HS-1793, a synthetic analogue, is found to inhibit the tumor growth and induce apoptosis via the activation of caspase 3, PARP cleavage, and altering of Bax/Bcl-2 ratio in a dose- and time-dependent manner when compared with resveratrol. It suppressed PI3K/Akt activation and enhanced the antitumor activity [170]. Similarly, another analogue of resveratrol, (E)-N-(2-(4-methoxystyryl) phenyl) furan-2-carboxamide (CS), showed similar cytotoxicity; however the cells showed sensitivity only 72 h posttreatment. This analogue enhanced the cytotoxicity via promoting the apoptotic protein activation including FADD, caspase-8, caspase-9, caspase-3, and PARP cleavage. This also resulted in the upregulation of tumor-suppressor proteins p53 and p21 [171]. Storniolo et al. [172] determined that the antioxidant activity of hydroxy analogue of resveratrol is due to the two benzene rings in the stilbene structure bonded together by central ethylene that is responsible for the inhibition of CRC cell growth, DNA synthesis, and inducing of cell cycle arrest. Resveratrol was also investigated to inhibit the expression of protein involved in developing MDR including MDR1, BRCP, and MRP1, and metabolic enzymes including GST and CYP3A4. Thus, resveratrol mediates the inhibition of ABC transporters, resulting in the decrease of overall efflux of drug and promoting apoptosis [173]. TNF-β, an inflammatory cytokine, shows pro-carcinogenic effects as well as promotes resistance in CRC cells. Resveratrol was determined to chemosensitize TNF-β to 5-FU. Furthermore, resveratrol also suppressed the formation of cancer stem cell markers including CD133, CD44, and ALDH1 that are induced by TNF-β. This was further accompanied by promoting apoptosis with the increase in the expression of caspase-3 and inhibiting the activity of MMP-9, NF-κB, and CXCR4 that are activated by TNF-β [174]. Therefore, resveratrol can be used in combinational therapies, combining it with chemo-drugs to prevent the obstacle of developing resistance and toxicity. For instance, resveratrol combined with 5-FU enhanced the anti-telomerase activity in CRC cell lines. The anticancer property potentiated with the inhibition in STAT3 and Akt signalling pathway. The STAT3 phosphorylation is inhibited by the binding of resveratrol to the promoter region of human telomerase reverse transcriptase (hTERT). The molecular mechanism as such in the combinational therapy is like resveratrol inducing cell cycle arrest at S-phase potentiated with apoptosis when treated with 5-FU [175]. Furthermore, resveratrol was also used in combination with other phytochemicals in order to enhance the cytotoxicity of the phytochemical drugs against CRC cells. Resveratrol was combined with curcumin for the first time by Gavrilas et al. [176]. Their data revealed that both the phytochemicals showed their inhibitory effect on multiple genes by modulating apoptotic related genes including FAS, CASP3, BID, CASP7, ZMAT3, and PMAIP1. The results obtained were more efficient when cancer cells were treated with combinatorial approach than as single treatment. In order to potentiate the therapeutic efficiency, improve the stability and bioavailability of the drug, researchers used nanotechnology to design nanoparticles encapsulated with these phytochemicals. More recently, the methylated derivative of resveratrol 3,5,4′-trimethoxy-trans-stilbene is loaded into PEG-PE micelles against CRC cells. This resulted in enhanced pharmacokinetic and pharmacodynamic potentialities with prolonged half-life and improved bioavailability [177]. Thus, considering these beneficial prospects in regard to combinational therapy and nanotechnology, future studies are still essential to address the pharmacological benefits and improvise the therapeutic strategies for the beneficiary of patients.

4.2 *Curcumin*

The hydrophobic polyphenol curcumin has the potentiality in inhibiting inflammation and progression of tumor cells [178]. The previous in vitro studies determine the antitumor efficacy of curcumin against CRC. Certainly, an oral intake of curcumin (4 g for 30 days) would decrease the ACF formed in colon for the prevention of CRC. The molecular mechanisms of curcumin involved in inhibiting the tumor progression target various signalling pathways including EGFR [179, 180], MAPK [181], AMP-COX-2 [182], and Wnt/β-catenin [183]. Furthermore, curcumin was found to modulate the expression of NBR2/AMPK/mTOR pathways. NBR2 is a noncoding sequence existing beside BRCA1, a tumor-suppressor gene. It was also determined that NBR2 was found to interact with AMPK and activate it whereas the deficiency of NBR2 reduces the glucose starvation [184]. Curcumin was found to significantly reduce the progression via regulating NBR2 levels and activating AMPK signalling. Moreover, the downstream mTOR is also downregulated by curcumin [185]. DJ-1, also called as Parkinson gene, activates PI3K/Akt signalling pathway via negatively controlling the activation of PTEN [186]. Thus, the expression of DJ-1 in CRC contributes cell proliferation and inhibition in apoptosis. Curcumin inhibits the expression of DJ-1 activating PTEN, thereby inhibiting PI3K/Akt signalling pathway and regulating progression of tumor cells [187]. YAP is another oncogenic protein that can be taken as a marker for CRC occurrence. The overexpression of YAP promotes cell proliferation and suppresses apoptosis causing loss of cell adhesion and malignancy. Curcumin inhibits YAP expression and activates autophagy pathway in CRC cells [188]. Additionally, curcumin also decreases the expression of IGF-1 receptors and insulin along with MYC expression. This resulted in inhibition of proliferation and movement of chemoresistant CRC cells [189]. Curcumin also plays a crucial role in sensitizing tumor cells to chemo-drug for the therapy of CRC. Curcumin along with 5-FU forms an effective treatment against chemoresistant CRC cells via the inhibition of NF-κB/PI3K/Src pathway and NF-κB-regulated gene products [190]. Cis-platinum combined with curcumin significantly induced apoptosis in CRC cell lines in a dose-dependent manner. They promoted the expression of Bax and downregulated Bcl-3. Additionally, NICD1 (Notch 1 intracellular domain) and Hes-1 (hairy and enhancer of split 1) expression was also significantly decreased with this combinational drug [191]. The analogues of curcumin are developed in order to enhance the efficacy of curcumin. Hexahydrocurcumin, IND-4, FLLL, C-5 curcumin analogue, 1-aroyl-3,5-bis (benzylidene)-4-piperidone, GO-Y030, C086, dehydrozingerone, dimeric 3,5-bis(arylidene)-4-piperidones, difluorinated curcumin, and curcumin diethyl disuccinate are few analogues synthesized for curcumin, which showed to be effective than parent curcumin against CRC cells [192]. Recently, a nitrogen-containing curcumin analogue, called as compound 19, was found to show inhibition against CRC epithelial cells. They exert anti-inflammatory nature by downregulating NF-κB, STAT3 activation, and induced cell cycle arrest at G1 phase. Moreover, the markers of CSCs including CD51 and CD133 are found reduced along with reduced STAT3 activity by binding at the hTERT promoter region. Additionally, they also inhibit the activation of CSC population including CD44, ALDHA1, and Oct-4. Thus, these analogues are more efficient to inhibit proliferation and metastasis and induce apoptosis in CRC cells [193]. Furthermore, with the bioavailability and stability of curcumin to be more effective against CRC therapy, researchers developed nanoparticles for the delivery of curcumin. Sabra et al. [194] developed cetuximab-conjugated altered citrus pectin-chitosan nanoparticle for the target delivery of curcumin to CRC cells. When compared, the delivery of curcumin enhanced the internalization and significantly reduced CRC cell proliferation. The cell cycle analysis also revealed that the nanoparticle efficiently induced cell cycle arrest at G2/M phase. Thus, the above data reflects novel and promising therapeutic strategies for CRC therapy. However, clinical and pharmacological evidences are still essential for determining efficacy of the drug.

4.3 Genistein

Genistein, the active ingredient of soy isoflavone, is a potent chemoprevention agent with various biological activities including antitumor, anti-cancerous, and antibacterial. Moreover, it is found to promote inhibition in various colon cancer cells via regulating various signalling pathways involved in progression. For instance, it was found to suppress the EGF-induced proliferation in colon cancer cells via the activation of FOXO3 and downregulation of PI3K/Akt pathway [195]. Furthermore, it was also suggested to induce apoptosis in CRC cell lines via reversing EMT and inhibiting Notch signalling pathway. This promoted the expression of E-cadherin and downregulated the expression of N-cadherin with the control of EMT markers including TWIST1, ZEB1, ZEB2, Snail1, Snail2/slug, and FOXC2. The apoptotic protein ratio of Bcl-2/Bax and caspase was promoted. Thus, the Notch-1 inactivation significantly downregulated the expression of NF-κB also [196]. This potentiated genistein as an antitumor agent. Lou et al. [197] also determined that genistein controls the expression of NF-κB in CRC cell lines in order to induce apoptosis by upregulating the expression of Bax and downregulating Bcl-2 in CRC cell lines, as NF-κB signalling pathway actively regulates the expression of genes responsible for survival. As suggested from the previous studies, activation of Akt was determined from CRC cell lines and the phosphorylated form of Akt is taken as the prognosis marker. Akt pathway plays a crucial role in preventing the cell cycle progression via inhibiting the degradation of cyclin D1 and promoting the expression of p21 and p27. Genistein was found to inhibit CRC cell proliferation via inhibiting the phosphorylation of Akt as well as inducing mitochondrial signalling cascades for apoptosis [198]. The activation of Akt pathway stimulates many substrates like mTOR and GSK3. Similarly, SGK1, a protein from AGC family of serine/threonine kinase, shares maximum similarity in amino acid sequence with the other members of signalling pathway including Akt and PKA. Moreover, the activation of SGK1 and PI3K/Akt pathway is associated with CRC progression and genistein was suggested to downregulate the expression of Akt and SGK1 and suppress Akt phosphorylation [199]. Furthermore, miR-95 was found to be upregulated in CRC cells that contributes to poor prognosis. Genistein was found to significantly decrease the expression of miR-95 in CRC cell lines [199]. This represents the protective ability of genistein in CRC. Zhang et al. [200] also found that genistein when taken in higher doses induces damage to DNA and blocks cell cycle causing cell cycle arrest at G2/M phase mediated by the upregulation of p53/p21 and GADD45α together with the downregulation of cdc2 and cdc25A.

Additionally it was also found to initiate programmed cell death. It attenuates the accumulation of β-catenin in nucleus and Wnt-related genes via inactivating Wnt/β-catenin signalling pathway to decrease ACF of colon, thus controlling the risk factors for the cause of CRC [201]. The epigenetic modification causing DNA methylation of CpG island also suppresses the activity of certain tumor-suppressor genes, such as Wnt inhibitory factor 1 (WIF1) whose methylation causes migration and invasion of CRC cells. Genistein was found to demethylate WIF1 in a dose-dependent manner. Additionally, it also controls the expression of certain proteins via downregulating MMP1 and MMP9 and upregulating metalloproteinase inhibitor 1 and E-cadherin significantly to induce apoptosis and prevent invasion [202]. Furthermore, including genistein in daily diet would potentiate the antioxidant activity and antitumor efficacy. It is also used in combinational therapy, combined with other chemo-drugs and phytochemicals. Pintova et al. [203] performed clinical trial for assessing the safety and tolerability when genistein is taken together with FOLFOX or FOLFOX-bevacizumab. The results suggested better efficacy when taken together and that they are without chemotherapy-related adverse events. However, further verifications through larger clinical trials are warranted. Moreover, there are derivatives of genistein developed against CRC cells. They are found to be more effective than the usual parent genistein. ME-143 alone or taken together with 5-FU and oxaliplatin showed similar results via inhibiting Wnt/β-catenin signalling pathway to inhibit the progression of CRC cells [204]. Similarly, Gen-27, another derivative of genistein, was found to prevent colitis-associated CRC (CAC) mediated via p65-CDX2-β-catenin. Where p65 was prevented from binding with the CDX2 at its silencer region and promoting its binding at the promoter region of APC and AXIN2 to inhibit the activation of β-catenin and TNF-α. This reflects the antitumor property of the derivative [205]. However, hydrophobicity remains as the common hurdle for the phytochemicals, and the usage of genistein as an anticancer material is also limited. This limitation can be overcome with the novel nano-formulations to improve the stability of genistein. For instance, hybrid nanomaterial was prepared by incorporating genistein into PEG silica nanoparticles. The physiochemical and biological properties of the nanohybrid were evaluated; the results suggested efficient antioxidant and antiproliferative properties when compared with normal genistein against CRC cells [206]. Further, potentiating therapeutic strategies are still to be concentrated to develop more novel techniques to develop the nanohybrid materials and future testing for their efficacy is also warranted.

5 Conclusion

Gastrointestinal cancers including esophagus, gastric, and CRC are especially associated with the Western lifestyle factors, most importantly the diet taken. Moreover, the prognosis of advanced gastrointestinal cancer remains poor; therefore safe and effective adjuvant therapy options are required. Despite the usage of regular administration of chemopreventive drugs, the cancer is not completely cured. Identifying valuable early markers of gastric intestinal cancer is extremely important for the diagnosis of cancer. This use of natural phytochemicals including EGCG, genistein, isothiocyanates, resveratrol, and curcumin is now worked by the researchers due to their antitumor, antioxidative, and antiproliferative properties. They participate actively in inactivating various signalling pathways involved in proliferation, invasion, and migration. Moreover, most of the tumor cases can be reduced or prevented altering the lifestyle. Including the fruits and vegetables in daily diet that possess lot of phytochemicals would be very effective in preventing cancer. Encouraging certain therapeutic strategies including molecular target and multi-targeted prevention of cancer in near future is highly advantageous. Nevertheless, the limitations in using phytochemicals are still not answered properly. Bioavailability of the phytochemicals is the common limitation determined since early days. There are lot of derivatives of phytochemicals synthesized till now and are found to be effective than the parent form. However, further clinical trials are still to be conducted to determine the safety and efficacy of the phytochemical drug used against cancer. The phytochemicals are used in combinational therapies to enhance the therapeutic efficacy of the chemo- and radiation drug to sensitize the tumor cells against these drugs; they are found effective in vitro and in vivo. Therefore, further clinical trials are still warranted to determine the safety and efficacy of the drug. More recently, the development of nano-chemoprevention is proposed to enhance the efficacy of the dietary phytochemicals in cancer prevention. Thus, taken together this reflects that the use of novel nanotechniques, molecular target therapies, and custom-tailored therapy regimens leads to efficient therapeutic management strategies for the better clinical outcome and for the beneficiary of patients suffering from cancers like gastrointestinal cancer diseases.

References

1. Siegel, R. L., Miller, K. D., & Jemal, A. (2019). Cancer statistics, 2019. *CA: a Cancer Journal for Clinicians, 69*(1), 7–34.
2. Bray, F., et al. (2018). Global cancer statistics 2018: GLOBOCAN estimates of incidence and mortality worldwide for 36 cancers in 185 countries. *CA: a Cancer Journal for Clinicians, 68* (6), 394–424.
3. Parkin, D. M., et al. (2005). Global cancer statistics, 2002. *CA: a Cancer Journal for Clinicians, 55*(2), 74–108.
4. Fitzmaurice, C., et al. (2018). Global, regional, and national cancer incidence, mortality, years of life lost, years lived with disability, and disability-adjusted life-years for 29 cancer groups, 1990 to 2016: A systematic analysis for the global burden of disease study. *JAMA Oncology, 4* (11), 1553–1568.
5. Nussbaumer, S., et al. (2011). Analysis of anticancer drugs: A review. *Talanta, 85*(5), 2265–2289.
6. Monsuez, J.-J., et al. (2010). Cardiac side-effects of cancer chemotherapy. *International Journal of Cardiology, 144*(1), 3–15.
7. Dropcho, E. J. (2011). The neurologic side effects of chemotherapeutic agents. *CONTINUUM: Lifelong Learning in Neurology, 17*(1), 95–112.

8. Lee, K. W., Bode, A. M., & Dong, Z. (2011). Molecular targets of phytochemicals for cancer prevention. *Nature Reviews Cancer, 11*(3), 211.
9. Howes, M.-J. R., & Simmonds, M. S. (2014). The role of phytochemicals as micronutrients in health and disease. *Current Opinion in Clinical Nutrition & Metabolic Care, 17*(6), 558–566.
10. Murakami, A. (2009). *Chemoprevention with phytochemicals targeting inducible nitric oxide synthase, in Food Factors for Health Promotion* (pp. 193–203). Basel: Karger Publishers.
11. Vidya Priyadarsini, R., & Nagini, S. (2012). Cancer chemoprevention by dietary phytochemicals: Promises and pitfalls. *Current Pharmaceutical Biotechnology, 13*(1), 125–136.
12. Surh, Y.-J. (2003). Cancer chemoprevention with dietary phytochemicals. *Nature Reviews Cancer, 3*(10), 768.
13. Straatman, J., et al. (2017). Techniques and short-term outcomes for total minimally invasive Ivor Lewis esophageal resection in distal esophageal and gastroesophageal junction cancers: pooled data from six European centers. *Surgical Endoscopy, 31*(1), 119–126.
14. Jenkins, G., et al. (2008). The bile acid deoxycholic acid has a non-linear dose response for DNA damage and possibly NF-κB activation in oesophageal cells, with a mechanism of action involving ROS. *Mutagenesis, 23*(5), 399–405.
15. Chiarion-Sileni, V., et al. (2007). Phase II trial of docetaxel, cisplatin and fluorouracil followed by carboplatin and radiotherapy in locally advanced oesophageal cancer. *British Journal of Cancer, 96*(3), 432–438.
16. Cooper, J. S., et al. (1999). Chemoradiotherapy of locally advanced esophageal cancer: Long-term follow-up of a prospective randomized trial (RTOG 85-01). *JAMA, 281*(17), 1623–1627.
17. Wagner, A. D., et al. (2006). Chemotherapy in advanced gastric cancer: A systematic review and meta-analysis based on aggregate data. *Journal of Clinical Oncology, 24*(18), 2903–2909.
18. Janmaat, M. L., et al. (2006). Predictive factors for outcome in a phase II study of gefitinib in second-line treatment of advanced esophageal cancer patients. *Journal of Clinical Oncology, 24*(10), 1612–1619.
19. Tew, W. Phase II trial of erlotinib for second-line treatment in advanced esophageal cancer. In Gastrointestinal Cancers Symposium, 2005. 2005.
20. Vanhoefer, U., et al. (2004). Phase I study of the humanized antiepidermal growth factor receptor monoclonal antibody EMD72000 in patients with advanced solid tumors that express the epidermal growth factor receptor. *Journal of Clinical Oncology, 22*(1), 175–184.
21. Daxenbichler, M. E., VanEtten, C. H., & Williams, P. H. (1979). Glucosinolates and derived products in cruciferous vegetables. Analysis of 14 varieties of Chinese cabbage. *Journal of Agricultural and Food Chemistry, 27*(1), 34–37.
22. Conaway, C. C., et al. (2005). Phenethyl isothiocyanate and sulforaphane and their N-acetylcysteine conjugates inhibit malignant progression of lung adenomas induced by tobacco carcinogens in A/J mice. *Cancer Research, 65*(18), 8548–8557.
23. Hecht, S. S. (1997). Approaches to chemoprevention of lung cancer based on carcinogens in tobacco smoke. *Environmental Health Perspectives, 105*(suppl 4), 955–963.
24. Xue, J.-H., et al. (2009). High glucose promotes intracellular lipid accumulation in vascular smooth muscle cells by impairing cholesterol influx and efflux balance. *Cardiovascular Research, 86*(1), 141–150.
25. Stoner, G. D., et al. (1999). Isothiocyanates and freeze-dried strawberries as inhibitors of esophageal cancer. *Toxicological Sciences: An Official Journal of the Society of Toxicology, 52*(suppl_1), 95–100.
26. Morse, M. A., et al. (1997). Mechanism of enhancement of esophageal tumorigenesis by 6-phenylhexyl isothiocyanate. *Cancer Letters, 112*(1), 119–125.
27. Sheerin, A., Thompson, K., & Goyns, M. (2002). Altered composition of the AP-1 transcription factor in immortalized compared to normal proliferating cells. *Cancer Letters, 177*(1), 83–87.
28. Stoner, G. D., & Wang, L.-S. (2012). Chemoprevention of esophageal squamous cell carcinoma with berries. In *Natural products in Cancer prevention and therapy* (pp. 1–20). Berlin: Springer.

29. Arcidiacono, P., et al. (2018). p63 is a key regulator of iRHOM2 signalling in the keratinocyte stress response. *Nature Communications, 9*(1), 1021.
30. Hirata, T., et al. (2019). 4-Methylthio-3-butenyl isothiocyanate (MTBITC) induced apoptotic cell death and G2/M cell cycle arrest via ROS production in human esophageal epithelial cancer cells. *The Journal of Toxicological Sciences, 44*(2), 73–81.
31. Langcake, P., & Pryce, R. (1976). The production of resveratrol by Vitis vinifera and other members of the Vitaceae as a response to infection or injury. *Physiological Plant Pathology, 9* (1), 77–86.
32. Catalgol, B., et al. (2012). Resveratrol: French paradox revisited. *Frontiers in Pharmacology, 3*, 141.
33. Chan, M. M.-Y. (2002). Antimicrobial effect of resveratrol on dermatophytes and bacterial pathogens of the skin. *Biochemical Pharmacology, 63*(2), 99–104.
34. Daroch, F., et al. (2001). In vitro antibacterial activity of Chilean red wines against Helicobacter pylori. *Microbios, 104*(408), 79–85.
35. Mahady, G. B., & Pendland, S. L. (2000). Resveratrol inhibits the growth of Helicobacter pylori in vitro. *The American Journal of Gastroenterology, 95*(7), 1849.
36. Mahady, G. B., Pendland, S. L., & Chadwick, L. R. (2003). Resveratrol and red wine extracts inhibit the growth of CagA+ strains of Helicobacter pylori in vitro. *The American Journal of Gastroenterology, 98*(6), 1440.
37. Aggarwal, B. B., et al. (2004). Role of resveratrol in prevention and therapy of cancer: Preclinical and clinical studies. *Anticancer Research, 24*(5A), 2783–2840.
38. Lackner, M., & Lass-Florl, C. (2013). Up-date on diagnostic strategies of invasive aspergillosis. *Current Pharmaceutical Design, 19*(20), 3595–3614.
39. Kundu, J. K., & Surh, Y.-J. (2008). Cancer chemopreventive and therapeutic potential of resveratrol: Mechanistic perspectives. *Cancer Letters, 269*(2), 243–261.
40. Harikumar, K. B., et al. (2010). Resveratrol, a multitargeted agent, can enhance antitumor activity of gemcitabine in vitro and in orthotopic mouse model of human pancreatic cancer. *International Journal of Cancer, 127*(2), 257–268.
41. Tang, Q., et al. (2013). Resveratrol-induced apoptosis is enhanced by inhibition of autophagy in esophageal squamous cell carcinoma. *Cancer Letters, 336*(2), 325–337.
42. Lin, Y., et al. (2014). A dietary pattern rich in lignans, quercetin and resveratrol decreases the risk of oesophageal cancer. *British Journal of Nutrition, 112*(12), 2002–2009.
43. McCormack, D., & McFadden, D. (2012). Pterostilbene and cancer: Current review. *Journal of Surgical Research, 173*(2), e53–e61.
44. Feng, Y., et al. (2016). Pterostilbene inhibits the growth of human esophageal cancer cells by regulating endoplasmic reticulum stress. *Cellular Physiology and Biochemistry, 38*(3), 1226–1244.
45. Beck, D., et al. (2013). Vemurafenib potently induces endoplasmic reticulum stress-mediated apoptosis in BRAFV600E melanoma cells. *Science Signaling, 6*(260), ra7-ra7.
46. Lakshmanan, A. P., et al. (2013). The hyperglycemia stimulated myocardial endoplasmic reticulum (ER) stress contributes to diabetic cardiomyopathy in the transgenic non-obese type 2 diabetic rats: A differential role of unfolded protein response (UPR) signaling proteins. *The International Journal of Biochemistry & Cell Biology, 45*(2), 438–447.
47. Tay, K. H., et al. (2014). Sustained IRE1 and ATF6 signaling is important for survival of melanoma cells undergoing ER stress. *Cellular Signalling, 26*(2), 287–294.
48. Khatiwada, J., et al. (2011). Green tea, phytic acid, and inositol in combination reduced the incidence of azoxymethane-induced colon tumors in Fischer 344 male rats. *Journal of Medicinal Food, 14*(11), 1313–1320.
49. Okello, E., et al. (2011). In vitro protective effects of colon-available extract of Camellia sinensis (tea) against hydrogen peroxide and beta-amyloid (Aβ (1–42)) induced cytotoxicity in differentiated PC12 cells. *Phytomedicine, 18*(8–9), 691–696.
50. Yang, G., et al. (2011). Green tea consumption and colorectal cancer risk: A report from the Shanghai Men's health study. *Carcinogenesis, 32*(11), 1684–1688.

51. Ye, F., et al. (2012). Suppression of esophageal cancer cell growth using curcumin,(−)-epigallocatechin-3-gallate and lovastatin. *World journal of gastroenterology: WJG, 18*(2), 126.
52. Liu, L., et al. (2015). Molecular mechanism of epigallocatechin-3-gallate in human esophageal squamous cell carcinoma in vitro and in vivo. *Oncology Reports, 33*(1), 297–303.
53. Liu, L., Zuo, J., & Wang, G. (2017). Epigallocatechin-3-gallate suppresses cell proliferation and promotes apoptosis in Ec9706 and Eca109 esophageal carcinoma cells. *Oncology Letters, 14*(4), 4391–4395.
54. Kato, K., et al. (2008). Effects of green tea polyphenol on methylation status of RECK gene and cancer cell invasion in oral squamous cell carcinoma cells. *British Journal of Cancer, 99* (4), 647.
55. Rocco, J. W., & Sidransky, D. (2001). p16 (MTS-1/CDKN2/INK4a) in cancer progression. *Experimental Cell Research, 264*(1), 42–55.
56. Meng, J., et al. (2017). Epigallocatechin-3-gallate inhibits growth and induces apoptosis in esophageal cancer cells through the demethylation and reactivation of the p16 gene. *Oncology Letters, 14*(1), 1152–1156.
57. Gao, Y., et al. (2013). Enhancement of (−)-epigallocatechin-3-gallate and theaflavin-3-3-′-digallate induced apoptosis by ascorbic acid in human lung adenocarcinoma SPC-A-1 cells and esophageal carcinoma Eca-109 cells via MAPK pathways. *Biochemical and Biophysical Research Communications, 438*(2), 370–374.
58. Liu, L., et al. (2017). Epigallocatechin-3-gallate promotes apoptosis and reversal of multidrug resistance in esophageal cancer cells. *Pathology-Research and Practice, 213*(10), 1242–1250.
59. Li, X., et al. (2019). Phase II trial of Epigallocatechin-3-Gallate in acute radiation-induced esophagitis for esophagus cancer. *Journal of Medicinal Food.*
60. Govindarajan, V., & Stahl, W. H. (1980). Turmeric—Chemistry, technology, and quality. *Critical Reviews in Food Science & Nutrition, 12*(3), 199–301.
61. Mirzaei, H., et al. (2018). MicroRNA: A novel target of curcumin in cancer therapy. *Journal of Cellular Physiology, 233*(4), 3004–3015.
62. Mirzaei, H., et al. (2017). Phytosomal curcumin: A review of pharmacokinetic, experimental and clinical studies. *Biomedicine & Pharmacotherapy, 85*, 102–112.
63. Mirzaei, H., et al. (2016). Can curcumin and its analogs be a new treatment option in cancer therapy? *Cancer Gene Therapy, 23*(11), 410–410.
64. Shehzad, A., Lee, J., & Lee, Y. S. (2013). Curcumin in various cancers. *BioFactors, 39*(1), 56–68.
65. Anand, P., et al. (2008). Curcumin and cancer: An "old-age" disease with an "age-old" solution. *Cancer Letters, 267*(1), 133–164.
66. Tajuddin, W. M., et al. (2019). Mechanistic understanding of Curcumin's therapeutic effects in lung cancer. *Nutrients, 11*(12), 2989.
67. Zhao, L., et al. (2015). Development of RGD-functionalized PEG-PLA micelles for delivery of curcumin. *Journal of Biomedical Nanotechnology, 11*(3), 436–446.
68. Jiang, G.-M., et al. (2015). Curcumin combined with FAPαc vaccine elicits effective antitumor response by targeting indolamine-2, 3-dioxygenase and inhibiting EMT induced by TNF-α in melanoma. *Oncotarget, 6*(28), 25932.
69. Zhang, F.-J., et al. (2015). Curcumin inhibits Ec109 cell growth via an AMPK-mediated metabolic switch. *Life Sciences, 134*, 49–55.
70. Lee, Y., & Kim, E.-K. (2013). AMP-activated protein kinase as a key molecular link between metabolism and clockwork. *Experimental & Molecular Medicine, 45*(7), e33–e33.
71. Hardie, D. G. (2013). AMPK: A target for drugs and natural products with effects on both diabetes and cancer. *Diabetes, 62*(7), 2164–2172.
72. Xiao, K., et al. (2013). Curcumin induces autophagy via activating the AMPK signaling pathway in lung adenocarcinoma cells. *Journal of Pharmacological Sciences*, 13085FP.

73. Li, X., et al. (2015). Curcumin induces apoptosis by PTEN/PI3K/AKT pathway in EC109 cells. *Zhongguo ying yong sheng li xue za zhi= Zhongguo yingyong shenglixue zazhi= Chinese Journal of Applied Physiology, 31*(2), 174–177.
74. Chemnitzer, O., et al. (2017). Response to TNF-α is increasing along with the progression in Barrett's esophagus. *Digestive Diseases and Sciences, 62*(12), 3391–3401.
75. Liu, Y., et al. (2018). The natural polyphenol curcumin induces apoptosis by suppressing STAT3 signaling in esophageal squamous cell carcinoma. *Journal of Experimental & Clinical Cancer Research, 37*(1), 1–12.
76. Wang, Y., et al. (2018). The curcumin analogs 2-pyridyl cyclohexanone induce apoptosis via inhibition of the JAK2–STAT3 pathway in human esophageal squamous cell carcinoma cells. *Frontiers in Pharmacology, 9*, 820.
77. Rahimi, H. R., et al. (2016). Novel delivery system for natural products: Nano-curcumin formulations. *Avicenna journal of phytomedicine, 6*(4), 383.
78. Pendleton, E. G., Jamasbi, R. J., & Geusz, M. E. (2019). Tetrahydrocurcumin, curcumin, and 5-fluorouracil effects on human esophageal carcinoma cells. *Anti-Cancer Agents in Medicinal Chemistry (Formerly Current Medicinal Chemistry-Anti-Cancer Agents), 19*(8), 1012–1020.
79. Sasaki, H., et al. (2011). Innovative preparation of curcumin for improved oral bioavailability. *Biological and Pharmaceutical Bulletin, 34*(5), 660–665.
80. Mizumoto, A., et al. (2019). Combination treatment with highly bioavailable curcumin and NQO1 inhibitor exhibits potent antitumor effects on esophageal squamous cell carcinoma. *Journal of Gastroenterology, 54*(8), 687–698.
81. Hosseini, S., et al. (2018). An in vitro study on curcumin delivery by nano-micelles for esophageal squamous cell carcinoma (KYSE-30). *Reports of Biochemistry & Molecular Biology, 6*(2), 137.
82. Martin, R. C., et al. (2015). Gold nanorods and curcumin-loaded nanomicelles for efficient in vivo photothermal therapy of Barrett's esophagus. *Nanomedicine, 10*(11), 1723–1733.
83. Rawla, P., & Barsouk, A. (2019). Epidemiology of gastric cancer: Global trends, risk factors and prevention. *Przeglad Gastroenterologiczny, 14*(1), 26.
84. Ustaalioğlu, B.B.Ö., et al., Capecitabine-cisplatin versus 5-fluorouracil/leucovorin in combination with radiotherapy for adjuvant therapy of lymph node positive locally advanced gastric cancer. 2018.
85. Lazăr, D. C., et al. (2016). New advances in targeted gastric cancer treatment. *World Journal of Gastroenterology, 22*(30), 6776.
86. Fan, B., et al. (2018). miR-17–92 cluster is connected with disease progression and oxaliplatin/capecitabine chemotherapy efficacy in advanced gastric cancer patients: A preliminary study. *Medicine, 97*(35).
87. Ryu, M.-H., et al. (2015). Multicenter phase II study of trastuzumab in combination with capecitabine and oxaliplatin for advanced gastric cancer. *European Journal of Cancer, 51*(4), 482–488.
88. Xu, R., et al. (2013). Results of a randomized and controlled clinical trial evaluating the efficacy and safety of combination therapy with Endostar and S-1 combined with oxaliplatin in advanced gastric cancer. *Oncotargets and Therapy, 6*, 925.
89. Van Cutsem, E., et al., Phase III study of docetaxel and cisplatin plus fluorouracil compared with cisplatin and fluorouracil as first-line therapy for advanced gastric cancer: A report of the V325 study group. 2006.
90. Wang, L., Sr. (2007). The effects of gemcitabine on cell apoptosis and cycle of gastric cancer. *Journal of Clinical Oncology, 25*(18_suppl), 15181.
91. De, R., et al. (2009). Antimicrobial activity of curcumin against Helicobacter pylori isolates from India and during infections in mice. *Antimicrobial Agents and Chemotherapy, 53*(4), 1592–1597.
92. Huang, F., et al. (2017). Curcumin inhibits gastric cancer-derived mesenchymal stem cells mediated angiogenesis by regulating NF-κB/VEGF signaling. *American Journal of Translational Research, 9*(12), 5538.

93. Qiang, Z., et al. (2019). Curcumin regulates the miR-21/PTEN/Akt pathway and acts in synergy with PD98059 to induce apoptosis of human gastric cancer MGC-803 cells. *Journal of International Medical Research, 47*(3), 1288–1297.
94. Liu, W.-H., et al. (2019). Curcumin inhibits proliferation, migration and invasion of gastric cancer cells via Wnt3a/β-catenin/EMT signaling pathway. *Zhongguo Zhong yao za zhi= Zhongguo zhongyao zazhi= China Journal of Chinese Materia Medica, 44*(14), 3107–3115.
95. Fu, H., et al. (2018). Curcumin regulates proliferation, autophagy, and apoptosis in gastric cancer cells by affecting PI3K and P53 signaling. *Journal of Cellular Physiology, 233*(6), 4634–4642.
96. Wang, L., et al. (2017). Curcumin suppresses gastric tumor cell growth via ROS-mediated DNA polymerase γ depletion disrupting cellular bioenergetics. *Journal of Experimental & Clinical Cancer Research, 36*(1), 47.
97. Xia, P., et al. (2015). Prognostic value of circulating CD133+ cells in patients with gastric cancer. *Cell Proliferation, 48*(3), 311–317.
98. Hatakeyama, K., et al. (2015). A novel splice variant of XIAP-associated factor 1 (XAF1) is expressed in peripheral blood containing gastric cancer-derived circulating tumor cells. *Gastric Cancer, 18*(4), 751–761.
99. Saito, H., et al. (2013). Increased apoptosis and elevated Fas expression in circulating natural killer cells in gastric cancer patients. *Gastric Cancer, 16*(4), 473–479.
100. Gu, X., et al. (2019). Curcumin inhibits liver metastasis of gastric cancer through reducing circulating tumor cells. *Aging (Albany NY), 11*(5), 1501.
101. Ye, C., et al. (2019). A novel curcumin derivative cl-6 exerts antitumor effect in human gastric cancer cells by inducing apoptosis through hippo–YaP signaling pathway. *Oncotargets and Therapy, 12*, 2259.
102. Silva, G., et al. (2018). Curcumin analog CH-5 suppresses the proliferation, migration, and invasion of the human gastric cancer cell line HGC-27. *Molecules, 23*(2), 279.
103. He, W., et al. (2019). Curcuminoid WZ35 synergize with cisplatin by inducing ROS production and inhibiting TrxR1 activity in gastric cancer cells. *Journal of Experimental & Clinical Cancer Research, 38*(1), 207.
104. Tsai, W. H., et al. (2018). EGFR-targeted photodynamic therapy by curcumin-encapsulated chitosan/TPP nanoparticles. *International Journal of Nanomedicine, 13*, 903.
105. Zhang, X., et al. (2015). Resveratrol protects against helicobacter pylori-associated gastritis by combating oxidative stress. *International Journal of Molecular Sciences, 16*(11), 27757–27769.
106. Jing, X., et al. (2016). Resveratrol induces cell cycle arrest in human gastric cancer MGC803 cells via the PTEN-regulated PI3K/Akt signaling pathway. *Oncology Reports, 35*(1), 472–478.
107. Miyoshi, K., & Hennighausen, L. (2003). β-Catenin: A transforming actor on many stages. *Breast Cancer Research, 5*(2), 63.
108. Dai, H., et al. (2018). Resveratrol inhibits the growth of gastric cancer via the Wnt/β-catenin pathway. *Oncology Letters, 16*(2), 1579–1583.
109. Yang, T., et al. (2018). Resveratrol inhibits Interleukin-6 induced invasion of human gastric cancer cells. *Biomedicine & Pharmacotherapy, 99*, 766–773.
110. Yang, Z., et al. (2019). Resveratrol suppresses the invasion and migration of human gastric cancer cells via inhibition of MALAT1-mediated epithelial-to-mesenchymal transition. *Experimental and Therapeutic Medicine, 17*(3), 1569–1578.
111. Gao, Q., et al. (2015). Resveratrol inhibits the hedgehog signaling pathway and epithelial-mesenchymal transition and suppresses gastric cancer invasion and metastasis. *Oncology Letters, 9*(5), 2381–2387.
112. Yang, Y., et al. (2018). Resveratrol induced apoptosis in human gastric carcinoma SGC-7901 cells via activation of mitochondrial pathway. *Asia-Pacific Journal of Clinical Oncology, 14*(5), e317–e324.

113. Wu, X., et al. (2018). Resveratrol induces apoptosis in SGC-7901 gastric cancer cells. *Oncology Letters, 16*(3), 2949–2956.
114. Xu, H., et al. (2018). Modulatory potential of curcumin and resveratrol on p53 post-translational modifications during gastric cancer. *Journal of Environmental Pathology, Toxicology and Oncology, 37*(2).
115. Xu, J., et al. (2017). Resveratrol reverses doxorubicin resistance by inhibiting epithelial-mesenchymal transition (EMT) through modulating PTEN/Akt signaling pathway in gastric cancer. *Journal of Experimental & Clinical Cancer Research, 36*(1), 19.
116. Kartal-Yandim, M., Adan-Gokbulut, A., & Baran, Y. (2016). Molecular mechanisms of drug resistance and its reversal in cancer. *Critical Reviews in Biotechnology, 36*(4), 716–726.
117. Nieth, C., et al. (2003). Modulation of the classical multidrug resistance (MDR) phenotype by RNA interference (RNAi). *FEBS Letters, 545*(2–3), 144–150.
118. Wu, C.-P., & Ambudkar, S. V. (2014). The pharmacological impact of ATP-binding cassette drug transporters on vemurafenib-based therapy. *Acta Pharmaceutica Sinica B, 4*(2), 105–111.
119. Kapse-Mistry, S., et al. (2014). Nanodrug delivery in reversing multidrug resistance in cancer cells. *Frontiers in Pharmacology, 5*, 159.
120. Borska, S., et al. (2012). In vitro effect of quercetin on human gastric carcinoma: Targeting cancer cells death and MDR. *Food and Chemical Toxicology, 50*(9), 3375–3383.
121. Karthikeyan, S., Hoti, S., & Prasad, N. R. (2014). Resveratrol modulates expression of ABC transporters in non-small lung cancer cells: Molecular docking and gene expression studies. *Journal of Cancer Science and Therapy, 6*(12), 497–504.
122. Belvedere, R., et al. (2016). Annexin A1 contributes to pancreatic cancer cell phenotype, behaviour and metastatic potential independently of formyl peptide receptor pathway. *Scientific Reports, 6*, 29660.
123. Mieszala, K., et al. (2018). Expression of genes and proteins of multidrug resistance in gastric cancer cells treated with resveratrol. *Oncology Letters, 15*(4), 5825–5832.
124. Hu, Y., et al. (2019). Anti-miRNA21 and resveratrol-loaded polysaccharide-based mesoporous silica nanoparticle for synergistic activity in gastric carcinoma. *Journal of Drug Targeting, 27*(10), 1135–1143.
125. Banerjee, S., et al. (2008). Multi-targeted therapy of cancer by genistein. *Cancer Letters, 269*(2), 226–242.
126. Li, Y., & Sarkar, F. H. (2002). Inhibition of nuclear factor κB activation in PC3 cells by genistein is mediated via Akt signaling pathway. *Clinical Cancer Research, 8*(7), 2369–2377.
127. Yuan-jing, F., Nan-shan, H., & Lian, X. (2009). Genistein synergizes with RNA interference inhibiting survivin for inducing DU-145 of prostate cancer cells to apoptosis. *Cancer Letters, 284*(2), 189–197.
128. Frey, R. S., Li, J., & Singletary, K. W. (2001). Effects of genistein on cell proliferation and cell cycle arrest in nonneoplastic human mammary epithelial cells: Involvement of Cdc2, p21waf/cip1, p27kip1, and Cdc25C expression. *Biochemical Pharmacology, 61*(8), 979–989.
129. Chang, K.-L., et al. (2004). Genistein arrests hepatoma cells at G2/M phase: Involvement of ATM activation and upregulation of p21waf1/cip1 and Wee1. *Biochemical Pharmacology, 67*(4), 717–726.
130. Ouyang, G., et al. (2009). Genistein induces G2/M cell cycle arrest and apoptosis of human ovarian cancer cells via activation of DNA damage checkpoint pathways. *Cell Biology International, 33*(12), 1237–1244.
131. Zhao, R., et al. (2009). Effects of selenite and genistein on G2/M cell cycle arrest and apoptosis in human prostate cancer cells. *Nutrition and Cancer, 61*(3), 397–407.
132. Park, C. E., et al. (2010). The antioxidant effects of genistein are associated with AMP-activated protein kinase activation and PTEN induction in prostate cancer cells. *Journal of Medicinal Food, 13*(4), 815–820.

133. Rahal, O. M., & Simmen, R. C. (2010). PTEN and p53 cross-regulation induced by soy isoflavone genistein promotes mammary epithelial cell cycle arrest and lobuloalveolar differentiation. *Carcinogenesis, 31*(8), 1491–1500.
134. Liu, Y.-L., et al. (2013). Genistein induces G2/M arrest in gastric cancer cells by increasing the tumor suppressor PTEN expression. *Nutrition and Cancer, 65*(7), 1034–1041.
135. Mazur, W. (1998). 11 Phytoestrogen content in foods. *Baillière's Clinical Endocrinology and Metabolism, 12*(4), 729–742.
136. Thompson, L.U., et al., Mammalian lignan production from various foods. 1991.
137. Takeshima, E., et al. (2009). NF-κB activation by Helicobacter pylori requires Akt-mediated phosphorylation of p65. *BMC Microbiology, 9*(1), 36.
138. Yang, J. J., et al. (2012). Interaction effects between genes involved in the AKT signaling pathway and phytoestrogens in gastric carcinogenesis: A nested case–control study from the Korean Multi-center Cancer Cohort. *Molecular Nutrition & Food Research, 56*(11), 1617–1626.
139. Tanabe, T., & Tohnai, N. (2002). Cyclooxygenase isozymes and their gene structures and expression. *Prostaglandins & Other Lipid Mediators, 68*, 95–114.
140. Li, Y., et al. (2011). Involvement of nuclear factor κB (NF-κB) in the downregulation of cyclooxygenase-2 (COX-2) by genistein in gastric cancer cells. *Journal of International Medical Research, 39*(6), 2141–2150.
141. Yu, D., et al. (2014). Genistein attenuates cancer stem cell characteristics in gastric cancer through the downregulation of Gli1. *Oncology Reports, 31*(2), 673–678.
142. Cho, L. Y., et al. (2015). Gene polymorphisms in the ornithine decarboxylase–polyamine pathway modify gastric cancer risk by interaction with isoflavone concentrations. *Gastric Cancer, 18*(3), 495–503.
143. Fearon, K., et al. (2011). Definition and classification of cancer cachexia: An international consensus. *The Lancet Oncology, 12*(5), 489–495.
144. Evans, W. J., et al. (2008). Cachexia: A new definition. *Clinical Nutrition, 27*(6), 793–799.
145. Yanagihara, K., et al. (2013). Inhibitory effects of isoflavones on tumor growth and cachexia in newly established cachectic mouse models carrying human stomach cancers. *Nutrition and Cancer, 65*(4), 578–589.
146. Huang, W., et al. (2014). Genistein-inhibited cancer stem cell-like properties and reduced chemoresistance of gastric cancer. *International Journal of Molecular Sciences, 15*(3), 3432–3443.
147. Verhey, K. J., & Hammond, J. W. (2009). Traffic control: Regulation of kinesin motors. *Nature Reviews Molecular Cell Biology, 10*(11), 765–777.
148. Sheng, Y., et al. (2018). Upregulation of KIF20A correlates with poor prognosis in gastric cancer. *Cancer Management and Research, 10*, 6205.
149. Cao, X., et al. (2016). 7-Difluoromethoxyl-5, 4′-di-n-octyl genistein inhibits the stem-like characteristics of gastric cancer stem-like cells and reverses the phenotype of epithelial-mesenchymal transition in gastric cancer cells. *Oncology Reports, 36*(2), 1157–1165.
150. Aditya, N., et al. (2013). Curcumin and genistein coloaded nanostructured lipid carriers: In vitro digestion and antiprostate cancer activity. *Journal of Agricultural and Food Chemistry, 61*(8), 1878–1883.
151. Lee, A., Fox, J., & Hazell, S. (1993). Pathogenicity of Helicobacter pylori: A perspective. *Infection and Immunity, 61*(5), 1601.
152. Cox, A. D., et al. (2014). Drugging the undruggable RAS: Mission possible? *Nature Reviews Drug Discovery, 13*(11), 828–851.
153. Graf, W., et al. (2020). Prognostic impact of BRAF and KRAS mutation in patients with colorectal and appendiceal peritoneal metastases scheduled for CRS and HIPEC. *Annals of Surgical Oncology, 27*(1), 293–300.
154. Mayor, S. (2006). NICE rules on chemotherapy drugs for colon and breast cancer. *BMJ, 332* (7549), 1052.

155. Li, Y.-H., et al. (2015). Role of phytochemicals in colorectal cancer prevention. *World journal of gastroenterology: WJG, 21*(31), 9262.
156. Liu, J., et al. (2018). MiR-106a-5p promotes 5-FU resistance and the metastasis of colorectal cancer by targeting TGFβR2. *International Journal of Clinical and Experimental Pathology, 11*(12), 5622.
157. Vymetalkova, V., et al. (2020). Expression quantitative trait loci in ABC transporters are associated with survival in 5-FU treated colorectal cancer patients. *Mutagenesis*.
158. Divisi, D., et al. (2006). Diet and cancer. *Acta Biomedica-Ateneo Parmense, 77*(2), 118.
159. Steinmetz, K. A., & Potter, J. D. (1996). Vegetables, fruit, and cancer prevention: A review. *Journal of the American Dietetic Association, 96*(10), 1027–1039.
160. Greenwald, P. (2005). Lifestyle and medical approaches to cancer prevention. In *Tumor Prevention and Genetics III* (pp. 1–15). Berlin: Springer.
161. Vainio, H., & Weiderpass, E. (2006). Fruit and vegetables in cancer prevention. *Nutrition and Cancer, 54*(1), 111–142.
162. Panaro, M. A., et al. (2012). Anti-inflammatory effects of resveratrol occur via inhibition of lipopolysaccharide-induced NF-κB activation in Caco-2 and SW480 human colon cancer cells. *British Journal of Nutrition, 108*(9), 1623–1632.
163. Gong, W., et al. (2017). The inhibitory effect of resveratrol on COX-2 expression in human colorectal cancer: A promising therapeutic strategy. *European Review for Medical and Pharmacological Sciences, 21*(5), 1136–1143.
164. Chang, C.-H., et al. (2017). Resveratrol-induced autophagy and apoptosis in cisplatin-resistant human oral cancer CAR cells: A key role of AMPK and Akt/mTOR signaling. *International Journal of Oncology, 50*(3), 873–882.
165. Li, D., et al. (2019). Resveratrol suppresses colon cancer growth by targeting the AKT/STAT3 signaling pathway. *International Journal of Molecular Medicine, 43*(1), 630–640.
166. Zeng, Y.-H., et al. (2017). Resveratrol inactivates PI3K/Akt signaling through upregulating BMP7 in human colon cancer cells. *Oncology Reports, 38*(1), 456–464.
167. Lao, L., Song, X., & Xu, J. (2017). *Effect of resveratrol in regulating proliferation and apoptosis of rectal cancer cells via up-regulating PTEN.* Zhongguo Zhong yao za zhi= Zhongguo zhongyao zazhi=. *China Journal of Chinese Materia Medica, 42*(9), 1730–1735.
168. Liu, Z., et al. (2019). Resveratrol induces p53 in colorectal cancer through SET7/9. *Oncology Letters, 17*(4), 3783–3789.
169. Karimi Dermani, F., et al. (2017). Resveratrol inhibits proliferation, invasion, and epithelial–mesenchymal transition by increasing miR-200c expression in HCT-116 colorectal cancer cells. *Journal of Cellular Biochemistry, 118*(6), 1547–1555.
170. Kim, D. H., et al. (2017). Resveratrol analogue, HS-1793, induces apoptotic cell death and cell cycle arrest through downregulation of AKT in human colon cancer cells. *Oncology Reports, 37*(1), 281–288.
171. Cheah, F. K., et al. (2018). Resveratrol analogue, (E)-N-(2-(4-methoxystyryl) phenyl) furan-2-carboxamide induces G 2/M cell cycle arrest through the activation of p53–p21 CIP1/WAF1 in human colorectal HCT116 cells. *Apoptosis, 23*(5–6), 329–342.
172. Storniolo, C. E., & Moreno, J. J. (2018). Resveratrol analogs with antioxidant activity inhibit intestinal epithelial cancer Caco-2 cell growth by modulating arachidonic acid cascade. *Journal of Agricultural and Food Chemistry, 67*(3), 819–828.
173. El-Readi, M. Z., et al. (2019). Resveratrol mediated cancer cell apoptosis, and modulation of multidrug resistance proteins and metabolic enzymes. *Phytomedicine, 55*, 269–281.
174. Buhrmann, C., et al. (2018). Resveratrol chemosensitizes TNF-β-induced survival of 5-FU-treated colorectal cancer cells. *Nutrients, 10*(7), 888.
175. Chung, S. S., et al. (2018). Combination of resveratrol and 5-fluorouracil enhanced anti-telomerase activity and apoptosis by inhibiting STAT3 and Akt signaling pathways in human colorectal cancer cells. *Oncotarget, 9*(68), 32943.

176. Gavrilas, L. I., et al. (2019). Pro-apoptotic genes as new targets for single and combinatorial treatments with resveratrol and curcumin in colorectal cancer. *Food & Function, 10*(6), 3717–3726.
177. Wu, J.-Y., et al. (2019). 3, 5, 4′-trimethoxy-trans-stilbene loaded PEG-PE micelles for the treatment of colon cancer. *International Journal of Nanomedicine, 14*, 7489.
178. Temraz, S., Mukherji, D., & Shamseddine, A. (2013). Potential targets for colorectal cancer prevention. *International Journal of Molecular Sciences, 14*(9), 17279–17303.
179. Chen, A., Xu, J., & Johnson, A. (2006). Curcumin inhibits human colon cancer cell growth by suppressing gene expression of epidermal growth factor receptor through reducing the activity of the transcription factor Egr-1. *Oncogene, 25*(2), 278–287.
180. Patel, B. B., et al. (2010). Curcumin targets FOLFOX-surviving colon cancer cells via inhibition of EGFRs and IGF-1R. *Anticancer Research, 30*(2), 319–325.
181. Binion, D. G., Otterson, M. F., & Rafiee, P. (2008). Curcumin inhibits VEGF-mediated angiogenesis in human intestinal microvascular endothelial cells through COX-2 and MAPK inhibition. *Gut, 57*(11), 1509–1517.
182. Greer, E. L., Banko, M. R., & Brunet, A. (2009). AMP-activated protein kinase and FoxO transcription factors in dietary restriction-induced longevity. *Annals of the New York Academy of Sciences, 1170*, 688.
183. Ryu, M.-J., et al. (2008). Natural derivatives of curcumin attenuate the Wnt/β-catenin pathway through down-regulation of the transcriptional coactivator p300. *Biochemical and Biophysical Research Communications, 377*(4), 1304–1308.
184. Liu, X., et al. (2016). LncRNA NBR2 engages a metabolic checkpoint by regulating AMPK under energy stress. *Nature Cell Biology, 18*(4), 431–442.
185. Yu, H., et al. (2019). Curcumin regulates the progression of colorectal cancer via LncRNA NBR2/AMPK pathway. *Technology in Cancer Research & Treatment, 18*, 1533033819870781.
186. Kim, R. H., et al. (2005). DJ-1, a novel regulator of the tumor suppressor PTEN. *Cancer Cell, 7*(3), 263–273.
187. Shang, H., et al. (2019). Over-expression of DJ-1 attenuates effects of curcumin on colorectal cancer cell proliferation and apoptosis. *European Review for Medical and Pharmacological Sciences, 23*, 3080–3087.
188. Zhu, J., et al. (2018). Curcumin induces autophagy via inhibition of yes-associated protein (YAP) in human colon cancer cells. *Medical Science Monitor: International Medical Journal of Experimental and Clinical Research, 24*, 7035.
189. Hosseini, S. A., Zand, H., & Cheraghpour, M. (2019). The influence of curcumin on the downregulation of MYC, insulin and IGF-1 receptors: A possible mechanism underlying the anti-growth and anti-migration in chemoresistant colorectal cancer cells. *Medicina, 55*(4), 90.
190. Shakibaei, M., et al. (2013). Curcumin enhances the effect of chemotherapy against colorectal cancer cells by inhibition of NF-κB and Src protein kinase signaling pathways. *PLoS One, 8* (2), e57218.
191. Chen, G.-P., et al. (2017). Curcumin combined with cis-platinum promote the apoptosis of human colorectal cancer HT29 cells and mechanism. *International Journal of Clinical and Experimental Pathology, 10*(12), 11496–11505.
192. Selvam, C., et al. (2019). Molecular mechanisms of curcumin and its analogs in colon cancer prevention and treatment. *Life Sciences*, 117032.
193. Chung, S. S., et al. (2019). A novel curcumin analog inhibits canonical and non-canonical functions of telomerase through STAT3 and NF-κB inactivation in colorectal cancer cells. *Oncotarget, 10*(44), 4516.
194. Sabra, R., Billa, N., & Roberts, C. J. (2019). Cetuximab-conjugated chitosan-pectinate (modified) composite nanoparticles for targeting colon cancer. *International Journal of Pharmaceutics, 572*, 118775.

195. Qi, W., et al. (2011). Genistein inhibits proliferation of colon cancer cells by attenuating a negative effect of epidermal growth factor on tumor suppressor FOXO3 activity. *BMC Cancer, 11*(1), 219.
196. Zhou, P., et al. (2017). Genistein induces apoptosis of colon cancer cells by reversal of epithelial-to-mesenchymal via a Notch1/NF-κB/slug/E-cadherin pathway. *BMC Cancer, 17* (1), 813.
197. Luo, Y., et al. (2014). Apoptotic effect of genistein on human colon cancer cells via inhibiting the nuclear factor-kappa B (NF-κB) pathway. *Tumor Biology, 35*(11), 11483–11488.
198. Qin, J., et al. (2016). Genistein induces activation of the mitochondrial apoptosis pathway by inhibiting phosphorylation of Akt in colorectal cancer cells. *Pharmaceutical Biology, 54*(1), 74–79.
199. Qin, J., et al. (2015). Genistein inhibits human colorectal cancer growth and suppresses miR-95, Akt and SGK1. *Cellular Physiology and Biochemistry, 35*(5), 2069–2077.
200. Zhang, Z., et al. (2013). Genistein induces G2/M cell cycle arrest and apoptosis via ATM/p53-dependent pathway in human colon cancer cells. *International Journal of Oncology, 43*(1), 289–296.
201. Zhang, Y., et al. (2013). Genistein, a soya isoflavone, prevents azoxymethane-induced up-regulation of WNT/β-catenin signalling and reduces colon pre-neoplasia in rats. *British Journal of Nutrition, 109*(1), 33–42.
202. Zhu, J., Ren, J., & Tang, L. (2018). Genistein inhibits invasion and migration of colon cancer cells by recovering WIF1 expression. *Molecular Medicine Reports, 17*(5), 7265–7273.
203. Pintova, S., et al. (2019). Genistein combined with FOLFOX or FOLFOX–Bevacizumab for the treatment of metastatic colorectal cancer: Phase I/II pilot study. *Cancer Chemotherapy and Pharmacology, 84*(3), 591–598.
204. Pintova, S., et al. (2017). ME-143 is superior to genistein in suppression of WNT signaling in colon cancer cells. *Anticancer Research, 37*(4), 1647–1653.
205. Du, Q., et al. (2016). Chemopreventive activity of GEN-27, a genistein derivative, in colitis-associated cancer is mediated by p65-CDX2-β-catenin axis. *Oncotarget, 7*(14), 17870.
206. Pool, H., et al. (2018). Development of genistein-PEGylated silica hybrid nanomaterials with enhanced antioxidant and antiproliferative properties on HT29 human colon cancer cells. *American Journal of Translational Research, 10*(8), 2306.

Chapter 2
Role of Phytochemicals on Growth and Metastasis of GI Cancer

Krishnamurthy Nakuluri and Gowru Srivani

Abstract Cancer metastasis is a multistage phenomenon, which can be prevented by the administration of various phytochemicals. Phytochemicals inhibit or prevent cancer initiation, promotion, progression, as well as metastasis by employing anti-oxidant, anti-inflammatory effects mediated via NF-kκB, Nrf2, and AP-1 signaling. Besides, phytochemicals also mediate apoptosis in tumor cells and inhibition of cancer growth. The dietary phytochemicals are abundant in fruits and vegetables that appear to be consisting of beneficial effects against cancer metastasis and induce apoptosis and arrest cell growth by multiple mechanisms.

Keywords Phytochemicals · Gastrointestinal cancer · Metastasis · Epithelial-mesenchymal transition

Abbreviations

APC	Adenomatous polyposis coli
CRC	Colorectal cancer
EGF	Epidermal growth factor
EGFR	Epidermal growth factor receptor
EMT	Epithelial-mesenchymal transition
GC	Gastric cancer
HGF	Hepatocyte growth factor
HIF-1α	Hypoxia-inducible factor-1 alpha
IBD	Inflammatory bowel disease
IL	Interleukins

K. Nakuluri (✉)
Dept. of Pediatrics, School of Medicine, University of California, San Francisco (UCSF), San Francisco, CA, USA

G. Srivani
Department of Biosciences and Biotechnology, Banasthali University, Banasthali, Rajasthan, India

G. P. Nagaraju (ed.), *Phytochemicals Targeting Tumor Microenvironment in Gastrointestinal Cancers*, https://doi.org/10.1007/978-3-030-48405-7_2

MAPK	Mitogen-activated protein kinase
MET	Mesenchymal growth factor
MMP9	Matrix metalloproteinase
NF-κB	Nuclear factor kappa-B
PDGF	Platelet-derived growth factor
ROS	Reactive oxygen species
TGF-β	Transforming growth factor-β

1 Introduction

Cancer is an abnormal or uncontrolled cell growth in the body, which can invade other body tissues through metastasis. Cancer metastasis is a multistep phenomenon that begins with initiation succeeded by promotion as well as progression. Cancer initiation, promotion, and progression comprise a sequence of epigenetic as well as genetic modifications influencing oncogenes as well as tumor-suppressor genes. Kusama suggested the notion of "chronology of cancer" to relate the character of cancers through the amplitude of time [1]. Previous reports with the evidence of the numerous processes that take place in cancer patients over time disclose aspects of cancer, going from cancer pathogenesis to spreading, progression, and metastasis. The most potent causative agents of cancer are tobacco smoke, which contains mutagens, such as benzopyrene and dimethyl nitrosamine. The most familiar gastrointestinal cancer associated with tobacco smoking is esophageal cancer. The principal reason to spread cancer to other body parts is its metastasis characteristics, by which cancer cells pass through locally by migrating into neighboring normal tissue. Various types of tumor cells can invade distant parts of the body, to lymph nodes, tissues, or organs, which is called metastatic cancer or stage IV cancer. The cancer cells could circulate into blood, lymphatic, or beyond body cavities, to generate secondary tumors. Nevertheless, not all cancers are metastatic, and yet in metastatic cancer, not all cells within it are accomplished of metastasizing [2]. Metastatic cancer cells comprise several specialized features: they go through an epithelial-mesenchymal transition (EMT) and become invasive, resistant to programmed cell death and anoikis, and gain the ability to spread and colonize secondary sites [3]. The "seed-and-soil" hypothesis is suggested by Stephen Paget, since metastasis relies on the connection between the selected cancer cells (seeds) and the microenvironment (soil) [4]. This concept illustrates various steps of cancer metastasis: acquiring of invasive phenotype relies on tumor cellular connection along with signals from the stromal cells [5], and also subsequent dormancy/growth of tumor cells on secondary sites also reckoned on microenvironment [6, 7].

Previous reports have classified EMT into different subcategories, each with very distinct functional outcomes [8]. Type 1 EMT is undergone during regular physiological developmental processes such as embryogenesis, implantation, and organ development; type 2 EMT is essential to tissue reconstruction and organ fibrosis, whereas type 3 EMT is associated with cancer progression and metastasis. Although it has been studied that EMT occurs in cancers [9], the role of EMT as a crucial mechanism for the acquisition of the malignant phenotype by epithelial cancer cells is unknown [10]. Cancer cells acquire mesenchymal phenotype and express mesenchymal markers including α-SMA, FSP1, vimentin, as well as desmin [11]. These cells are also identified in the invasive tumor cells which are capable of following intravasation, blood circulation, extravasation, and finally colonization. EMT-transited cells can generate tumors at secondary sites which are similar to the primary tumor, with the desertion of the mesenchymal phenotype. The exuviating of the mesenchymal phenotype at the time of secondary tumor generation is termed as a MET. This EMT-MET mechanistic model is critical in explaining the metastasis of tumor cells: EMT mediates altered cell phenotype that enables the evasion of epithelial cancer cells from their structural restrictions enforced by tissue architecture, while MET switches these modifications and promotes colonization in secondary sites [12].

Recent reports reinforce the concept that tumor-microenvironment interplay is significant in the advancement of metastasis. For example, fully malignant cancer cells can be regressed to typical phenotype by revealing them to nonpermissive stroma [13]. Thus, other than the cellular context, tumor-related stroma may provide signals that mediate EMT. These signals include HGF, EGF, PDGF, and TGFβ and are delineated to be accountable for the stimulation of EMT-mediating factors ("Snail, Slug, ZEB1, Twist, Goosecoid, and FOXC2"). Besides, MAPK, PI3KAkt, Smads, RhoB, β-catenin, Ras, c-Fos, and integrins are also demonstrated to induce EMT. As reported from previous studies, the effects of phytochemicals on carcinogenesis are anti-inflammatory and antioxidant properties and genomic stability that prevail to be principal targets in chemoprevention [14, 15]. They have strongly associated with the induction of apoptosis and growth suppression of cancer cells. EGFR plays a significant role in various cancers, including colorectal cancer, by altering several signaling pathways [16]. The elevated expression levels and function of EGFR are strongly connected with the metastatic ability of colon cancer cells. Previous reports reveal that curcumin suppresses colon cancer cell growth by decreasing the ERK/Egr-1/EGFR signaling cascade and reduces the EGFR expression. Curcumin was also shown to block the development of chemoresistant colon cancer cells through suppression of EGFR and IGF-1R.

Various phytochemicals, predominantly curcumin, resveratrol, EGCG, and other polyphenolic compounds, have been shown to have synergistic and beneficial effects against several GI cancers.

2 Gastrointestinal Cancer

Gastrointestinal (GI) cancer is majorly a result of metastasis, which is an indication of a malignant tumor disposed through a multistep process in which cancer cells disseminate consecutively from the original site to other organs. For GI cancers, the prevalent or routine target site for metastasis includes lymph nodes, liver, peritoneal, and, subsequently, lung and other sites of the body, which are predominant causes of GI cancer-associated mortality. The mechanism of gastrointestinal cancer metastasis is categorized into local angiogenesis, diversity of tumor cells, interplay and cascade of signaling, reduced expression of E-cadherin, and EMT. Several studies have evidenced that the "anatomical/mechanical" and "seed-and-soil" hypotheses are extensively approved to describe the tumor metastatic spread [17–20]. The seed-and-soil hypothesis describes that specific tumor cells may show a predisposition to particular target organs of metastasis [21–23]. Previous studies revealed that N-desulfated heparin is efficient in blocking metastasis of gastric cancer through inhibiting tumor bFGF expression and tumor angiogenesis [24, 25]. The potential candidate biomarkers for GI cancer and diagnosis of tumor metastasis include EGFR, miR-21, ki-67 antigen, and urinary free amino acids [25].

Previous studies have shown that CaA inhibits MEK1 and TOPK activities and binds directly to either MEK1 or TOPK in an ATP-noncompetitive fashion [26]. CaA is known to suppress ERK phosphorylation, AP-1, and NF-κB transactivation and consequently block TPA-, EGF-, and H-Ras-mediated transformation of epidermal cells. Coffee intake was also correlated with a compelling depletion of ERK phosphorylation in cancer patients. These previous reports indicate that coffee and CaA target MEK1 and TOPK to inhibit metastasis and new cancer cell transformation [27]. Recent reports reveal that Triphala extract (naringin, quercetin, homoorientin, and isorhamnetin) suppresses proliferation and induces apoptosis in colon cancer stem cells via suppressing c-Myc/cyclin D1 and elevating Bax/Bcl-2 ratio [28]. Previous studies revealed that the herbal cocktail THL induces cell death in several cancer cells [28]. THL inhibits metastasis and angiogenesis by blocking several biological and pathological processes in tumor cells. Besides, THL could also directly suppress tube formation of endothelial cells and the migration, invasion, and also THL could suppress the secretion of pro-angiogenic factors by tumor cells [29].

3 Gastric Cancer

Gastric cancer (GC) is the fourth most recurrent cancer globally and it lies second among cancer mortality [30]. Gastric cancer metastatic spread is very lethal, which accumulates to trigger altered physiological homeostasis. GC prevails when cells in the lining of the stomach grow in an uncontrolled manner and progressively leads to the formation of a tumor. Previous reports reveal that the percentage of metastasis in gastric cancer patients has increased to over 40% [31–33]. These cancer cells infiltrate normal tissues and invade other parts of the body. About 80–85% of gastric cancers appear to be generated from the lining of the stomach, which is called adenocarcinoma. The other cancers that may appear in the stomach include stromal tumors, lymphoma, and gastrointestinal and carcinoid tumors, among others. Previous reports revealed that curcumin inhibits *H. pylori* infection by obstructing its

Table 2.1 List of phytochemicals and cell cycle arrest

Phytochemical	Source	Cell line investigated	Cell cycle phase	Reference
Curcumin	*Curcuma longa*	COLO	G0/G1	[88]
Resveratrol	Grapes, peanuts	HCT-116, Caco2	G1/S	[89]
Curcumin	Curcuma longa	HT-29	G2/M	[56]
Berberine	Berberis, coptis	SW480	G0/G1	[56]
Quercetin	Fruits, vegetables, nut	HT-29	G0/G1	[11]
6-Gingerol	Ginger	SW480	G2/M	[84]
Berberine	Berberis and coptis	LoVo	G2/M	[90]
Piperine	*Piper nigrum* and *Piper longum*	HRT-18	G0/G	[77]
Crocetin	*Crocus sativus* L.	HCT116 p53 (-/-)	G2/M	[87]
Crocetin	*Crocus sativus* L.	HCT116 wild type	G0/G1	[87]

growth, and the therapeutic efficacy of curcumin further evidenced by using various gastric cancer cells [34, 35]. Curcumin also safeguards against GC by downregulation of NF-κB and NF-κB-induced anti-apoptotic genes in human gastric cancer [35]. Resveratrol suppresses cell cycle progression by stimulating cell cycle blocking at the G0/G1 stage via suppressing kinase C-mediated manner and stimulating cell death in multiple gastric adenocarcinoma cell lines (Table 2.1) [35, 36]. Besides, resveratrol also controls cell proliferation, which is connected with the MEK1/2-ERK1/2-c-Jun signaling cascade, crucial signaling involved in growth and proliferation of GC cells [37].

4 Colorectal Cancer

In colorectal cancer (CRC), cancer cells broken down from a tumor in colon or rectum disseminate to body and they metastasize to the liver, lungs, or any other organs. The usual site of metastasis for colon cancer or rectal cancer is the liver but it also spreads to the brain, bones, liver, or spinal cord. The previous family history of CRC or chronic IBD is the predominant contributor to the progression of CRC. Besides, sedentary lifestyle, smoking and alcohol abuse, and diets with less fiber and a higher red meat or fat are crucial roots of CRC progression and development [38]. Most CRC cases are identified in the final phases of the cancer metastasis, which causes curative therapy for cancer patients [39]. The predominant CRC cases are the consequences of genetic and epigenetic modifications [40–42]. Previous studies demonstrated the essential role of p53 in tumor repression; 50% of CRC are due to mutations in p53, which stimulates invasion, cell proliferation, metastasis, and resistance to several anticancer therapeutics. Besides, mutations in the adenomatous polyposis coli (APC) gene in CRC assist the impairment of β-catenin and trigger the Wnt signaling that activates cyclin D1 and c-Myc, which contribute favorable settings for cellular proliferation [43]. In CRC, induction of NF-κB stimulates genes important for production of pro-inflammatory factors and cytokines, crucial for CRC cell propagation [44]. Further, the PI3K/Akt pathway stimulates cancer cell proliferation through suppression of cell death and induction of cell cycle [45].

Phytochemicals are abundantly present in vegetables, fruits, grains, herbs, and spices, which are health-promoting and disease-preventing features. Previous reports revealed that phytochemicals present in diet prevent the CRC progression, and clinical reports have shown the beneficial health effects of the intake of fruits and vegetables [46–50]. Inflammation in CRC tumors is associated with altered genomic instability and expression levels of several oncogenes and tumor-suppressor genes [51]. The repeated episodes of inflammation in tumor microenvironment stimulate the proliferation and survival of cancer cells, elevated angiogenesis, and tumor metastasis [52, 53]. NF-κB implicated in tumor initiation and progression and deletion of IKKb is associated with decreased tumor incidence [54]. NF-κB signaling pathway is significant in guiding cancer-associated inflammation including gastrointestinal cancer [54]. NF-κB signaling cascade is regulated by chemopreventive compounds such as phytochemicals. Several phytochemical compounds have been used as effective anticancer agents that inhibit the development of DNA mutation caused by carcinogens. Keap1–Nrf2 axis in redox signaling plays a significant role, involving phytochemicals as antioxidants. Several dietary phytochemicals including PEIC and sulforaphane are strong stimulators of phase II/detoxifying genes, and this induction is in a Nrf2-dependent manner.

Curcumin was previously shown to have potent antioxidant, anti-inflammatory, and anticancer characteristics [55]. Previous reports revealed that curcumin mediates cell death in HT29 cells through the calpain/caspase-12 apoptotic signaling pathway [56]. β-Catenin is familiar to play a notable role in controlling cell proliferation in CRC, which stimulates the expression of *c-myc* and cyclin D1 [57]. Curcumin inhibits β-catenin response transcription without changing intracellular levels of β-catenin. Curcumin blocks Wnt/β-catenin pathway-mediated *c-myc* expression to impair cell adhesion in colon cancer cells [58]. Curcumin also arrests cell cycle in CRC cells by increasing the expression levels of p53 and p21 (Table 2.1) [59]. Besides, curcumin stimulates ROS production in p53-mutated cancer cells, which leads to cell cycle block and apoptosis through stimulation of ROS-mediated mitochondrial pathway [60]. Numerous studies demonstrated that curcumin inhibits colon cancer by targeting EGFR, MAPK, AMPK-COX-2, and Wnt/β-catenin signaling pathways [16, 57, 61–63]. EGFR plays an important role in various cancers including colon cancer by regulating numerous signaling pathways [16]. In fact, previous studies showed that the upregulation of EGFR is strongly correlated with the metastatic capacity of colon cancer cells. It is demonstrated that curcumin suppresses colon cancer cell growth by downregulating the ERK/Egr-1/EGFR signaling and reduced levels of EGFR [61].

Resveratrol, which is present in grapes, has been familiar with its anticancer and anti-inflammatory properties [64]. It controls energy metabolism, plays a significant role in the inhibition of tumor cell growth, and mediates cell death. It also inhibits the pentose phosphate pathway, besides suppressing talin and FAK expression, and it also represses cell growth and stimulation of apoptosis in CRC cells [65]. Previous reports have shown that resveratrol impedes cell proliferation signaling pathways [66–69]. It also remarkably decreases the expression of glycolytic enzymes in Caco-2 cells, increases the activity of citrate synthase, and decreases the intake of glucose [70, 71]. Resveratrol has also been studied in conjugation with etoposide in CRC cells; synergistic beneficial effects have been noticed on cell growth suppression through decreasing MAPK signaling and a rise in apoptosis via activation of p53 [67–69]. Besides, the mixture of resveratrol and grape seed extract was previously reported to block Wnt/β-catenin signaling as well as elevate mitochondrial dependent cell death in in vitro and in vivo models [69]. It was demonstrated that resveratrol suppresses through downregulation of HIF-1α and MMP-9 expression in colon carcinoma cells [72, 73].

Capsaicin is a vital constituent of red pepper, which mediates cell death in colon cancer cells by blocking cells at G0/G1 stage, which is connected with the increased levels of Bax in concurrence with PARP cleavage [73, 74]. Capsaicin alters the expression of cell cycle proteins, including reduced cyclin D1, and elevates the expression of p21, both Bax [74]. Besides, capsaicin upregulates p53 and reduces cell death which is reported in p53-knockdown cells that suggests the significant role of p53 in capsaicin-mediated cell death [74].

Colchicine is an alkaloid obtained from *Colchicum autumnale* that has been shown to terminate cancer metastasis by its antimitotic activity [75]. Previous reports indicate that colchicine mediates apoptosis via ROS production, MMP loss, triggering caspase-3 activation and augmented Bax, and reduced Bcl-2 expression levels in tumor cells [76]. Piperine, which is an amide alkaloid extracted from pepper, is shown to block the cell cycle and suppress CRC cell proliferation unrestrained p53 status [77]. Besides, piperine also mediates cell death by suppressing the cell survival PI3K/Akt signaling and increases inositol-requiring enzyme-1α, and CHOP, which leads to loss of MMPs, cytochrome c release, and PARP cleavage that suggest the significant role of piperine-mediated programmed cell death [78]. Berberine is an alkaloid found in several medicinal plants that have been familiar for its anticancer properties in various cancers including neuroblastoma, prostate cancer, and osteosarcoma [79, 80]. Previous reports have demonstrated that berberine mediates through caspase-dependent and -independent mechanisms [81–83]. 6-Gingerol is a well-known widely studied phytochemical for its cytotoxic properties in several kinds of cancers, including colon cancer. It also suppresses the proliferation of cancer cells by blocking cell cycle at G2/M phase and mediates cell death through stimulation of caspases and PARP degradation [84]. Flavonoids were also previously demonstrated to show anticancer, anti-inflammatory, and antioxidant characteristics.

Casticin is a flavonoid that is shown to cause cell death in colon cancer cells by cell cycle arrest at G2/M stage (Table 2.1) [38]. It also increases the ROS production, downregulates MMP expression levels, ameliorates the liberation of cytochrome c, and stimulates various caspases. Besides, it also enhances TRAIL, Fas, FasL, and FADD as has been reported after treating with casticin [85]. Quercetin is very familiar for its antioxidant, antiproliferative, and anti-inflammatory properties; previous reports have shown that treatment with quercetin reduces cell viability, blocks cell cycle at G1 stage, and mediates cell death in colon cancer cells [11, 86]. Quercetin also suppresses the PI3K-induced cell survival signaling through phosphorylation of Akt [86].

A recent study demonstrated that coffee phenolic phytochemicals suppress colon cancer-induced cell-mediated lung metastasis through inhibiting phosphorylation of ERKs [26]. CaA actively inhibits MEK1 as well as TOPK actions, and binds to MEK1 or TOPK in an ATP-noncompetitive mode [26, 38]. These previous studies show that CaA targets MEK1 or TOPK to block metastasis [26]. Carotenoids such as zeaxanthin, lycopenes, luteins, and β-carotenes are the principal constituents present in saffron and have been used to treat various cancers. Crocetin is a potent carotenoid that can induce apoptosis in colon cancer cells. The wild-type p53 transactivates Bax together with increased levels of p53-induced death domain protein that cleaves and triggers Bid through caspase-2 [87]. But in p53 knockout cells stimulation of the p53 paralogue p73 was noticed, which increases Fas to cleave Bid via FADD-caspase-8 pathway [87].

5 Esophageal Cancer

Esophageal cancers are one of the major familial cancers and have the most frequent cancer-associated mortality [91]. As long as symptoms are absent, patients with esophageal cancers are not aware of their cancer status until the metastatic stages of cancer [92]. In spite of development in present-day cancer therapies, including radiation therapy, chemotherapy, and surgery, patients with esophageal cancer are not often cured of the disease [93]. The predominant risk factors contributing to the cancer are chewing and smoking tobacco products, drinking alcohol, regular intake of salt pickle or moldy foods, and consumption of lesser fruits and vegetables [94–96]. Recent reports have shown the helpful effects of various phytochemicals, including curcumin, resveratrol, and isothiocyanates, to counteract esophageal cancer.

Curcumin is known for its anticancer, anti-inflammatory characteristics; numerous reports have revealed that it suppresses the NF-κB expression in esophageal cancers [97, 98]. NF-κB is a pro-inflammatory factor, which intricates in the initiation, progression, and development of tumors, and elevated NF-κB activity is associated with a significant increase in cell proliferation, invasion, metastasis, angiogenesis, inhibition of cell death, as well as chemoresistance in several types of cancers [97, 99, 100]. Curcumin also safeguards in opposition to bile acid-mediated increased NF-κB expression in esophageal cells, and sequentially decreases the expression of several NF-κB downstream genes such as IL-8 [101]. Besides, cancer patients supplemented with curcumin reported showing reduced IL-8 expression, indicating that curcumin plays a significant role as a possible chemopreventive candidate to counteract esophageal cancer [101]. Recent studies revealed that it also mediates apoptosis and blocks cell cycle by targeting Notch signaling. It is established that Notch signaling is upregulated in esophageal cancer and it could be a plausible target ascribed to its crucial role in cancer cell proliferation, programmed cell death, stem cell maintenance, and renewal in esophageal cancer [102–104].

EGCG is a polyphenol, which is the most abundant and active component in tea with strong antioxidant and anti-inflammatory potential properties [102]. It was previously reported that the intake of black and green tea reduced esophageal tumorigenesis which is possibly owing to inhibition of tumor occurrence and multiplicity [105]. EGCG mediates anticarcinogenic activities via several mechanisms, including the suppression of MAPK activator protein-1 and cell transformation, and also blocks EGFR phosphorylation [106–109]. Besides, EGCG is known to mediate cell cycle blocking at G0/G1, cell death, and suppression of DNA methyltransferase (DNMT) activity [110–113].

6 Conclusion

Gastroenterological cancers are associated with diet and lifestyle factors. Despite significant development and progression in diagnosis and cancer therapy, the prevalence of colorectal cancer and various other cancers is increasing worldwide. Due to the greater prevalence of resistance and dreadful side effects to be concerned with chemotherapeutics, there is a crucial prerequisite to instigate greater effective drugs. Plant-based phytochemicals are familiar sources of several compounds that are presently used as chemotherapeutics. The substantial data from several reports have revealed the effect of phytochemicals to identify signaling pathways implicated in the suppression or inhibition of tumor metastasis. Numerous phytochemicals such as curcumin, resveratrol, isothiocyanates, and EGCG have been demonstrated to contain antioxidant, anti-inflammatory, and anticancer effects by blocking various molecules or controlling signaling cascades, allowing to safeguard against the progression of gastroenterological cancers.

References

1. Murakami, K., & Matsubara, H. (2018). Chronology of gastrointestinal cancer. *Surgery Today, 48*(4), 365–370.
2. Hart, I. R., & Fidler, I. J. (1981). The implications of tumor heterogeneity for studies on the biology and therapy of cancer metastasis. *Biochimica et Biophysica Acta (BBA) - Reviews on Cancer, 651*(1), 37–50.
3. Eccles, S. A., & Welch, D. R. (2007). Metastasis: Recent discoveries and novel treatment strategies. *Lancet, 369*(9574), 1742–1757.
4. Fidler, I. J. (2003). The pathogenesis of cancer metastasis: The 'seed and soil' hypothesis revisited. *Nature Reviews Cancer, 3*(6), 453–458.

5. Karnoub, A. E., Dash, A. B., Vo, A. P., Sullivan, A., Brooks, M. W., Bell, G. W., Richardson, A. L., Polyak, K., Tubo, R., & Weinberg, R. A. (2007). Mesenchymal stem cells within tumour stroma promote breast cancer metastasis. *Nature, 449*(7162), 557–563.
6. Chambers, A. F. (2009). Influence of diet on metastasis and tumor dormancy. *Clinical & Experimental Metastasis, 26*(1), 61–66.
7. Cameron, M. D., Schmidt, E. E., Kerkvliet, N., Nadkarni, K. V., Morris, V. L., Groom, A. C., Chambers, A. F., & MacDonald, I. C. (2000). Temporal progression of metastasis in lung: Cell survival, dormancy, and location dependence of metastatic inefficiency. *Cancer Research, 60* (9), 2541–2546.
8. Kalluri, R., & Weinberg, R. A. (2009). The basics of epithelial-mesenchymal transition. *The Journal of Clinical Investigation, 119*(6), 1420–1428.
9. Tarin, D. (2005). The fallacy of epithelial mesenchymal transition in neoplasia. *Cancer Research, 65*(14), 5996–6001.
10. Thiery, J. P. (2002). Epithelial–mesenchymal transitions in tumour progression. *Nature Reviews Cancer, 2*(6), 442–454.
11. Yang, L., Liu, Y., Wang, M., Qian, Y., Dong, X., Gu, H., Wang, H., Guo, S., & Hisamitsu, T. (2016). Quercetin-induced apoptosis of HT-29 colon cancer cells via inhibition of the Akt-CSN6-Myc signaling axis. *Molecular Medicine Reports, 14*(5), 4559–4566.
12. Hugo, H., Ackland, M. L., Blick, T., Lawrence, M. G., Clements, J. A., Williams, E. D., & Thompson, E. W. (2007). Epithelial—mesenchymal and mesenchymal—epithelial transitions in carcinoma progression. *Journal of Cellular Physiology, 213*(2), 374–383.
13. Bissell, M. J., Kenny, P. A., & Radisky, D. C. (2005). Microenvironmental regulators of tissue structure and function also regulate tumor induction and progression: The role of extracellular matrix and its degrading enzymes. *Cold Spring Harbor Symposia on Quantitative Biology, 70*, 343–356.
14. Ho, E., Clarke, J. D., & Dashwood, R. H. (2009). Dietary sulforaphane, a histone deacetylase inhibitor for cancer prevention. *The Journal of Nutrition, 139*(12), 2393–2396.
15. Bode, A. M., & Dong, Z. (2004). Targeting signal transduction pathways by chemopreventive agents. *Mutation Research/Fundamental and Molecular Mechanisms of Mutagenesis, 555*(1), 33–51.
16. Patel, B. B., Gupta, D., Elliott, A. A., Sengupta, V., Yu, Y., & Majumdar, A. P. N. (2010). Curcumin targets FOLFOX-surviving colon cancer cells via inhibition of EGFRs and IGF-1R. *Anticancer Research, 30*(2), 319–325.
17. Langley, R. R., & Fidler, I. J. (2011). The seed and soil hypothesis revisited--the role of tumor-stroma interactions in metastasis to different organs. *International Journal of Cancer, 128*(11), 2527–2535.
18. Riihimäki, M., Hemminki, A., Fallah, M., Thomsen, H., Sundquist, K., Sundquist, J., & Hemminki, K. (2014). Metastatic sites and survival in lung cancer. *Lung Cancer, 86*(1), 78–84.
19. Weiss, L., Grundmann, E., Torhorst, J., Hartveit, F., Moberg, I., Eder, M., Fenoglio-Preiser, C., Napier, J., Horne, C., & Lopez, M. (1986). Haematogenous metastatic patterns in colonic carcinoma: An analysis of 1541 necropsies. *The Journal of Pathology, 150*(3), 195–203.
20. Viadana, E., Bross, I., & Pickren, J. (1978). The metastatic spread of cancers of the digestive system in man. *Oncology, 35*(3), 114–126.
21. Aparicio, S., & Caldas, C. (2013). The implications of clonal genome evolution for cancer medicine. *New England Journal of Medicine, 368*(9), 842–851.
22. Cummings, M. C., Simpson, P. T., Reid, L. E., Jayanthan, J., Skerman, J., Song, S., McCart Reed, A. E., Kutasovic, J. R., Morey, A. L., Marquart, L., et al. (2014). Metastatic progression of breast cancer: Insights from 50 years of autopsies. *The Journal of Pathology, 232*(1), 23–31.
23. Schreiber, R. D., Old, L. J., & Smyth, M. J. (2011). Cancer immunoediting: Integrating immunity's roles in cancer suppression and promotion. *Science, 331*(6024), 1565–1570.
24. Chen, J.-L., Fan, J., Chen, M.-X., Dong, Y., & Gu, J.-Z. (2012). Effect of non-anticoagulant N-desulfated heparin on basic fibroblast growth factor expression, angiogenesis, and

metastasis of gastric carcinoma in vitro and in vivo. *Gastroenterology Research and Practice, 2012*, 752940–752940.

25. Chen, J.-L., Gurski, R. R., Takahashi, K., & Andersson, R. (2012). Gastrointestinal cancer metastasis. *Gastroenterology Research and Practice, 2012*, 415498–415498.
26. Kang, N. J., Lee, K. W., Kim, B. H., Bode, A. M., Lee, H.-J., Heo, Y.-S., Boardman, L., Limburg, P., Lee, H. J., & Dong, Z. (2011). Coffee phenolic phytochemicals suppress colon cancer metastasis by targeting MEK and TOPK. *Carcinogenesis, 32*(6), 921–928.
27. Vadde, R., Radhakrishnan, S., Reddivari, L., & Vanamala, J. K. P. (2015). Triphala extract suppresses proliferation and induces apoptosis in human colon cancer stem cells via suppressing c-Myc/cyclin D1 and elevation of Bax/Bcl-2 ratio. *BioMed Research International, 2015*, 649263–649263.
28. Chia, J.-S., Du, J.-L., Hsu, W.-B., Sun, A., Chiang, C.-P., & Wang, W.-B. (2010). Inhibition of metastasis, angiogenesis, and tumor growth by Chinese herbal cocktail Tien-Hsien liquid. *BMC Cancer, 10*, 175–175.
29. Ferlay, J., Shin, H. R., Bray, F., Forman, D., Mathers, C., & Parkin, D. M. (2010). Estimates of worldwide burden of cancer in 2008: GLOBOCAN 2008. *International Journal of Cancer, 127*(12), 2893–2917.
30. Bernards, N., Creemers, G.-J., Nieuwenhuijzen, G., Bosscha, K., Pruijt, J., & Lemmens, V. (2013). No improvement in median survival for patients with metastatic gastric cancer despite increased use of chemotherapy. *Annals of Oncology, 24*(12), 3056–3060.
31. Thomassen, I., van Gestel, Y. R., van Ramshorst, B., Luyer, M. D., Bosscha, K., Nienhuijs, S. W., Lemmens, V. E., & de Hingh, I. H. (2014). Peritoneal carcinomatosis of gastric origin: A population-based study on incidence, survival and risk factors. *International Journal of Cancer, 134*(3), 622–628.
32. Hundahl, S. A. (2002). Staging, stage migration, and patterns of spread in gastric cancer. *Seminars in Radiation Oncology, 12*(2), 141–149.
33. Yu, L.-L., Wu, J.-G., Dai, N., Yu, H.-G., & Si, J.-M. (2011). Curcumin reverses chemoresistance of human gastric cancer cells by downregulating the NF-κB transcription factor. *Oncology Reports, 26*(5), 1197–1203.
34. De, R., Kundu, P., Swarnakar, S., Ramamurthy, T., Chowdhury, A., Nair, G. B., & Mukhopadhyay, A. K. (2009). Antimicrobial activity of curcumin against Helicobacter pylori isolates from India and during infections in mice. *Antimicrobial Agents and Chemotherapy, 53* (4), 1592–1597.
35. Atten, M. J., Attar, B. M., Milson, T., & Holian, O. (2001). Resveratrol-induced inactivation of human gastric adenocarcinoma cells through a protein kinase C-mediated mechanism 11 Abbreviations: COX-1, cyclooxygenase-1; COX-2, cyclooxygenase-2; PKC, protein kinase C; ERK1/ERK2, mitogen-activated protein kinases; NA, nitrosamine(s); TCA, trichloroacetic acid; and PMSF, phenylmethylsulfonyl fluoride. *Biochemical Pharmacology, 62*(10), 1423–1432.
36. Atten, M. J., Godoy-Romero, E., Attar, B. M., Milson, T., Zopel, M., & Holian, O. (2005). Resveratrol regulates cellular PKC α and δ to inhibit growth and induce apoptosis in gastric cancer cells. *Investigational New Drugs, 23*(2), 111–119.
37. Aquilano, K., Baldelli, S., & Rotilio, G. (2009). Ciriolo MR: Trans-resveratrol inhibits H2O2-induced adenocarcinoma gastric cells proliferation via inactivation of MEK1/2-ERK1/2-c-Jun signalling axis. *Biochemical Pharmacology, 77*(3), 337–347.
38. Ahmed, K., Zaidi, S. F., Cui, Z.-G., Zhou, D., Saeed, S. A., & Inadera, H. (2019). Potential proapoptotic phytochemical agents for the treatment and prevention of colorectal cancer. *Oncology Letters, 18*(1), 487–498.
39. Hafström, L., Johansson, H., & Ahlberg, J. (2012). Does diagnostic delay of colorectal cancer result in malpractice claims? A retrospective analysis of the Swedish board of malpractice from 1995-2008. *Patient Safety in Surgery, 6*(1), 13–13.
40. Boland, C. R., & Goel, A. (2010). Microsatellite instability in colorectal cancer. *Gastroenterology, 138*(6), 2073–2087.e2073.

41. Lao, V. V., & Grady, W. M. (2011). Epigenetics and colorectal cancer. *Nature Reviews. Gastroenterology & Hepatology, 8*(12), 686–700.
42. Pino, M. S., & Chung, D. C. (2010). The chromosomal instability pathway in colon cancer. *Gastroenterology, 138*(6), 2059–2072.
43. Testa, U., Pelosi, E., & Castelli, G. (2018). Colorectal cancer: Genetic abnormalities, tumor progression, tumor heterogeneity, clonal evolution and tumor-initiating cells. *Medical Sciences (Basel), 6*(2), 31.
44. Wang, S., Liu, Z., Wang, L., & Zhang, X. (2009). NF-kappaB signaling pathway, inflammation and colorectal cancer. *Cellular & Molecular Immunology, 6*(5), 327–334.
45. Vivanco, I., & Sawyers, C. L. (2002). The phosphatidylinositol 3-kinase–AKT pathway in human cancer. *Nature Reviews Cancer, 2*(7), 489.
46. Fung, T. T., Hu, F. B., Wu, K., Chiuve, S. E., Fuchs, C. S., & Giovannucci, E. (2010). The Mediterranean and dietary approaches to stop hypertension (DASH) diets and colorectal cancer. *The American Journal of Clinical Nutrition, 92*(6), 1429–1435.
47. Nomura, A. M. Y., Wilkens, L. R., Murphy, S. P., Hankin, J. H., Henderson, B. E., Pike, M. C., & Kolonel, L. N. (2008). Association of vegetable, fruit, and grain intakes with colorectal cancer: The multiethnic cohort study. *The American Journal of Clinical Nutrition, 88*(3), 730–737.
48. van Duijnhoven, F. J., Bueno-De-Mesquita, H. B., Ferrari, P., Jenab, M., Boshuizen, H. C., Ros, M. M., Casagrande, C., Tjønneland, A., Olsen, A., Overvad, K., et al. (2009). Fruit, vegetables, and colorectal cancer risk: The European Prospective Investigation into Cancer and Nutrition. *The American Journal of Clinical Nutrition, 89*(5), 1441–1452.
49. González-Vallinas, M., González-Castejón, M., Rodríguez-Casado, A., & Ramírez de Molina, A. (2013). Dietary phytochemicals in cancer prevention and therapy: A complementary approach with promising perspectives. *Nutrition Reviews, 71*(9), 585–599.
50. Lee, K. W., Bode, A. M., & Dong, Z. (2011). Molecular targets of phytochemicals for cancer prevention. *Nature Reviews Cancer, 11*(3), 211–218.
51. Mantovani, A., Allavena, P., Sica, A., & Balkwill, F. (2008). Cancer-related inflammation. *Nature, 454*(7203), 436.
52. Mantovani, A. (2010). Molecular pathways linking inflammation and cancer. *Current Molecular Medicine, 10*(4), 369–373.
53. Colotta, F., Allavena, P., Sica, A., Garlanda, C., & Mantovani, A. (2009). Cancer-related inflammation, the seventh hallmark of cancer: Links to genetic instability. *Carcinogenesis, 30* (7), 1073–1081.
54. Greten, F. R., Eckmann, L., Greten, T. F., Park, J. M., Li, Z.-W., Egan, L. J., Kagnoff, M. F., & Karin, M. (2004). IKKβ links inflammation and tumorigenesis in a mouse model of colitis-associated cancer. *Cell, 118*(3), 285–296.
55. Tong, W., Wang, Q., Sun, D., & Suo, J. (2016). Curcumin suppresses colon cancer cell invasion via AMPK-induced inhibition of NF-κB, uPA activator and MMP9. *Oncology Letters, 12*(5), 4139–4146.
56. Singh, N., Shrivastav, A., & Sharma, R. K. (2009). Curcumin induces caspase and calpain-dependent apoptosis in HT29 human colon cancer cells. *Molecular Medicine Reports, 2*(4), 627–631.
57. Ryu, M.-J., Cho, M., Song, J.-Y., Yun, Y.-S., Choi, I.-W., Kim, D.-E., Park, B.-S., & Oh, S. (2008). Natural derivatives of curcumin attenuate the Wnt/β-catenin pathway through down-regulation of the transcriptional coactivator p300. *Biochemical and Biophysical Research Communications, 377*(4), 1304–1308.
58. Jaiswal, A. S., Marlow, B. P., Gupta, N., & Narayan, S. (2002). β-Catenin-mediated transactivation and cell–cell adhesion pathways are important in curcumin (diferuylmethane)-induced growth arrest and apoptosis in colon cancer cells. *Oncogene, 21* (55), 8414.

59. Irving, G. R. B., Karmokar, A., Berry, D. P., Brown, K., & Steward, W. P. (2011). Curcumin: The potential for efficacy in gastrointestinal diseases. *Best Practice & Research Clinical Gastroenterology, 25*(4), 519–534.
60. Watson, J. L., Hill, R., Yaffe, P. B., Greenshields, A., Walsh, M., Lee, P. W., Giacomantonio, C. A., & Hoskin, D. W. (2010). Curcumin causes superoxide anion production and p53-independent apoptosis in human colon cancer cells. *Cancer Letters, 297*(1), 1–8.
61. Chen, A., Xu, J., & Johnson, A. (2006). Curcumin inhibits human colon cancer cell growth by suppressing gene expression of epidermal growth factor receptor through reducing the activity of the transcription factor Egr-1. *Oncogene, 25*(2), 278.
62. LeRoith, D., & Roberts, C. T. (2003). The insulin-like growth factor system and cancer. *Cancer Letters, 195*(2), 127–137.
63. Binion, D. G., Otterson, M. F., & Rafiee, P. (2008). Curcumin inhibits VEGF-mediated angiogenesis in human intestinal microvascular endothelial cells through COX-2 and MAPK inhibition. *Gut, 57*(11), 1509–1517.
64. Bertelli, A., Ferrara, F., Diana, G., Fulgenzi, A., Corsi, M., Ponti, W., Ferrero, M., & Bertelli, A. (1999). Resveratrol, a natural stilbene in grapes and wine, enhances intraphagocytosis in human promonocytes: A co-factor in anti-inflammatory and anticancer chemopreventive activity. *International Journal of Tissue Reactions, 21*(4), 93–104.
65. Vanamala, J., Radhakrishnan, S., Reddivari, L., Bhat, V. B., & Ptitsyn, A. (2011). Resveratrol suppresses human colon cancer cell proliferation and induces apoptosis via targeting the pentose phosphate and the talin-FAK signaling pathways - a proteomic approach. *Proteome Science, 9*(1), 49–49.
66. Buhrmann, C., Shayan, P., Popper, B., Goel, A., & Shakibaei, M. (2016). Sirt1 is required for resveratrol-mediated chemopreventive effects in colorectal cancer cells. *Nutrients, 8*(3), 145–145.
67. Chen, H., Jin, Z.-L., & Xu, H. (2016). MEK/ERK signaling pathway in apoptosis of SW620 cell line and inhibition effect of resveratrol. *Asian Pacific Journal of Tropical Medicine, 9*(1), 49–53.
68. Yuan, S.-X., Wang, D.-X., Wu, Q.-X., Ren, C.-M., Li, Y., Chen, Q.-Z., Zeng, Y.-H., Shao, Y., Yang, J.-Q., & Bai, Y. (2016). BMP9/p38 MAPK is essential for the antiproliferative effect of resveratrol on human colon cancer. *Oncology Reports, 35*(2), 939–947.
69. Saud, S. M., Li, W., Morris, N. L., Matter, M. S., Colburn, N. H., Kim, Y. S., & Young, M. R. (2014). Resveratrol prevents tumorigenesis in mouse model of Kras activated sporadic colorectal cancer by suppressing oncogenic Kras expression. *Carcinogenesis, 35*(12), 2778–2786.
70. Baur, J. A., & Sinclair, D. A. (2006). Therapeutic potential of resveratrol: The in vivo evidence. *Nature Reviews Drug Discovery, 5*(6), 493.
71. Fouad, M., Agha, A., Merzabani, M. A., & Shouman, S. (2013). Resveratrol inhibits proliferation, angiogenesis and induces apoptosis in colon cancer cells: Calorie restriction is the force to the cytotoxicity. *Human & Experimental Toxicology, 32*(10), 1067–1080.
72. Wu, H., Liang, X., Fang, Y., Qin, X., Zhang, Y., & Liu, J. (2008). Resveratrol inhibits hypoxia-induced metastasis potential enhancement by restricting hypoxia-induced factor-1α expression in colon carcinoma cells. *Biomedicine & Pharmacotherapy, 62*(9), 613–621.
73. Lopez de las Hazas, M.-C., Piñol, C., Macià, A., & Motilva, M.-J. (2017). Hydroxytyrosol and the colonic metabolites derived from virgin olive oil intake induce cell cycle arrest and apoptosis in colon cancer cells. *Journal of Agricultural and Food Chemistry, 65*(31), 6467–6476.
74. Jin, J., Lin, G., Huang, H., Xu, D., Yu, H., Ma, X., Zhu, L., Ma, D., & Jiang, H. (2014). Capsaicin mediates cell cycle arrest and apoptosis in human colon cancer cells via stabilizing and activating p53. *International Journal of Biological Sciences, 10*(3), 285–295.
75. Risinger, A. L., Giles, F. J., & Mooberry, S. L. (2009). Microtubule dynamics as a target in oncology. *Cancer Treatment Reviews, 35*(3), 255–261.

76. Huang, Z., Xu, Y., & Peng, W. (2015). Colchicine induces apoptosis in HT-29 human colon cancer cells via the AKT and c-Jun N-terminal kinase signaling pathways. *Molecular Medicine Reports, 12*(4), 5939–5944.
77. Yaffe, P. B., Doucette, C. D., Walsh, M., & Hoskin, D. W. (2013). Piperine impairs cell cycle progression and causes reactive oxygen species-dependent apoptosis in rectal cancer cells. *Experimental and Molecular Pathology, 94*(1), 109–114.
78. Yaffe, P. B., Power Coombs, M. R., Doucette, C. D., Walsh, M., & Hoskin, D. W. (2015). Piperine, an alkaloid from black pepper, inhibits growth of human colon cancer cells via G1 arrest and apoptosis triggered by endoplasmic reticulum stress. *Molecular Carcinogenesis, 54* (10), 1070–1085.
79. Wang, Y., Liu, Q., Liu, Z., Li, B., Sun, Z., Zhou, H., Zhang, X., Gong, Y., & Shao, C. (2012). Berberine, a genotoxic alkaloid, induces ATM-Chk1 mediated G2 arrest in prostate cancer cells. *Mutation Research/Fundamental and Molecular Mechanisms of Mutagenesis, 734*(1), 20–29.
80. Yan, K., Zhang, C., Feng, J., Hou, L., Yan, L., Zhou, Z., Liu, Z., Liu, C., Fan, Y., Zheng, B., et al. (2011). Induction of G1 cell cycle arrest and apoptosis by berberine in bladder cancer cells. *European Journal of Pharmacology, 661*(1), 1–7.
81. Tillhon, M., Guamán Ortiz, L. M., Lombardi, P., & Scovassi, A. I. (2012). Berberine: New perspectives for old remedies. *Biochemical Pharmacology, 84*(10), 1260–1267.
82. Wang, L., Liu, L., Shi, Y., Cao, H., Chaturvedi, R., Calcutt, M. W., Hu, T., Ren, X., Wilson, K. T., Polk, D. B., et al. (2012). Berberine induces caspase-independent cell death in colon tumor cells through activation of apoptosis-inducing factor. *PLoS One, 7*(5), e36418–e36418.
83. Guamán Ortiz, L. M., Tillhon, M., Parks, M., Dutto, I., Prosperi, E., Savio, M., Arcamone, A. G., Buzzetti, F., Lombardi, P., & Scovassi, A. I. (2014). Multiple effects of berberine derivatives on colon cancer cells. *BioMed Research International, 2014*, 924585–924585.
84. Radhakrishnan, E. K., Bava, S. V., Narayanan, S. S., Nath, L. R., Thulasidasan, A. K. T., Soniya, E. V., & Anto, R. J. (2014). [6]-Gingerol induces caspase-dependent apoptosis and prevents PMA-induced proliferation in colon cancer cells by inhibiting MAPK/AP-1 signaling. *PLoS One, 9*(8), e104401–e104401.
85. Shang, H. S., Liu, J. Y., Lu, H. F., Chiang, H. S., Lin, C. H., Chen, A., Lin, Y. F., & Chung, J. G. (2017). Casticin induced apoptotic cell death and altered associated gene expression in human colon cancer Colo 205 cells. *Environmental Toxicology, 32*(8), 2041–2052.
86. Kim, H.-J., Kim, S.-K., Kim, B.-S., Lee, S.-H., Park, Y.-S., Park, B.-K., Kim, S.-J., Kim, J., Choi, C., & Kim, J.-S. (2010). Apoptotic effect of quercetin on HT-29 colon cancer cells via the AMPK signaling pathway. *Journal of Agricultural and Food Chemistry, 58*(15), 8643–8650.
87. Ray, P., Guha, D., Chakraborty, J., Banerjee, S., Adhikary, A., Chakraborty, S., Das, T., & Sa, G. (2016). Crocetin exploits p53-induced death domain (PIDD) and FAS-associated death domain (FADD) proteins to induce apoptosis in colorectal cancer. *Scientific Reports, 6*, 32979–32979.
88. Dasiram, J. D., Ganesan, R., Kannan, J., Kotteeswaran, V., & Sivalingam, N. (2017). Curcumin inhibits growth potential by G1 cell cycle arrest and induces apoptosis in p53-mutated COLO 320DM human colon adenocarcinoma cells. *Biomedicine & Pharmacotherapy, 86*, 373–380.
89. Lin, W., & Tongyi, S. (2014). Role of Bax/Bcl-2 family members in green tea polyphenol induced necroptosis of p53-deficient Hep3B cells. *Tumor Biology, 35*(8), 8065–8075.
90. Cai, Y., Xia, Q., Luo, R., Huang, P., Sun, Y., Shi, Y., & Jiang, W. (2014). Berberine inhibits the growth of human colorectal adenocarcinoma in vitro and in vivo. *Journal of Natural Medicines, 68*(1), 53–62.
91. Parkin, D. M., Bray, F., Ferlay, J., & Pisani, P. (2005). Global cancer statistics, 2002. *CA: a Cancer Journal for Clinicians, 55*(2), 74–108.
92. Jemal, A., Siegel, R., Ward, E., Murray, T., Xu, J., & Thun, M. J. (2007). Cancer statistics, 2007. *CA: a Cancer Journal for Clinicians, 57*(1), 43–66.

93. Subramaniam, D., Ponnurangam, S., Ramamoorthy, P., Standing, D., Battafarano, R. J., Anant, S., & Sharma, P. (2012). Curcumin induces cell death in esophageal cancer cells through modulating Notch signaling. *PLoS One, 7*(2), e30590–e30590.
94. Stoner, G. D., Kresty, L. A., Carlton, P. S., Siglin, J. C., & Morse, M. A. (1999). Isothiocyanates and freeze-dried strawberries as inhibitors of esophageal cancer. *Toxicological Sciences: An Official Journal of the Society of Toxicology, 52*(suppl_1), 95–100.
95. Wynder, E. L., & Bross, I. J. (1961). A study of etiological factors in cancer of the esophagus. *Cancer, 14*(2), 389–413.
96. Block, G., Patterson, B., & Subar, A. (1992). Fruit, vegetables, and cancer prevention: A review of the epidemiological evidence. *Nutrition and Cancer, 18*(1), 1–29.
97. Tian, F., Song, M., Xu, P., Liu, H., & Xue, L. (2008). Curcumin promotes apoptosis of esophageal squamous carcinoma cell lines through inhibition of NF-kappaB signaling pathway. *Ai zheng= Aizheng=Chinese Journal of Cancer, 27*(6), 566–570.
98. Hartojo, W., Silvers, A. L., Thomas, D. G., Seder, C. W., Lin, L., Rao, H., Wang, Z., Greenson, J. K., Giordano, T. J., Orringer, M. B., et al. (2010). Curcumin promotes apoptosis, increases chemosensitivity, and inhibits nuclear factor kappaB in esophageal adenocarcinoma. *Translational Oncology, 3*(2), 99–108.
99. Kunnumakkara, A. B., Guha, S., Krishnan, S., Diagaradjane, P., Gelovani, J., & Aggarwal, B. B. (2007). Curcumin potentiates antitumor activity of gemcitabine in an orthotopic model of pancreatic cancer through suppression of proliferation, angiogenesis, and inhibition of nuclear factor-κB-regulated gene products. *Cancer Research, 67*(8), 3853–3861.
100. Arlt, A., Gehrz, A., Müerköster, S., Vorndamm, J., Kruse, M.-L., Fölsch, U. R., & Schäfer, H. (2003). Role of NF-κB and Akt/PI3K in the resistance of pancreatic carcinoma cell lines against gemcitabine-induced cell death. *Oncogene, 22*(21), 3243.
101. Rawat, N., Alhamdani, A., McAdam, E., Cronin, J., Eltahir, Z., Lewis, P., Griffiths, P., Baxter, J. N., & Jenkins, G. J. (2012). Curcumin abrogates bile-induced NF-κB activity and DNA damage in vitro and suppresses NF-κB activity whilst promoting apoptosis in vivo, suggesting chemopreventative potential in Barrett's oesophagus. *Clinical and Translational Oncology, 14* (4), 302–311.
102. Woo, S.-M., Kim, J., Han, H.-W., Chae, J.-I., Son, M.-Y., Cho, S., Chung, H.-M., Han, Y.-M., & Kang, Y.-K. (2009). Notch signaling is required for maintaining stem-cell features of neuroprogenitor cells derived from human embryonic stem cells. *BMC Neuroscience, 10*, 97–97.
103. Peters, J. H., & Avisar, N. (2010). The molecular pathogenesis of Barrett's esophagus: Common signaling pathways in embryogenesis metaplasia and neoplasia. *Journal of Gastrointestinal Surgery, 14*(1), 81–87.
104. Mendelson, J., Song, S., Li, Y., Maru, D. M., Mishra, B., Davila, M., Hofstetter, W. L., & Mishra, L. (2011). Dysfunctional transforming growth factor-β signaling with constitutively active Notch signaling in Barrett's esophageal adenocarcinoma. *Cancer, 117*(16), 3691–3702.
105. Chen, J. (1992). The effects of Chinese tea on the occurrence of esophageal tumors induced by N-nitrosomethylbenzylamine in rats. *Preventive Medicine, 21*(3), 385–391.
106. Shimizu, M., Deguchi, A., Lim, J. T. E., Moriwaki, H., Kopelovich, L., & Weinstein, I. B. (2005). (−)-Epigallocatechin gallate and polyphenon E inhibit growth and activation of the epidermal growth factor receptor and human epidermal growth factor receptor-2 signaling pathways in human colon cancer cells. *Clinical Cancer Research, 11*(7), 2735–2746.
107. Dong, Z., Ma, W.-Y., Huang, C., & Yang, C. S. (1997). Inhibition of tumor promoter-induced activator protein 1 activation and cell transformation by tea polyphenols, (−)-epigallocatechin gallate, and theaflavins. *Cancer Research, 57*(19), 4414–4419.
108. Chung, J. Y., Park, J. O., Phyu, H., Dong, Z., & Yang, C. S. (2001). Mechanisms of inhibition of the Ras-MAP kinase signaling pathway in 30.7 b Ras 12 cells by tea polyphenols (−)-epigallocatechin-3-gallate and theaflavin-3, 3′-digallate. *The FASEB Journal, 15*(11), 2022–2024.

109. Chung, J. Y., Huang, C., Meng, X., Dong, Z., & Yang, C. S. (1999). Inhibition of activator protein 1 activity and cell growth by purified green tea and black tea polyphenols in H-ras-transformed cells: Structure-activity relationship and mechanisms involved. *Cancer Research, 59*(18), 4610–4617.
110. Fang, M. Z., Wang, Y., Ai, N., Hou, Z., Sun, Y., Lu, H., Welsh, W., & Yang, C. S. (2003). Tea polyphenol (−)-epigallocatechin-3-gallate inhibits DNA methyltransferase and reactivates methylation-silenced genes in cancer cell lines. *Cancer Research, 63*(22), 7563–7570.
111. Ahmad, N., Feyes, D. K., Agarwal, R., Mukhtar, H., & Nieminen, A.-L. (1997). Green tea constituent epigallocatechin-3-gallate and induction of apoptosis and cell cycle arrest in human carcinoma cells. *JNCI: Journal of the National Cancer Institute, 89*(24), 1881–1886.
112. Gupta, S., Hussain, T., & Mukhtar, H. (2003). Molecular pathway for (−)-epigallocatechin-3-gallate-induced cell cycle arrest and apoptosis of human prostate carcinoma cells. *Archives of Biochemistry and Biophysics, 410*(1), 177–185.
113. Ahmad, N., Cheng, P., & Mukhtar, H. (2000). Cell cycle dysregulation by green tea polyphenol epigallocatechin-3-gallate. *Biochemical and Biophysical Research Communications, 275* (2), 328–334.

Chapter 3
Cancer Stem Cells as Therapeutic Targets for Gastrointestinal Cancers

Jyothi Priya Mandala, Srinivas Pittala, and Gowru Srivani

Abstract Gastrointestinal cancers are the most severe malignancies in the world and tend to be the most prominent cause of cancer mortality. Gastrointestinal (GI) cancer leads to malignant gastrointestinal tract diseases and accessory gastrointestinal organs, namely the esophagus, uterus, kidney, pancreas, small intestine, colon rectum, and anus. And it is believed that "cancer stem cells (CSCs)" are responsible for tumor growth and drug resistance; therefore, radiation tolerance, aggressive growth, metastasis, and tumor relapse are the main causes of cancer-related deaths. Because gastrointestinal CSCs are also considered as resistant to traditional treatments, effective and innovative treatment of cancer is crucial. So, targeting gastrointestinal CSCs is quite difficult. CSCs in a gastrointestinal tumor are identified for the first time in colorectal cancer. Many gastrointestinal cancers are identified later in the esophagus, stomach, liver, and pancreas. Consequently, current basic and translational studies are primarily designed at gaining a better understanding of the biology and these approaches are used to target CSCs. Therefore, recent developments and advancements in the field of GI CSCs can continue to provide new insights into gastrointestinal cancer and its treatment approaches for GI cancer eradication. Hence this chapter reflects on the modern advancements by using CSCs as the main target to eradicate gastrointestinal cancers. Knowledge about CSCs can help to develop new clinical strategies and markers for gastrointestinal cancers.

Keywords Cancer stem cells · Gastrointestinal cancer · Esophagus · Pancreas

---

J. P. Mandala (✉)
Bhagwan Mahavir Medical Research Centre, Hyderabad, India

Department of Genetics, Osmania University, Hyderabad, India

S. Pittala
Department of Life Sciences and the National Institute for Biotechnology in the Negev, Ben-Gurion University of the Negev, Beer-Sheva, Israel

G. Srivani
Department of Biosciences and Biotechnology, Banasthali University, Banasthali, Rajasthan, India

G. P. Nagaraju (ed.), *Phytochemicals Targeting Tumor Microenvironment in Gastrointestinal Cancers*, https://doi.org/10.1007/978-3-030-48405-7_3

Abbreviations

ALDH1	Aldehyde dehydrogenase 1
BetA	Betulinic acid
CaMK2	Calmodulin kinase
Cdc42	Cell division control protein 42
CRC	Colorectal cancer
CSCs	Cancer stem cells
CXCR4	C-X-C chemokine receptor type 4
DHH	Desert Hedgehog
DVL	Dishevelled phosphorylation
EGF	Epidermal growth factor
ESA	Epithelial specific antigen
GI	Gastrointestinal cancer
GLI	Glioma-associated oncogene
GPR	G-protein-coupled receptor
GSK-3	Glycogen synthase kinase 3
IFNα	Interferon-α
IHH	Indian Hedgehog
IL-6	Interleukin-6
JNK	Jun kinase
Lgr5	Leucine-rich repeat-containing G-protein-coupled receptor 5
MSCs	Mesenchymal stem cells
OS	Overall survival
PDGF	Platelet-derived growth factor
RAC	Ras-related C3 botulinum toxin substrate
SHH	Sonic Hedgehog
TCF	T-cell-specific transcription factor
TGF-β	Transforming growth factor-β
TNF	Tumor necrosis factor

1 Introduction

Cancer is associated with high mortality and morbidity and among all cancers, gastrointestinal cancers remain a great burden worldwide [1]. Despite critical developments in anticancer treatments over the past few decades, patients' overall survival (OS) rate remains insufficient [2]. The high mortality rates in gastrointestinal cancers are due to late diagnosis, high morbidity, and accessibility of not many focused-on treatments [3]. The incidence rate of colorectal cancer (CRC) is recorded in the top 10 for the tumor; however, five gastrointestinal cancers, including colorectal, pancreatic, hepatic, biliary, and esophageal cancers, are in the top 10 for tumor death rates in the USA [4]. The use of a few therapeutic methods such as surgery, endoscopic care, chemotherapy, and radiation will improve the recovery of gastrointestinal cancer patients. The adequacy of these drugs depends on the cancer state, metastasis, radiation/chemotherapy tolerance, and recurrence, all of which are believed to be induced by CSCs. Therefore, additional medicinal choices need to be developed for these diseases. But recent postulation suggests that cancer stem cells (CSCs) are a small subpopulation of cells which have self-regeneration and uncontrolled proliferation capacity that causes cancers. The cancer stem cells are found in several forms of tumors and could be effective therapeutic targets [5]. In addition to their self-renewal ability, CSCs have the potential to metastasize and recur to cancer [6, 7]. This (stochastic) theory of clonal evolution proposes that many cancers are usually driven by CSCs via self-renewal property, leading to an increase in the population of CSCs that can be further changed through genetic or epigenetic changes [8, 9]. CSCs have been known for years in a wide range of solid tumors including GI cancers [10]. The $CD44^{+}CD24$ cancer stem cells of breast cancer were first reported in solid tumors [7]. The main gastrointestinal CSC study was reported in $CD133^{+}$, $CD44^{+}$, $ALDH1^{+}$, and CRC fraction [4, 11]. These cells are crucial for tumor improvement and harbor the transformations needed to start a tumor. But reports demonstrate that CSCs may originate from differentiated mature cells, progenitor cells, and/or pools of transdifferentiated stem cells [10, 11]. It was also suggested that the cell fusion, chromosomal rearrangement, and/or horizontal gene transfer processes that often include tissue repair processes can also play an important role in tumor initiation, growth, and origin of CSCs [6, 11]. The deregulation of the key regulatory signaling pathways like Hedgehog, TGF-β, Wnt, and Notch is involved in normal homeostasis of the tissue, which is also involved in the advancement and development of CSCs in tumors [12, 13].

2 Cancer Stem Cells in Gastrointestinal Cancers

The current treatment methods (including chemotherapy, radiotherapy, and other specific therapies) only affect the rapidly dividing segregated cancer cells, while cancer stem cells (CSCs) or otherwise known as tumor-initiating cells, which are considered to be the vital origin cells of cancer, will usually avoid and endure these treatments [14]. CSCs become the best target for cancer due to their capacity for self-renewal and uncontrolled proliferation ability [15]. But there is a need for possible application of CSCs in the therapy of GI cancer. In addition, inadequate diagnosis of colorectal cancer (CRC) and metastasis of the liver are the major reasons for GI cancer mortality [16]. Early diagnosis and distant metastasis of any primary cancer are based on specific and accurate tumor markers. Dr. ZY Jiao has demonstrated the importance of colorectal CSCs, which helps in metastasis of liver in patients with CRC, and he reported the use of colorectal CSCs in the prevention of metastasis and also improvements in therapeutic treatments [17]. From a therapeutic standpoint, the complete eradication of colorectal CSCs would be an ideal approach. Betulinic acid

(BetA) is a broad-acting natural compound introduced by Dr. Lisette Potze et al. in this special issue [18]. The authors have demonstrated that BetA can induce a quick method for eradicating CSCs of the colon by reducing their clonogenic ability [18]. Indeed, this complex permits other experimental studies in future, especially animal studies [18]. Mesenchymal stem cells (MSCs) contain self-renewal potential to retain multi-potency nature. These MSCs show immunomodulatory effects during inflammatory conditions [19]. MSCs secrete numerous factors, which dcreases inflammation, improves tissue repairing capacity, promotes angiogenesis. These roles may further be improved by altering other genes found in MSCs [19]. As a result, increasing numbers of researchers are trying to improve the therapeutic effectiveness by using genetic engineering methods in MSCs. Many MSC-based cell therapies have shown to be reliable and useful in certain diseases, such as cirrhosis, graft-versus-host disease, and osteoarthritis, but the efficacy has been lacking in most of the diseases [20]. Further investigations to study the beneficial ability of MSCs in GI cancers are probably warranted. In this respect, Dr. YL Zhou et al. reported the issues and the trials related to this method for the understanding of the beneficial ability of MSCs in gastric cancer [21].

Generally, suitable reports have shown up-to-date information on common GI cancers in the field of CSCs for readers. The information in this report certainly provides clinicians and translation researchers with insights into improved curative methods for GI cancers.

2.1 Colorectal Cancer

CRC cells that expressed CD133 were first reported to have a CSC phenotype in 2007 [35]. Lgr5, a marker of intestinal stem cells that express upon upregulation of the Wnt signals, leads to the transformation of intestinal stem cells into CSCs [36]. Additionally, tumorigenicity reduction in CRC cells by Lgr5 knockdown was observed in some studies [37]. CD44 or CD166 is a colon CSC marker [38]; other CSC markers are ALDH1, Lgr5, and EpCAM [39]. Those are not only classified as CSCs, but they are also still found in regular stem cells. Cancer stem cells were known to express Dclk1 but they do not express in regular intestinal stem cells [40]. Epigenetic pathways generally regulate CSCs, wherein promoter methylation regulates CD133 marker [41], and in turn Lgr5's DNA methylation is involved in CRC tumorigenesis [42]. Furthermore, studies reported that regulatory stemness gene expression was inhibited by miRNAs [43]. Cellular niches, a microenvironment formed by adjacent cells such as vascular endothelial cells or fibroblasts, play an important role in the development and maintenance of ordinary stem cells. Myofibroblasts stimulate colon-stemming CSCs by secreting growth factors in hepatocytes or type I collagen [44]. Alternatively, endothelial vascular cells which secrete Jagged-1 stimulate the CSC phenotype in CRC [45]. A method was reported from existing CRC cell lines which produce CRC-like stem cells [46]. In brief, a group of identified factors (OCT3/4, SOX2, and KLF4) were retrovirally transfected and induced pluripotent stem cells from CRC cells, and these induced cells had CSC properties. This methodology will promote the study on colon CSC which supports the growth of new therapies focused on CSC.

2.2 *Pancreatic Cancer*

The most severe histological type of pancreatic cancer is pancreatic ductal adenocarcinoma. It is a complex genetic disease and its progression includes the sequential growth of numerous genetic mutations, containing inactivated CDKN2A, SMAD4, and TP53 and active KRAS which are already detectible in premalignant lesions. Met^+, $CD133^+$, $CXCR4^+$, and $CD24^+CD44^+EpCAM^+$ are unique markers in pancreatic CSC isolation [47]. An alternate CSC recognition strategy in PDAC is focused on the activity of enhanced ALDH1 and improved efflux capability in Hoechst 33342. In CSCs of pancreas many signaling pathways like the Hedgehog, Notch, Wnt, and phosphatidylinositol-3 kinase/Akt (protein kinase B) are activated. Hedgehog inhibition reduced pancreatic CSC phenotypes and tumorigenesis [48]. Moreover, several miRNAs are important when regulating the phenotypes of CSC. However, in PDAC patients miR-221 and microRNA-21 are overexpressed, and downregulation occurs simultaneously with antisense oligos that leads to reduced development, chemoresistance, and metastasis [49]. An increased expression of miR-21 is associated with inadequate diagnosis in patients of PDAC. In contrast, tumor suppressors, miR-34, miR-200a, and miRNAs, are reduced in PDAC, and their repair activity inhibits cancer [50]. Mutant KRAS control in PDAC cancer stem cells is a really difficult process [51]. Although the ablation of KRAS contributed to the regression of the tumor, PDAC cells developed resistance and showed tumorigenic capacity with elevated expressions of CD133 and CD44 [4]. Endured KRAS ablation in CSC-like cells was strongly mitochondrial and showed inhibition of tumorigenesis and elevated sensitivity to inhibitors of oxidative phosphorylation.

2.3 *Liver Cancer*

HCC and intrahepatic cholangiocarcinoma are two major liver cancers. Cholangiocytes and hepatocytes are differentiated by progenitor cells called bipotential hepatic cells; these two kinds of cancers originate from the progenitor cells, while the latest studies reported that a trans-differentiation process from intrahepatic cholangiocarcinoma results in the development of cholangiocytes from hepatocytes [52]. In this chapter, we discuss the CSCs within HCC. Most normal hepatocytes multiply and maintain liver function after surgical removal and cause severe liver injury. In contrast, hepatic progenitor cells are induced in chronic liver diseases and are differentiated into cholangiocytes or hepatocytes. Because HCC usually progresses with chronic liver diseases, regularly expressed hepatic progenitor cell markers are present in this manner, in which hepatic progenitor is related to hepatocarcinogenesis. The pharmacological blockage of interleukin-6 decreases a link between HCC and chronic inflammation in hepatitis [53]. Hepatic CSC marker isolation involves EpCAM, CD44, CD90, CD13, OV6, CD24, and CD133 [54]. Most normal progenitor hepatic cells express markers present on it, in which OV6$^+$ cells and CD90$^+$ are metastatic in nature, whereas CD133$^+$, EpCAM$^+$, CD13$^+$, and CD24$^+$ are chemoresistant [55, 56]. In turn, nonmetastatic EpCAM$^+$-co-injected cells metastasize from metastatic CD90$^+$ cells into the lungs [57]. Hepatocarcinogenesis includes many signaling pathways like Hedgehog, Wnt, P53, Akt, insulin-like growth factor-1 receptor, Notch, and TGF-β. Such pathways are triggered in common and chronic liver diseases. For example, cell cycle signaling regulators are Wnt signals and CD24- and STAT3-mediated Nanog regulator triggered by EpCAM [4, 53]. Protein nestin is a class IV intermediate filament that controls CSC tumorigenesis in liver and cellular plasticity in a p53-dependent manner. Likewise, liver CSCs' self-renewal process is controlled by a transcription factor Twist2 which is CD24 dependent [58, 59]. A study reported that CD133$^+$ HCC cells upregulate families like miR-181, let-7, and miR-130b, while downregulating miR-150, which regulates phenotypes of cancer stemness. The self-renewal and tumorigenesis regulated by increasing miR-130b levels lead to decrease in tumor protein P53 expression stimulating nuclear protein-1 [60]. Inhibition of let-7 or miR-181 reduces invasive capacity and motility [61]. Overexpression of miR-150 substantially decreases CD133$^+$ liver CSCs [62].

2.4 Esophageal Cancer

Esophageal adenocarcinoma and ESCC are two subtypes of cancer. Esophageal cancer treatment is done by the combined use of chemotherapy drugs or with radiation in any case, if ordinary medications are not truly successful. ESCC cell line as a single clone source for isolating esophageal CSCs [63]. There have been similar characteristics of stem cells, the ESCC cells being more radioresistant than their parental cells. High-level expression was observed in b1-integrin, b-catenin, and Oct3/4 in SP cells which are radioresistant cancer cells of the esophagus [64]. The latest findings show the connection between the miR-296 [65] and miR-200c [66] miRNA expression, in the chemoresistance of ESCC. The esophageal tumorigenesis involves many genetic alterations. PIK3CA inhibition decreases CSC proliferation in ESCC. In cells that have a PIK3CA mutation, the inhibition of phosphatidylinositol-3 kinase was more successful than controls. Likewise, WNT10A overexpression enhances the ability to self-renew and causes a higher CSC population, indicating invasion, and WNT10A mediates migration in ESCC [67]. CD44, aldehyde dehydrogenase 1, and Lgr5 are helpful in esophageal CSC categorization. High level of CD44 expression in cancer cells shows characteristics of EMT. The initiation of EMT via TGF-β by the receptor epidermal growth factor plays a vital role in this signaling [68].

2.5 *Gastric Cancer*

The first discovered CSCs in GC occurred when cell lines of GC were analyzed. [69] EpCAM and CD44 are two markers used for isolating cancer stem cells from GC cell lines or resected tumors. In addition, CD54 and CD44 present in peripheral blood of GC patients help in the isolation of gastric CSCs. $Lgr5^+$ stem cells present in the stomach were the source for isolating gastric CSC [70]. Increased levels of $Lgr5^+$ in patients of GC show median survivability [71]. Induction of hyperplasia and manipulation of all progenitor cells and $Lgr5^+$ stem cells are due to *Helicobacter pylori* colonization [72]. Gastric CSCs are believed to derive from regular stem cells in the tissue. *Helicobacter pylori* leads to chronic infection; however, induction of inflammation led to the regenerating gastric tissue made with bone marrow, although acute inflammation does not contribute to the induction of bone marrow-derived cells [73]. In the pyloric gland, stem cells that express villin and $villin^+$ gastric stem cells may be transformed into GC cells [74]. KLF4 may play a crucial role in the initiation and progression of GC in gastric $villin^+$ stem cells [74]. Furthermore, CSC candidate markers might be ALDH1, CD90, CD71, and CD133. By inducing EMT, microRNAs may control the properties of gastric CSCs [75].

3 Signaling Pathways of Cancer Stem Cells in GI Cancer

Some major signaling mechanisms involved in CSCs are TGF-β-signals, Hedgehog, Notch, and Wnt/β-catenin; these pathways have been associated with CSC maintenance in GI cancers [11, 76] (Table 3.1).

3.1 *Wnt Signaling*

Self-renewal of gastrointestinal epithelial cells controls the growth and reproduction by the Wnt signaling pathway which is crucial in embryogenesis [77]. Epigenetic and genetic changes observed in GI cancers are due to abnormality in the pathway of Wnt [78, 79]. This pathway has also been used in recent years to control stem cell biology in adult gastrointestinal organs [80]. The noncanonical (Wnt/calcium), canonical (Wnt/β-catenin), and noncanonical planar cell polarity (PCP) are the three branches classified in the Wnt pathway [77]. The canonical pathway requires Wnt ligand binding to the receptor Frizzled (FZD) as well as the low-density lipoprotein receptor associated with protein 5/6 co-receptor (LRP5/6) to activate intracellular signaling by β-catenin nuclear translocation. When a Wnt ligand binds to the FZD receptor the signaling process begins and induces dishevelled phosphorylation (DVL) that further recruits Axin to deconstruct the degradation complex and it tends to monitor and control β-catenin and trigger a β-catenin T-cell-specific

Table 3.1 Unique markers of gastrointestinal cancer stem cells

Tumor type (references)	Regulatory pathways	Markers of cancer stem cells according to tumor type
Colorectal cancer [22–25]	Wnt signals, epigenetic pathways	Lgr5$^+$/GPR49$^+$ CD133$^+$/ CD44$^{+/}$ALDH1$^+$ CD44$^+$/CD24$^+$ EpCAM$^+$/CD44$^+$ CD166$^+$
Metastatic colon [26]	EGF signaling, Ras-ERK, PI3K/Akt kinase pathway PI3K/Akt and, STAT3-dependent signaling	CD133$^+$/CD26$^+$
Gastric cancer [27]	Wnt/β-catenin and (NF)-kB	CD44$^+$
Liver cancer [28–31]	Hedgehog, Wnt, P53, Akt, insulin-like growth factor-1 receptor, Notch, and TGF-β	CD13$^+$ D90$^+$/CD45$^-$ EpCAM$^+$ CD133$^+$/CD49$^+$
Pancreatic cancer [32, 33]	Hedgehog, Notch, Wnt, and phosphatidylinositol-3 kinase/act (protein kinase B)	CXCR4$^+$ CD133$^+$/CD44+/CD24$^+$/ ESA$^+$
Esophageal cancer [34]	TGF-β	CD44$^+$/ALDH1$^+$

ESA epithelial specific antigen, *ALDH1* aldehyde dehydrogenase-1, *Lgr5* leucine-rich repeat-containing G-protein-coupled receptor 5, *EpCAM* epithelial cell adhesion molecule, *GPR* G-protein-coupled receptor, *CXCR4* C-X-C chemokine receptor type 4

transcription factor (TCF)-lymphoid enhancer-binding factor (LEF) transactivation complex [81, 82]. Without Wnt ligand binding, cytoplasmic β-catenin is phosphorylated by a degradation complex and degrades within the proteasomes. This degradation complex is constituted by the tumor suppressor adenomatous polyposis coli (APC), the scaffolding protein AXIN, CK1 (casein kinase 1), and GSK-3 (glycogen synthase kinase 3). In general, noncanonical Wnt pathways are associated with differentiation, cell polarity, and migration. By recruiting and activating DVL, Wnt ligands bind to the FZD receptor in the noncanonical PCP pathway and activate various GTPases such as Ras homologous gene family member A (RhoA), Ras-related C3 botulinum toxin substrate (RAC), and cell division control protein 42 (Cdc42). Wnt ligands bind to both the FZD receptor and alternative receptors of the tyrosine kinase family also known as RYK (receptor-like tyrosine kinase) or ROR (tyrosine kinase-like orphan receptor) in the noncanonical calcium-dependent Wnt signal. This signaling pathway promotes cell migration and canonical Wnt signaling inhibition through intracellular calcium flux and calmodulin kinase (CaMK2), Jun kinase (JNK), and PKCα activation. Notch activation can also enhance active β-catenin levels by regulating the endo-lysosomal degradation of β-catenin after translation [83]. The equilibrium between β-catenin delocalization distinction and self-renewal in several adult CSCs is mainly regulated by the "canonical" Wnt/β-catenin pathway [11]. This process allows the control of stem cells (SCs) and their instability may lead to the expansion of CSCs. A recent study shows that CD133 and EpCAM have been described as specific transcription targets for hepatocellular carcinoma (HCC) in the signaling of Wnt/β-catenin [55]. In particular, the depletion of EpCAM in HCC stem cells interfered with proliferation, colony formation, and migration [55]. Further, β-catenin siRNA knockdown inhibits CSCs [84]. Wnt/β-catenin signaling activation occurs in the intestine after Apc mutation leading to the disease of the familial adenomatous polyposis (FAP) [85]. One of the early incidents during carcinogenic cases in the most intermittent colorectal cancers was due to Apc gene complete impairment. In addition, intense Apc mutant polyposis mice (Apc1322 T) was associated with increased Lgr5 expression, and other stem cell markers like Bmi1, CD44, and Musashi1 [86]. Deleting the main gene Wnt CD44 in Apcmin/+ mice also reduces intestinal tumorigenesis [87]. All these findings related to Wnt signaling provide information on gastrointestinal tumorigenesis for cancer stem cell model and it also helps in maintaining the CSC role to enhance progression of cancer.

3.2 *Signaling of Transforming Growth Factor-β (TGF-β)*

In all the signaling pathways the transforming growth factor-β (TGF-β) shows a key role in regulating the gastrointestinal epithelial cells' development, differentiation, survival, and fate [88]. TGF-β functions as a tumor suppressor in a normal and healthy environment, by cell proliferation inhibition, autophagy suppression, and apoptosis-triggering processes. Change in their response to TGF-β develops tumors and use it as a powerful promoter of cell motility, invasion, metastasis, and CSC preservation [89]. TGF-β is an important inducer in the transformation of mesenchymal-epithelial (EMT) by regulating transcriptional activation of the protein family Snail and TWIST, the EMT system's key regulators [90, 91]. One of the most frequently altered signaling pathways is TGF-β signaling in GI cancers [92]. And it plays an important role in the maintenance of CSCs in human kidney, pancreatic, gastric, and colorectal cancers [4]. Kim et al. recently stated its importance of control in the development of colon cancer by stimulating nuclear translocation of β-catenin showing a correlation between TGF-β1 and ALDH1 [11].

3.3 *Notch Signaling Pathway*

The Notch pathways play an important role including cell homeostasis and differentiation during embryogenesis, and are of major importance in many areas of cancer biology, from CSC to angiogenesis, and tumor immunity [93, 94]. The pathway of Notch signaling is usually complicated and multidimensional, imitating its functions in various functional processes [95, 96]. Notch mediates a number of biological processes through four Notch receptors (Notch-1–4) and five Notch ligands such as Delta-like ligands 1, 3, and 4, and Jagged-1 and Jagged-2 [97]. Cell-to-cell contact for canonical Notch signaling is usually necessary for the activation of Notch, where Notch can be separated by multiple enzymes through a series of proteolytic enzyme cleavages, resulting in the release and activation of target gene Notch [97]. Notch's key genes include NF-κβ, c-Myc, cyclin D1, Akt, and mTOR and the endothelial vascular (VEGF) growth factor [98]. The different GI cancers express Notch receptors and ligands differently. Also, noncanonical Notch signaling has begun to be delineated independently of ligand-receptor interaction and some of its roles are essential for GI cancer [99]. Cross talk with Wnt and/or Hedgehog (HH) signaling may also be used to determine the overall effect of signaling in Notch adding an additional layer of complexity [13]. For example, Notch signaling activation as a suppressor may have occurred in HCC tumor but it can play an oncogenic role in both colon and pancreatic cancer [100]. In fact, the key role of Notch signaling in the extending of CSCs has been demonstrated. In pancreatic CSCs, Notch-1 and -2 are overexpressed and associated with reduced CD44 [101].

3.4 JAK–STAT3 Pathway

The signal transducer and transcription activator 3 (STAT3) significantly contribute to the regulation of cell-related processes mediated to producing and progressing cancer, including proliferation, angiogenesis, cell survival, and immune function [102]. In many GI cancer types, including colorectal cancer, dysregulated STAT3 has been identified [103]. Consider that the activation cycle for the STAT3 starts with Janus kinases (JAKs) which are phosphorylated to specific signals such as interleukin-6 (IL-6), interferon-α (IFNα), tumor necrosis factor (TNF), epidermal growth factor (EGF), and platelet-derived growth factor (PDGF) [104]. Nevertheless, the JAK–STAT3 mechanisms are of interest not only for cancer-related immune cells but also for CSCs [104]. In this way, CSCs of hepatocellular cancers EpCAM$^+$/CD133$^+$ and ALDH$^+$/CD133 and CSC of colon cancers demonstrate the increased activity of IL-6/STAT3 which is a causative interplay in the niche spreading in CSCs [11, 105]. Recent evidence suggests that STAT3-signaling feedback activation plays an important role in mediating drug resistance to a wide spectrum of anticancer treatments and IL6/STAT3 pathway inhibitors can be used to eradicate CSCs [11, 105].

3.5 Hedgehog (HH) Signaling Pathway

The regulation of cell destiny specifications and the patterns are due to the Hedgehog (HH) signaling which is involved in embryonic development, normal tissue repair, and EMT [106]. In mammals with HH ligands, there are three proteins: sonic Hedgehog (SHH), Indian Hedgehog (IHH), and desert Hedgehog (DHH). Such proteins bind to the transmembrane receptor Patched-1, which induces the internalization and prevents its suppression of the transmembrane protein Smoothened (SMO) and thereby activates the signaling pathway [107]. Subsequent signaling by SMO leads to activation and nuclear localization of transcription glioma-associated oncogene (GLI) factor that helps to produce HH target genes such as c-myc, cyclin D1, VEGF, BCL2, and Split (HES) family protein enhancer [108]. The development, survival, and angiogenesis involve such target genes [109]. CSCs are influenced by the HH signaling, according to the emerging results from gastrointestinal tumors [48]. Activated HH signals have been identified in the CSCs, which was demonstrated later by relatively high colorectal cancer expression of GLI1, GLI2, PTCH1, and Hedgehog interacting protein (HIP) [110]. Moreover, in colorectal cancer the progression of CCSs with the target gene SNAIL1 is linked to EMT and involved in metastasis [110]. In addition, cyclopamine and siRNA of SMO, GLI1, and GLI2 inhibited the HH pathway activation, reduced the tumor cell growth, and induced apoptosis [111]. EMT-clonogenic growth possibilities have also been studied in pancreatic CSCs and cyclopamine inhibits each functional property and leads to the formation of the metastatic disease [112]. In fact, CD133 + liver CSCs are strongly expressed as genes participating in the hedgehog pathway [113].

3.6 *mTOR Pathway*

Recent reports have shown that the mTOR pathways are important for GI cancer pathogenesis [114]. PIK3 mutations occur in a number of cancers including gastric and colorectal cancers [115]. Many human cancers, like GC, are related to poor prognosis of Akt activation [114]. Aktl and Akt2 were particularly observed for gastric, pancreatic, and colorectal cancers [116]. mTOR complex 1 (mTORC1) and mTOR complex 2 (mTORC2) are increased during cancer progressions in hepatic, pancreas, gastric, and colorectal cancers. They also control EMTs, motility, and metastasis [117, 118]. Radioresistance is also associated with EMT and CSC phenotypes by activating the PI3 K/Akt/mTOR signals [119]. Recent studies of colon cancer cells have also shown that PI3 K/Akt/mTOR inhibits proliferation of the CSC in colon and lowers stemness, as observed by CD133 and Lgr5 expression [120]. mTOR inhibition also reduces ALDH1, a marker for colorectal CSCs [121]. Similarly, the inhibition of mTORC2 has led to decreased EpCAM expression in the liver CSCs that have little or no tumorigenicity [122]. Matsumoto et al. and Yang et al. also show that mTOR inhibition increases CD133^{+} subpopulation and activates the CD133 shift to the CD133^{+} in vitro population, by using gastrointestinal tumor cells [123].

Classic signaling pathways described above play an important role in GI and CSC self-renewal [124]. Considering the growing reports that GI cancer is a disease driven by multipotent, self-renewing CSCs, it is essential that we understand how these signaling pathways synchronize events and the development and evolution of

CSC. This will lead to a more successful early diagnosis of cancer and the development of treatment approaches to reduce recurrence and/or cancer therapy.

4 Therapeutic Resistance Mechanisms

Chemotherapy and radiotherapy are key components of GI cancer treatment, namely esophageal, gastric, hepatic, pancreatic, and rectal cancer. Unfortunately, following such therapies, disease recurrence and worsening frequently occur, with increasing evidence including CSCs for these adverse effects. Mechanisms by which CSCs survive when establishing standard cancer therapies include increased DNA repair, dormancy maintenance, drug efflux, and redox capacity.

4.1 Senescence Maintenance

Radiation and traditional chemotherapy kill cancer cells by causing DNA damage that most effectively induces cell death in rapidly dividing cells with inactive replication of DNA. While this effectively helps to separate cancer cells rapidly, CSCs are often quiescent, reducing the cytotoxic effects of radiation and chemotherapy on these cells. In addition, stemlike $CD44^{+}$ cells sustain a quiescent condition in prostate cancer [14]. This CSCs engage in DNA repair mechanisms in this quiescent state before progressing into the mitotic phase of the cell cycle [125]. Likewise, in experiments with cell lines of gastric, colon, and esophageal cancer, chemotherapy treatment enriches a stemlike population of cells with a quiescent state [126]. In the EC9706 line of esophageal cancer cells, this subgroup of stem cells display increased resistance to DNA damage compared to non-stem cancer cells [127]. These examples together highlight the demand for innovative methods of targeting and killing CSCs that do not rely on cell proliferation.

4.2 DNA Damage Checkpoint Repair

As above, the proliferation rate of CSCs provides an innate defense against genotoxic cancer therapies. Similarly, CSCs also increased DNA repair efficiency, further reducing the efficacy of these conventional cancer therapies. Glioma treatment with ionizing radiation for example enriches CD133 + CSCs. CD133 + glioma cells express greater checkpoint activation of ataxia-telangiectasia-mutated (ATM) Rad17, Chk1, and Chk2 checkpoint proteins in response to DNA damage, resulting in cell cycle arrest. This radioresistance is opposed by inhibition of checkpoint kinases [128]. Similarly, other DNA damage response targets including ATM, ATR, Chk1, and PARP1 have increased levels of glioblastoma CSCs [129].

4.3 Increased Redox Capacity

Radiation therapy induces DNA damage by reactive oxygen species (ROS) production, where ROS reaches the cell's antioxidant capacity [130]. CSCs produce extremely ROS scavengers, such as glutathione (GSH), which results in resistance to DNA damage induced by ROS. To support this, GSH pharmacological reduction induces radiosensitivity in CSCs [131]. The CD44 variant isoforms (CD44v), strongly expressed in carcinomas of the epithelial form and GI CSCs, are implicated in intracellular GSH control [132]. CD44v-expressed cells play a vital role in the tumor-beginning process and have increased resistance to H_2O_2, cisplatin, and docetaxel in order to play a crucial role in the initiation of tumors. This indicates that the control and enhancement of the cellular antioxidant ability of CSC CD44v play a role not only in tumorigenesis but also in resistance to chemotherapeutic treatment strategies and in maintaining ROS levels below those of non-stem cells [133].

4.4 Efflux of Drug

In addition, preventing or repairing chemoradiation-induced DNA damage, CSCs have the capability to export toxic chemicals and drugs. This is induced by proteins that transport from the cell membrane, the most common being the ATP-binding cassette (AC) transporter family. Such hydrophobic chemotherapy drugs are eliminated by transport proteins from the cytosol to the extracellular space [134]. Studies of CSCs from various types of solid cancers revealed superior efflux ability compared to non-cancer stem cells. For example, two drug transporters, MDR1 and BRCP1, are overexpressed by $CD133^+$ glioma CSCs compared with $CD133^-$ cells [126, 135]. In fact, enhanced production of the MDR1 transporter protein ABCG2 in colorectal CSCs in these cells conferred chemoresistance [136].

5 Targeting of CSCs

CSCs are armed with numerous mechanisms for avoiding conventional cancer therapy, limiting the effectiveness of these therapeutic strategies and enabling CSCs to promote the recurrence of metastatic diseases. So ideal antitumor therapies should target both the proliferating population of cancer cells and CSCs. In this case, therapies designed to eliminate CSCs have attempted to remove these cells through either activate differentiation or targeted eradication [137, 138].

5.1 Differentiation Induction

Differentiation therapies are based on the principle that differentiation of CSCs contributes to a loss of self-renewal capabilities and properties of drug resistance, hence making them susceptible to regular therapies. The best known example of treatment designed to induce differentiation of CSCs is the treatment of APL. ATRA, a retinoid, has helped turn APL into one of the most treatable leukemia forms. ATRA targets PML/RAR-α, a differentiation suppressor, which induces cell differentiation [139]. Retinoids were also used in head-and-neck and lung cancer in addition to their use in APL, where differentiation induction was used as a chemical prevention tool for precancerous lesions [140]. In GI cancer ATRA induces differentiation in the cell lines of colon cancer [141]. Furthermore, ATRA treatment of patient xenografts resulting from stomach cancers causes CSC differentiation and apoptosis, decreasing tumorigenicity [142]. Clinically, ATRA substantially improves precancerous gastric dysplasia when combined with omeprazole and sucralfate [143]. Furthermore, the use of ATRA in traditional gastric cancer treatment increases survival rate compared to standard therapy alone [144]. While ATRA has failed to demonstrate therapeutic effectiveness in the diagnosis of other GI tumors, ATRA provides a framework and proof of concept for the future use of differentiation therapy in specific cases. Certain compounds cause differentiation in comparison to ATRA, like PPAR-γ agonists. PPAR-γ is an important regulator of differentiation in many cell types, particularly those involved in lipid homeostasis, controlling preadipocyte and fibroblast terminal differentiation [145]. Most of the work with PPAR-γ has been done in cancer cell lines to date. PPAR-γ agonists, such as pioglitazone, exit the cell cycle by inducing terminal differentiation [146]. Of interest to GI, Sarraf et al. worked on tumors in colonic adenocarcinoma and he showed the enhanced expression of PPAR-γ in adenocarcinoma. Additionally, treatment with PPAR-γ agonist troglitazone leads to the differentiation of colon cancer cells, measured by increased carcinoembryonic antigen expression (CEA) [147]. In addition, knockdown of PPAR-γ in mice promoted tumor growth by decreasing cancer cell differentiation [148]. Such findings showed that there are mechanisms that can be controlled for cell differentiation in GI tract cancers. Nevertheless, significant work is required in this field before therapies reach the clinic since most experiments have been performed in vitro in cancer cell lines.

5.2 Targeted Elimination

Besides therapies that induce differentiation, treatment of CSCs can also be performed by targeting stem cells for elimination. As previously described, CSCs have distinct surface marker expression profiles, creating opportunities for pharmacotherapeutic strategies targeting these different CSC properties. Targeted removal may also be done through targeting pathways that give therapeutic resistance or survival benefits to CSCs.

6 Targeting of Cell Surface Receptors

The classification of CSCs by cell surface markers is observed in many GI cancers, including the pancreatic liver and colon [54, 149, 150]. Identification and selective targeting of CSC-specific cell surface markers enable the administration of highly potent cytotoxic agents with minimal systemic toxicity, as compared to traditional chemotherapeutics that target all rapidly dividing cells. There are two possible ways to remove such markers: immunotherapy and drug carriers.

6.1 Immunotherapy

Targeting CSCs that use the immune system provides benefits compared to standard therapies. First, along with other antibody treatments, immune cells exhibit antigen-specific cytotoxic activity, providing a more focused approach to CSC targeting. Second, in conventional treatments, such as chemotherapy and radiation, toxicity depends in part on the phase of the cell cycle [151]. Since CSCs are relatively quiescent compared to non-CSCs, immunotherapeutic strategies can provide a way of eliminating CSCs irrespective of proliferation status [152]. Finally, immunotherapy can produce long-lasting memory responses that might be effective in challenging a cancer relapse. Numerous immunotherapy strategies are listed below, targeting CSCs in gastrointestinal malignancies.

6.1.1 Chimeric Antigen Receptor T-Cell Therapy

With the recent US FDA approval of tisagenlecleucel and axicabtagene for refractory B-cell malignancies, chimeric antigen receptor (CAR)T cells have turned into an exciting immunotherapeutic approach to cancer treatment [153]. In addition, CAR T cells are T cells engineered to express an artificial receptor that consists of a targeting domain generated from an antibody linked to intracellular signals [153]. Therefore, CARs derived from antibodies which target surface antigens on CSCs represent a potential therapeutic approach. Details of a phase I study of CAR T cells guided against CD133 in patients with hepatocellular, pancreatic, and colorectal carcinomas have recently been reported [154]. Of the 23 cases, 3 had limited recovery and 14 had stable illnesses. Analysis of biopsied tissues also shows that $CD133^{+}$ cells were decreased. While EpCAM is a less selective CSC marker, CAR T cells target this marker. Ang et al.'s report found that anti-EpCAM CAR T cells increased survival with human rectal tumors in xenograft mouse models

[155]. Clinical trials are currently ongoing to test anti-EpCAM CAR T cells in various gastrointestinal malignancies (NCT03013712).

6.1.2 Vaccines

Ning et al. found that vaccination with dendritic cells pulsed with CSC lysates identified by high dehydrogenase expression (ALDH) was capable of generating in vivo CSC-specific T cells and antibody responses [156]. In addition, dendritic cells pulsed with tumor lysates from ALDH cells showed increased inhibition of tumor growth compared to whole-tumor lysates and reduced metastases in squamous cell and melanoma tumor models. It indicates that autologous tumor cell vaccines targeting CSCs may have a greater effect on antitumors. Phase I/II clinical trials delivering CSC vaccines in the liver (NCT02089919), colorectal (NCT02176746), and pancreatic (NCT02074046) cancers were performed based on the Ning et al. methodology. Reports of these studies are still to be published.

6.1.3 Other Immune Cells

Although most efforts targeting CSCs have based on exploiting the adaptive immune system, it is increasingly recognized that innate immune cells often identify CSCs. Tallerico et al.'s in vitro experiments showed that natural killer (NK) cells in colorectal tumors preferentially lysed CSCs over non-CSCs [157]. Cytotoxic effect against CSCs was associated with enhanced expression of NK-activating ligands NKp30 and NKp44 and reduced expression on CSC surfaces of inhibitory ligands such as MHC class I compared to non-CSC cells. In melanoma and glioblastoma, similar reports of CSC-specific killing by NK cells were published [157, 158]. In addition, recent studies by Ames et al. have shown NK cells' ability to target pancreatic CSCs in vivo. The adoptive migration of NK cells was observed using mice with human pancreatic tumor xenografts to decrease percentages of ALDH high cells which act synergistically with radiation to inhibit tumor growth [159, 160]. However, γδ T cells in various malignancies often show anti-CSC activation [161]. In colorectal cancer, Todaro et al. documented that zoledronate caused the aggregation of metabolites of mevalonate in CSCs, making them targets for the destruction of cells by γδ T cells [161]. Alternative methods using NK and γδ T cells for targeting CSCs are independent of antigen processing and expression of MHC.

6.2 Drug Carriers

Apart from immunological strategies, the delivery of cytotoxic agents on the surface of cells is a possible method for the eradication of CSCs. One such successful therapy is the development of aptamers, which are small single-stranded DNA or RNA, about 20 times smaller than antibodies. These aptamers bind to their targets with great affinity and are internalized by cells [162]. In 2010 Shigdar et al. created the first RNA aptamer targeting a CSC surface marker. This aptamer was designed to interact with the molecule of epithelial cell adhesion (EpCAM), a transmembrane glycoprotein commonly overexpressed in both solid tumors and CSCs. It was associated with several cell lines of cancer including KATO III (gastric carcinoma) and T47D (cell line of colon adenocarcinoma) [163]. More recently, two RNA aptamers were found to target CD133AC133 epitope, a CSC marker in the colon and pancreas [164, 165]. Among other cells, HT-29 (human colorectal cancer cell line) and Hep3B (hepatocellular carcinoma cell line) internalized these CD133 aptamers. They also demonstrated a superior ability to penetrate HT-29 tumor spheres compared to an antibody CD133 [166]. A recent study showed that an aptamer directed at the CD44 surface receptor, a specific CSC marker, has been internalized via breast cancer cell lines [167]. While this report did not show the internalization of the aptamer in GI cells, it is important to note that CD44 was previously used as a marker for GI CSCs [165]. As aptamers are usually less immunogenic and have low toxicity, they hold excellent potential as a drug delivery mechanism with less systemic toxicity than conventional therapies. The exciting potential of these conjugates has not been proved to be effective in vivo at this point and further work is required before systematic delivery [168]. Antibody-drug conjugates are a promising therapeutic choice, like nanocarriers such as aptamers, which would enable cytotoxic agents to be administered to specific cells in the absence of systemic toxicity. Antibody-drug conjugates require internalization accompanied by lysosomal processing and cleavage to activate the drug. It causes only those cells which show the antigen to be given therapy [169]. Such conjugates can be used together with normal chemotherapy and radiation to produce improved results. In addition, this concept was used in the treatment of acute myeloid leukemia, where a gemtuzumab ozogamicin conjugate targeting $CD33^+$ leukemia cells was paired with conventional chemotherapy to increase survival rate [170]. Antibody-drug conjugates targeting CSC surface markers are under study. Two antibody conjugates have recently been established that target LGR5, a marker of CSCs in colon cancer. In a mouse model, a study shows within in vivo antitumor efficacy and safety. Although much more work should be done until therapies such as these are safe for humans, this study provided evidence of the idea that antibody-drug conjugates can be targeted at CSC surface markers [171].

6.3 *Targeting Resistance Mechanisms*

Another potential mechanism for eradicating CSCs is to target the machinery that mediates standard therapy resistance. Two fields where this has been examined in CSCs include inhibition of ABC transporters and targeting of antioxidant systems.

6.3.1 Transporters

As previously described, ABC transporters allow CSCs to avoid conventional chemotherapy by effluxing chemotherapeutic agents. Therapy designed to disrupt these transporters makes CSCs sensitive to standard chemotherapy. The best studied technique for inhibiting the role of ABC transporters is through direct modulators, three generations of which exist. Despite showing promise versus leukemia cells in vitro, in phase I clinical trial the first known modulator, verapamil, failed to improve vinblastine toxicity [172]. Second-generation inhibitors seem to be optimistic, but resulted in lower clearance of chemotherapy and increased toxicity in clinical trials [173]. Third-generation inhibitors have shown more promise as a possible multidrug resistance therapy [173]. Certain approaches targeted at transcriptional regulation of ABC carriers or signaling pathways involving ABC carriers are in their infancy and will need further improvement [173].

6.3.2 Antioxidant Systems

Another therapeutic approach to disarm mechanisms of resistance to CSCs is through targeting antioxidant systems, increasing oxidative stress in radiation and chemotherapy setting. The most important potential target is GSH, a metabolite that defends the cells from oxidative damage [174]. In squamous head-and-neck carcinoma, inhibition of xCT, a cysteine transport mediator required for the synthesis of GSH, leads to apoptosis in CD44v-expressing stemlike cells [175]. CD44v interacts and stabilizes xCT, promoting cysteine uptake enabling synthesis of GSH. Subsequently, CD44v ablation destabilizes xCT and decreases GSH. CD44v ablation in a mouse model of gastric cancer resulted in a loss of cell surface expression and a decline in intracellular GSH, thereby suppressing tumor growth [176]. These studies show that extracting aspects of the cell defense system from ROS will influence cell viability.

6.4 Antitelomerase Therapy

The shortening of telomeres is a major regulator of cell death. In most tissues, telomerase that helps maintain the length of the telomere is suppressed before birth and maintains normal telomere-dependent cell mortality. Lifetime telomerase activity is relegated to the selection of stem cell populations, thus allowing immortality. Unlike ordinary stem cells, CSCs remain immortal and capable of self-renewal, largely due to telomerase expression which enables them to avoid replicative senescence. Besides CSCs, most tumor cells express any level of telomerase activity [177]. This makes telomerase an outstanding target therapy because it can influence all differentiated cancer cells and CSCs. There are currently two methods of guiding telomerase therapy. The first BIBR1532 antitelomerase compound was effective but it failed to advance to the clinical trial level. More recently, the GRN163L compound has progressed to the clinical trial level and has proven effective in multiple tissues of mouse xenografts [178]. In the field of GI cancer, GRN163L showed the efficacy of human hepatoma impairing tumor growth in vivo in mouse xenografts. When GRN163L was granted prechemotherapy, chemosensitivity to doxorubicin was increased in vitro [179]. There is also a decrease in telomerase expression in cells isolated from surgical specimens of the Barrett's esophagus treated with GRN163L. In addition, telomere shortening is observed resulting in eventual in vitro apoptosis. In vivo treatment with GRN163L decreased the volume of tumors in a mouse xenograft model [180]. In fact, GRN163L enhanced the sensitivity to radiation in the esophageal squamous cell carcinoma cell lines, leading to increased apoptosis [181]. Although these studies suggest promise for a potential therapeutic for GI cancer, to date 19 clinical trials using GRN163L have been conducted, but none have been targeted for GI cancers [182]. The second antitelomerase treatment method is through immunotherapy. Vaccines targeted at TERT, a catalytic component of telomerase, will require $CD8^+$ T cells to destroy tumor cells while largely avoiding toxicity to normal tissues with little to no expression of telomerase [183]. There was potential in the area of pancreatic cancer therapy that GV1001, a telomerase vaccine, would prove effective in patients with advanced-stage pancreatic cancer. However, given in combination with chemotherapy, in a phase III clinical trial, GV1001 showed no improvement in overall survival [184]. Further study in the field of telomerase immunotherapy and telomerase-inhibiting therapy is required to understand its potential for targeting CSCs.

7 Targeting Tumor Microenvironment

Specific activation of CSCs is a first-line clinical technique for combating these cells. Furthermore, other therapeutic approaches are also suggested as knowledge of the tumor microenvironment is rapidly increasing, which could establish a gap for developing and protecting CSCs from cancer therapy. Tumor microenvironment cells comprise fibroblast, myofibroblast, adipocyte, mesenchymal stem cells, and immune cells, such as macrophages and neutrophils, as well as endothelial cells forming the blood vessel walls and moving through the tumor [185]. CXCR4, the stromal cell receptor associated with factor-1 (CXCL12/SDF-1α), makes tumor progression, angiogenesis, and drug tolerance easier. However, expression of CXCR4 is a prognostic factor in several GI carcinomas, including gastrointestinal carcinoma [185]. The association of adhesive tumor/stroma will disrupt CXCR4 antagonists, such as analogs plerixafor (AMD3100) and T14003, which can make stem cells responsive to cytotoxic drugs [186]. In both clinical studies and gastrointestinal cancer mouse models, a new approach to targeting the CXCR4-CXCL12 axis is being investigated [185]. Developing more efficient anticancer methods often means inhibiting the angiogenic process needed to vascularize and grow tumors.

Likewise, the development and observation of antiangiogenic agents that could interact with a VEGF-VEGFR pathway were carried out to effectively combat tumor growth in in vivo animal models, including anti-VEGF or VEGFR antibodies, VEGFR antagonists, and soluble truncated VEGFR form [187].

8 The New Approach to Preclinical Therapy Assessment

In our opinion, preclinical evaluation of efficient treatment of CSC involves confirmation, and this test can be conducted in a variety of ways, each representing different intensity levels, and which more accurately demonstrates clinical conditions. Grafting and cell culture models are the conventional way to test the success of the treatment against CSCs. These initiatives may be inaccurate because culturally adapted cells cannot imitate actual primary CSC properties.

9 Cell Line, Patient-Derived Xenograft (PDX), and Tumoroids

The traditional new drug screening by using cell line-derived xenograft or syngeneic mouse models could not predict the successful development of oncological drugs because 97% of novel treatments were successful in in vivo xenograft studies but were unsuccessful in clinical trials [188]. In contrast, a small fraction of fresh tumor tissue from the patient is transplanted into an immunodeficient mouse tumor model [188]. This procedure allows for faster cell movement and effective tumor growth and position control. PDX models can be preferable to traditional line xenografts because they are similar to parental tumors. Detailed examination of PDX mice reveals that histology and gene expression profiles are maintained with SNPs and copy number variants, and PDX models efficiently screen the drug efficacy [188].

Another new cell culture technology, known as "organoids" and "tumoroids," was recently developed and allowed to derive from adult stem cells and tumors (especially CSCs), respectively [189]. The structures are the same as organ/tumor in vivo and can develop fast and in relatively great amounts in structural and developmental processes. While many works have been done on the production of tissue repair organoids/tumoroids, more detailed implementation includes high-throughput therapeutic testing, from cell signals and analyses to palliative chemotherapy sensitization and to optimization of treatment protocols in personalized medicinal products. Therefore, without the complications associated with organism growth, gene knockout and knock-in can be done. This form of preclinical models in vitro helps researchers to predict clinical reaction trends and to conduct customized clinical trials.

10 Conclusion

Many gastrointestinal tumors are likely to generate a small population of self-regenerating cells called CSCs. Moreover, it does not show enough evidence in order to determine the relationships between CSCs sorted according to different methods. As previously mentioned, supposed CSC is isolated by their markers. Anticancer therapy is usually assessed for its ability to shrink tumors. If these treatments do not eliminate CSCs, there could be a relapse and tumors may establish more resistance through CSCs. Targeted therapies against these molecules could provide new ways of eradicating malignant cancer phenotypes without disturbing ordinary stem cells. CSC-targeted therapy has arisen as a method of treatment that could revolutionize cancer therapy and have a significant impact on reducing recurrence and metastatic diseases. Furthermore, many CSC-targeted therapies are more specific and would allow less systemic toxicity than traditional chemotherapy and radiation therapy. There are several major obstacles to implementing CSC-targeted therapies. Many of the treatments mentioned above are not specific to CSCs but are typically inherent in stem cells. In fact, there is a huge amount of cross-talking between signaling pathways, and the impact of interrupting such paths in normal cell populations remains unclear. Therapies targeted at CSC-specific cell surface markers offer an interesting opportunity to avoid this issue, as they can provide selective therapy with reduced systemic toxicity. This can be accomplished in many forms, including drug carrier mechanisms and immunotherapies, such as vaccinations and CAR-T-cell therapies. Stem cells have only been identified in a small number of GI cancers. Therefore, there is the possibility of stem cell subsets that do not express known markers. In addition, there are potential surface marker profiles between stem cells that may vary across various patients. The substantial effort will be required to reliably identify stem cell markers among various GI cancer profiles before these therapies can progress to a clinically impactful stage. More work is needed to recognize CSCs and consider their survival mechanisms, resistant therapeutic properties, and cell signaling pathways. However, this is an exciting therapeutic approach that will involve a lot of research and investment in the coming years to fulfill its promise of revolutionizing cancer therapy.

References

1. Xu, M., Shao, X., Kuai, X., Zhang, L., Zhou, C., & Cheng, Z. (2019). Expression analysis and implication of Rab1A in gastrointestinal relevant tumor. *Scientific Reports, 9*(1), 13384.
2. DeSantis, C. E., Lin, C. C., Mariotto, A. B., Siegel, R. L., Stein, K. D., Kramer, J. L., et al. (2014). Cancer treatment and survivorship statistics, 2014. *CA: a Cancer Journal for Clinicians, 64*(4), 252–271.
3. Ferlay, J., Soerjomataram, I., Dikshit, R., Eser, S., Mathers, C., Rebelo, M., et al. (2015). Cancer incidence and mortality worldwide: Sources, methods and major patterns in GLOBOCAN 2012. *International Journal of Cancer, 136*(5), E359–EE86.

4. Taniguchi, H., Moriya, C., Igarashi, H., Saitoh, A., Yamamoto, H., Adachi, Y., et al. (2016). Cancer stem cells in human gastrointestinal cancer. *Cancer Science, 107*(11), 1556–1562.
5. Clarke, M. F., Dick, J. E., Dirks, P. B., Eaves, C. J., Jamieson, C. H. M., Jones, D. L., et al. (2006). Cancer stem cells--perspectives on current status and future directions: AACR workshop on cancer stem cells. *Cancer Research, 66*(19), 9339–9344.
6. Pardal, R., Clarke, M. F., & Morrison, S. J. (2003). Applying the principles of stem-cell biology to cancer. *Nature Reviews. Cancer, 3*(12), 895–902.
7. Zhang, M., Li, Z., Zhang, X., & Chang, Y. (2014). Cancer stem cells as a potential therapeutic target in breast cancer. *Stem Cell Investigation, 1*, 14.
8. Feinberg, A. P. (2007). Phenotypic plasticity and the epigenetics of human disease. *Nature, 447*(7143), 433–440.
9. Feinberg, A. P., & Tycko, B. (2004). The history of cancer epigenetics. *Nature Reviews. Cancer, 4*(2), 143–153.
10. Reya, T., Morrison, S. J., Clarke, M. F., & Weissman, I. L. (2001). Stem cells, cancer, and cancer stem cells. *Nature, 414*(6859), 105–111.
11. Ahmad, R., Dhawan, P., & Singh, A. B. (2016). Cancer stem cell and gastrointestinal cancer: Current status, targeted therapy and future implications. *Biochemical Pharmacology (Los Angel), 5*(2), 202.
12. Massagué, J., Blain, S. W., & Lo, R. S. (2000). TGF-beta signaling in growth control, cancer, and heritable disorders. *Cell, 103*(2), 295–309.
13. Takebe, N., Miele, L., Harris, P. J., Jeong, W., Bando, H., Kahn, M., et al. (2015). Targeting notch, hedgehog, and Wnt pathways in cancer stem cells: Clinical update. *Nature Reviews. Clinical Oncology, 12*(8), 445–464.
14. Zhao, J. (2016). Cancer stem cells and chemoresistance: The smartest survives the raid. *Pharmacology & Therapeutics, 160*, 145–158.
15. De Francesco, E. M., Sotgia, F., & Lisanti, M. P. (2018). Cancer stem cells (CSCs): Metabolic strategies for their identification and eradication. *The Biochemical Journal, 475*(9), 1611–1634.
16. Valderrama-Treviño, A. I., Barrera-Mera, B., Ceballos-Villalva, J. C., & Montalvo-Javé, E. E. (2017). Hepatic metastasis from colorectal cancer. *Euroasian J Hepatogastroenterology, 7*(2), 166–175.
17. Anderson, E. C., Hessman, C., Levin, T. G., Monroe, M. M., & Wong, M. H. (2011). The role of colorectal cancer stem cells in metastatic disease and therapeutic response. *Cancers (Basel), 3*(1), 319–339.
18. Sousa, J. L. C., Freire, C. S. R., Silvestre, A. J. D., & Silva, A. M. S. (2019). Recent developments in the functionalization of betulinic acid and its natural analogues: A route to new bioactive compounds. *Molecules, 24*(2), 355.
19. Ullah, I., Subbarao, R. B., & Rho, G. J. (2015). Human mesenchymal stem cells - current trends and future prospective. *Bioscience Reports, 35*(2), e00191.
20. Tsuchiya, A., Kojima, Y., Ikarashi, S., Seino, S., Watanabe, Y., Kawata, Y., et al. (2017). Clinical trials using mesenchymal stem cells in liver diseases and inflammatory bowel diseases. *Inflammation Regeneration, 37*, 16.
21. Lin, W., Huang, L., Li, Y., Fang, B., Li, G., Chen, L., et al. (2019). Mesenchymal stem cells and cancer: Clinical challenges and opportunities. *BioMed Research International, 2019*, 2820853.
22. Vermeulen, L., Todaro, M., de Sousa, M. F., Sprick, M. R., Kemper, K., Perez Alea, M., et al. (2008). Single-cell cloning of colon cancer stem cells reveals a multi-lineage differentiation capacity. *Proceedings of the National Academy of Sciences of the United States of America., 105*(36), 13427–13432.
23. Yeung, T. M., Gandhi, S. C., Wilding, J. L., Muschel, R., & Bodmer, W. F. (2010). Cancer stem cells from colorectal cancer-derived cell lines. *Proceedings of the National Academy of Sciences of the United States of America., 107*(8), 3722–3727.

24. Dalerba, P., Dylla, S. J., Park, I. K., Liu, R., Wang, X., Cho, R. W., et al. (2007). Phenotypic characterization of human colorectal cancer stem cells. *Proceedings of the National Academy of Sciences of the United States of America., 104*(24), 10158–10163.
25. Ricci-Vitiani, L., Lombardi, D. G., Pilozzi, E., Biffoni, M., Todaro, M., Peschle, C., et al. (2007). Identification and expansion of human colon-cancer-initiating cells. *Nature, 445* (7123), 111–115.
26. Pang, R., Law, W. L., Chu, A. C., Poon, J. T., Lam, C. S., Chow, A. K., et al. (2010). A subpopulation of CD26+ cancer stem cells with metastatic capacity in human colorectal cancer. *Cell Stem Cell, 6*(6), 603–615.
27. Takaishi, S., Okumura, T., Tu, S., Wang, S. S., Shibata, W., Vigneshwaran, R., et al. (2009). Identification of gastric cancer stem cells using the cell surface marker CD44. *Stem Cells (Dayton, Ohio), 27*(5), 1006–1020.
28. Kimura, O., Takahashi, T., Ishii, N., Inoue, Y., Ueno, Y., Kogure, T., et al. (2010). Characterization of the epithelial cell adhesion molecule (EpCAM)+ cell population in hepatocellular carcinoma cell lines. *Cancer Science, 101*(10), 2145–2155.
29. Haraguchi, N., Ishii, H., Mimori, K., Tanaka, F., Ohkuma, M., Kim, H. M., et al. (2010). CD13 is a therapeutic target in human liver cancer stem cells. *The Journal of Clinical Investigation, 120*(9), 3326–3339.
30. Yang, Z. F., Ho, D. W., Ng, M. N., Lau, C. K., Yu, W. C., Ngai, P., et al. (2008). Significance of CD90+ cancer stem cells in human liver cancer. *Cancer Cell, 13*(2), 153–166.
31. Rountree, C. B., Senadheera, S., Mato, J. M., Crooks, G. M., & Lu, S. C. (2008). Expansion of liver cancer stem cells during aging in methionine adenosyltransferase 1A-deficient mice. *Hepatology (Baltimore, Md)., 47*(4), 1288–1297.
32. Hermann, P. C., Huber, S. L., Herrler, T., Aicher, A., Ellwart, J. W., Guba, M., et al. (2007). Distinct populations of cancer stem cells determine tumor growth and metastatic activity in human pancreatic cancer. *Cell Stem Cell, 1*(3), 313–323.
33. Li, C., Heidt, D. G., Dalerba, P., Burant, C. F., Zhang, L., Adsay, V., et al. (2007). Identification of pancreatic cancer stem cells. *Cancer Research, 67*(3), 1030–1037.
34. Zhao, J. S., Li, W. J., Ge, D., Zhang, P. J., Li, J. J., Lu, C. L., et al. (2011). Tumor initiating cells in esophageal squamous cell carcinomas express high levels of CD44. *PLoS One, 6*(6), e21419.
35. Paschall, A. V., & Liu, K. (2015). Epigenetic and immune regulation of colorectal cancer stem cells. *Current Colorectal Cancer Reports, 11*(6), 414–421.
36. Morgan, R. G., Mortensson, E., & Williams, A. C. (2018). Targeting LGR5 in colorectal cancer: Therapeutic gold or too plastic? *British Journal of Cancer, 118*(11), 1410–1418.
37. Al-Kharusi, M. R. A., Smartt, H. J. M., Greenhough, A., Collard, T. J., Emery, E. D., Williams, A. C., et al. (2013). LGR5 promotes survival in human colorectal adenoma cells and is upregulated by PGE2: Implications for targeting adenoma stem cells with NSAIDs. *Carcinogenesis, 34*(5), 1150–1157.
38. Todaro, M., Francipane, M. G., Medema, J. P., & Stassi, G. (2010). Colon cancer stem cells: Promise of targeted therapy. *Gastroenterology, 138*(6), 2151–2162.
39. Vázquez-Iglesias, L., Barcia-Castro, L., Rodríguez-Quiroga, M., Páez de la Cadena, M., Rodríguez-Berrocal, J., & Cordero, O. J. (2019). Surface expression marker profile in colon cancer cell lines and sphere-derived cells suggests complexity in CD26(+) cancer stem cells subsets. *Biology Open, 8*(7), bio041673.
40. Sarkar, S., Popov, V. L., O'Connell, M. R., Stevenson, H. L., Lee, B. S., Obeid, R. A., et al. (2017). A novel antibody against cancer stem cell biomarker, DCLK1-S, is potentially useful for assessing colon cancer risk after screening colonoscopy. *Laboratory Investigation, 97*(10), 1245–1261.
41. Gopisetty, G., Xu, J., Sampath, D., Colman, H., & Puduvalli, V. K. (2013). Epigenetic regulation of CD133/PROM1 expression in glioma stem cells by Spl/myc and promoter methylation. *Oncogene, 32*(26), 3119–3129.

42. Su, S., Hong, F., Liang, Y., Zhou, J., Liang, Y., Chen, K., et al. (2015). Lgr5 methylation in cancer stem cell differentiation and prognosis-prediction in colorectal cancer. *PLoS One, 10* (11), e0143513-e.
43. Khan, A. Q., Ahmed, E. I., Elareer, N. R., Junejo, K., Steinhoff, M., & Uddin, S. (2019). Role of miRNA-regulated cancer stem cells in the pathogenesis of human malignancies. *Cell, 8*(8), 840.
44. Poltavets, V., Kochetkova, M., Pitson, S. M., & Samuel, M. S. (2018). The role of the extracellular matrix and its molecular and cellular regulators in cancer cell plasticity. *Frontiers in Oncology, 8*, 431.
45. Lu, J., Ye, X., Fan, F., Xia, L., Bhattacharya, R., Bellister, S., et al. (2013). Endothelial cells promote the colorectal cancer stem cell phenotype through a soluble form of Jagged-1. *Cancer Cell, 23*(2), 171–185.
46. Francipane, M. G., Bulanin, D., & Lagasse, E. (2019). Establishment and characterization of 5-fluorouracil-resistant human colorectal cancer stem-like cells: Tumor dynamics under selection pressure. *International Journal of Molecular Sciences, 20*(8), 1817.
47. Pelosi, E., Castelli, G., & Testa, U. (2017). Pancreatic cancer: Molecular characterization, clonal evolution and cancer stem cells. *Biomedicine, 5*(4), 65.
48. Sari, I. N., Phi, L. T. H., Jun, N., Wijaya, Y. T., Lee, S., & Kwon, H. Y. (2018). Hedgehog signaling in cancer: A prospective therapeutic target for eradicating cancer stem cells. *Cell, 7* (11), 208.
49. Brunetti, O., Russo, A., Scarpa, A., Santini, D., Reni, M., Bittoni, A., et al. (2015). MicroRNA in pancreatic adenocarcinoma: Predictive/prognostic biomarkers or therapeutic targets? *Oncotarget, 6*(27), 23323–23341.
50. Słotwiński, R., Lech, G., & Słotwińska, S. M. (2018). MicroRNAs in pancreatic cancer diagnosis and therapy. *Central European Journal of Immunology, 43*(3), 314–324.
51. Di Carlo, C., Brandi, J., & Cecconi, D. (2018). Pancreatic cancer stem cells: Perspectives on potential therapeutic approaches of pancreatic ductal adenocarcinoma. *World Journal of Stem Cells, 10*(11), 172–182.
52. Doffou, M., Adams, G., Bowen, W. C., Paranjpe, S., Parihar, H. S., Nguyen, H., et al. (2018). Oct4 is crucial for transdifferentiation of hepatocytes to biliary epithelial cells in an in vitro organoid culture model. *Gene Expression, 18*(1), 51–62.
53. Wang, N., Wang, S., Li, M.-Y., Hu, B.-G., Liu, L.-P., Yang, S.-L., et al. (2018). Cancer stem cells in hepatocellular carcinoma: An overview and promising therapeutic strategies. *Therapeutic Advances in Medical Oncology, 10*, 1758835918816287.
54. Qiu, L., Li, H., Fu, S., Chen, X., & Lu, L. (2018). Surface markers of liver cancer stem cells and innovative targeted-therapy strategies for HCC. *Oncology Letters, 15*(2), 2039–2048.
55. Flores-Téllez, T. N., Villa-Treviño, S., & Piña-Vázquez, C. (2017). Road to stemness in hepatocellular carcinoma. *World Journal of Gastroenterology, 23*(37), 6750–6776.
56. Xiao, Y., Lin, M., Jiang, X., Ye, J., Guo, T., Shi, Y., et al. (2017). The recent advances on liver cancer stem cells: Biomarkers, separation, and therapy. *Analytical Cellular Pathology (Amsterdam), 2017*, 5108653.
57. Yoshida, M., Yamashita, T., Okada, H., Oishi, N., Nio, K., Hayashi, T., et al. (2017). Sorafenib suppresses extrahepatic metastasis de novo in hepatocellular carcinoma through inhibition of mesenchymal cancer stem cells characterized by the expression of CD90. *Scientific Reports, 7*(1), 11292.
58. Liu, A. Y., Cai, Y., Mao, Y., Lin, Y., Zheng, H., Wu, T., et al. (2013). Twist2 promotes self-renewal of liver cancer stem-like cells by regulating CD24. *Carcinogenesis, 35*(3), 537–545.
59. Xiang, Y., Yang, T., Pang, B.-Y., Zhu, Y., & Liu, Y.-N. (2016). The progress and prospects of putative biomarkers for liver cancer stem cells in hepatocellular carcinoma. *Stem Cells International, 2016*, 7614971.
60. Shahbazi, J., Lock, R., & Liu, T. (2013). Tumor protein 53-induced nuclear protein 1 enhances p53 function and represses tumorigenesis. *Frontiers in Genetics, 4*, 80.

61. Meng, F., Glaser, S. S., Francis, H., DeMorrow, S., Han, Y., Passarini, J. D., et al. (2012). Functional analysis of microRNAs in human hepatocellular cancer stem cells. *Journal of Cellular and Molecular Medicine, 16*(1), 160–173.
62. Zhang, J., Luo, N., Luo, Y., Peng, Z., Zhang, T., & Li, S. (2012). microRNA-150 inhibits human CD133-positive liver cancer stem cells through negative regulation of the transcription factor c-Myb. *International Journal of Oncology, 40*(3), 747–756.
63. Wang, Y., Zhang, C., Zhu, H., Tang, J., Zhang, S., Luo, J., et al. (2017). CD90 positive cells exhibit aggressive radioresistance in esophageal squamous cell carcinoma. *Journal of Thoracic Disease, 9*(3), 610–620.
64. Wu, Q., Wu, Z., Bao, C., Li, W., He, H., Sun, Y., et al. (2019). Cancer stem cells in esophageal squamous cell cancer. *Oncology Letters, 18*(5), 5022–5032.
65. Zheng, Z., Ke, X., Wang, M., He, S., Li, Q., Zheng, C., et al. (2013). Human microRNA hsa-miR-296-5p suppresses enterovirus 71 replication by targeting the viral genome. *Journal of Virology, 87*(10), 5645–5656.
66. Komatsu, S., Ichikawa, D., Kawaguchi, T., Miyamae, M., Okajima, W., Ohashi, T., et al. (2016). Circulating miR-21 as an independent predictive biomarker for chemoresistance in esophageal squamous cell carcinoma. *American Journal of Cancer Research, 6*(7), 1511–1523.
67. Long, A., Giroux, V., Whelan, K. A., Hamilton, K. E., Tétreault, M.-P., Tanaka, K., et al. (2015). WNT10A promotes an invasive and self-renewing phenotype in esophageal squamous cell carcinoma. *Carcinogenesis, 36*(5), 598–606.
68. Sato, F., Kubota, Y., Natsuizaka, M., Maehara, O., Hatanaka, Y., Marukawa, K., et al. (2015). EGFR inhibitors prevent induction of cancer stem-like cells in esophageal squamous cell carcinoma by suppressing epithelial-mesenchymal transition. *Cancer Biology & Therapy, 16* (6), 933–940.
69. Zhang, X., Hua, R., Wang, X., Huang, M., Gan, L., Wu, Z., et al. (2016). Identification of stem-like cells and clinical significance of candidate stem cell markers in gastric cancer. *Oncotarget, 7*(9), 9815–9831.
70. Wang, B., Chen, Q., Cao, Y., Ma, X., Yin, C., Jia, Y., et al. (2016). LGR5 is a gastric cancer stem cell marker associated with stemness and the EMT signature genes NANOG, NANOGP8, PRRX1, TWIST1, and BMI1. *PLoS One, 11*(12), e0168904-e.
71. Bu, Z., Zheng, Z., Zhang, L., Li, Z., Sun, Y., Dong, B., et al. (2013). LGR5 is a promising biomarker for patients with stage I and II gastric cancer. *Chinese Journal of Cancer Research, 25*(1), 79–89.
72. Sigal, M., Rothenberg, M. E., Logan, C. Y., Lee, J. Y., Honaker, R. W., Cooper, R. L., et al. (2015). Helicobacter pylori activates and expands Lgr5(+) stem cells through direct colonization of the gastric glands. *Gastroenterology, 148*(7), 1392–404.e21.
73. Takaishi, S., Okumura, T., & Wang, T. C. (2008). Gastric cancer stem cells. *Journal of Clinical Oncology, 26*(17), 2876–2882.
74. Zhao, Y., Feng, F., & Zhou, Y.-N. (2015). Stem cells in gastric cancer. *World Journal of Gastroenterology, 21*(1), 112–123.
75. Pan, Y., Shu, X., Sun, L., Yu, L., Sun, L., Yang, Z., et al. (2017). miR-196a-5p modulates gastric cancer stem cell characteristics by targeting Smad4. *International journal of oncology., 50*(6), 1965–1976.
76. Pelullo, M., Zema, S., Nardozza, F., Checquolo, S., Screpanti, I., & Bellavia, D. (2019). Wnt, Notch, and TGF-β pathways impinge on Hedgehog signaling complexity: An open window on cancer. *Frontiers in Genetics, 10*, 711.
77. Flanagan, D. J., Austin, C. R., Vincan, E., & Phesse, T. J. (2018). Wnt signalling in gastrointestinal epithelial stem cells. *Genes (Basel), 9*(4), 178.
78. Serman, L., Nikuseva Martic, T., Serman, A., & Vranic, S. (2014). Epigenetic alterations of the Wnt signaling pathway in cancer: A mini review. *Bosnian Journal of Basic Medical Sciences, 14*(4), 191–194.

79. You, J. S., & Jones, P. A. (2012). Cancer genetics and epigenetics: Two sides of the same coin? *Cancer Cell, 22*(1), 9–20.
80. Liu, Q., & Jin, L. H. (2017). Organ-to-organ communication: A Drosophila gastrointestinal tract perspective. *Frontiers in Cell and Development Biology, 5*, 29.
81. Sharma, M., Castro-Piedras, I., Simmons, G. E., Jr., & Pruitt, K. (2018). Dishevelled: A masterful conductor of complex Wnt signals. *Cellular Signalling, 47*, 52–64.
82. MacDonald, B. T., & He, X. (2012). Frizzled and LRP5/6 receptors for Wnt/β-catenin signaling. *Cold Spring Harbor Perspectives in Biology, 4*(12), a007880.
83. Flentke, G. R., Garic, A., Hernandez, M., & Smith, S. M. (2014). CaMKII represses transcriptionally active beta-catenin to mediate acute ethanol neurodegeneration and can phosphorylate beta-catenin. *Journal of Neurochemistry, 128*(4), 523–535.
84. Li, K., Zhou, Z. Y., Ji, P. P., & Luo, H. S. (2016). Knockdown of beta-catenin by siRNA influences proliferation, apoptosis and invasion of the colon cancer cell line SW480. *Oncology Letters, 11*(6), 3896–3900.
85. Eshghifar, N., Farrokhi, N., Naji, T., & Zali, M. (2017). Tumor suppressor genes in familial adenomatous polyposis. *Gastroenterology and Hepatology from Bed to Bench, 10*(1), 3–13.
86. Lewis, A., Segditsas, S., Deheragoda, M., Pollard, P., Jeffery, R., Nye, E., et al. (2010). Severe polyposis in Apc(1322T) mice is associated with submaximal Wnt signalling and increased expression of the stem cell marker Lgr5. *Gut, 59*(12), 1680–1686.
87. Zeilstra, J., Joosten, S. P., Dokter, M., Verwiel, E., Spaargaren, M., & Pals, S. T. (2008). Deletion of the WNT target and cancer stem cell marker CD44 in Apc(Min/+) mice attenuates intestinal tumorigenesis. *Cancer Research, 68*(10), 3655–3661.
88. Mullen, A. C., & Wrana, J. L. (2017). TGF-β family signaling in embryonic and somatic stem-cell renewal and differentiation. *Cold Spring Harbor Perspectives in Biology, 9*(7), a022186.
89. Bellomo, C., Caja, L., & Moustakas, A. (2016). Transforming growth factor β as regulator of cancer stemness and metastasis. *British Journal of Cancer, 115*(7), 761–769.
90. Xu, J., Lamouille, S., & Derynck, R. (2009). TGF-beta-induced epithelial to mesenchymal transition. *Cell Research, 19*(2), 156–172.
91. Hao, Y., Baker, D., & Ten Dijke, P. (2019). TGF-β-mediated epithelial-mesenchymal transition and cancer metastasis. *International Journal of Molecular Sciences, 20*(11), 2767.
92. Luo, J., Chen, X.-Q., & Li, P. (2019). The role of TGF-β and its receptors in gastrointestinal cancers. *Translational Oncology, 12*(3), 475–484.
93. Huang, Q., Li, J., Zheng, J., & Wei, A. (2019). The carcinogenic role of the Notch signaling pathway in the development of hepatocellular carcinoma. *Journal of Cancer, 10*(6), 1570–1579.
94. Venkatesh, V., Nataraj, R., Thangaraj, G. S., Karthikeyan, M., Gnanasekaran, A., Kaginelli, S. B., et al. (2018). Targeting notch signalling pathway of cancer stem cells. *Stem Cell Investigation, 5*, 5.
95. Natsuizaka, M., Whelan, K. A., Kagawa, S., Tanaka, K., Giroux, V., Chandramouleeswaran, P. M., et al. (2017). Interplay between Notch-1 and Notch-3 promotes EMT and tumor initiation in squamous cell carcinoma. *Nature Communications, 8*(1), 1758.
96. Lee, H.-J., Kim, M.-Y., & Park, H.-S. (2015). Phosphorylation-dependent regulation of Notch-1 signaling: The fulcrum of Notch-1 signaling. *BMB Reports, 48*(8), 431–437.
97. Luca, V. C., Jude, K. M., Pierce, N. W., Nachury, M. V., Fischer, S., & Garcia, K. C. (2015). Structural biology. Structural basis for Notch-1 engagement of Delta-like 4. *Science, 347* (6224), 847–853.
98. Wang, Z., Li, Y., & Sarkar, F. H. (2010). Notch signaling proteins: Legitimate targets for cancer therapy. *Current Protein & Peptide Science, 11*(6), 398–408.
99. Huang, T., Zhou, Y., Cheng, A. S. L., Yu, J., To KF, & Kang, W. (2016). NOTCH receptors in gastric and other gastrointestinal cancers: Oncogenes or tumor suppressors? *Molecular Cancer, 15*(1), 80.

100. Lobry, C., Oh, P., & Aifantis, I. (2011). Oncogenic and tumor suppressor functions of Notch in cancer: it's NOTCH what you think. *The Journal of Experimental Medicine, 208*(10), 1931–1935.
101. Xu, Y.-F., Hannafon, B. N., & Ding, W.-Q. (2017). microRNA regulation of human pancreatic cancer stem cells. *Stem Cell Investigation, 4*, 5.
102. Loh, C.-Y., Arya, A., Naema, A. F., Wong, W. F., Sethi, G., & Looi, C. Y. (2019). Signal transducer and activator of transcription (STATs) proteins in cancer and inflammation: Functions and therapeutic implication. *Frontiers in Oncology, 9*, 4.
103. Hernández-Luna, M. A., López-Briones, S., & Luria-Pérez, R. (2019). The four horsemen in colon cancer. *Journal of Oncology, 2019*, 5636272.
104. Berishaj, M., Gao, S. P., Ahmed, S., Leslie, K., Al-Ahmadie, H., Gerald, W. L., et al. (2007). Stat3 is tyrosine-phosphorylated through the interleukin-6/glycoprotein 130/Janus kinase pathway in breast cancer. *Breast Cancer Research : BCR., 9*(3), R32.
105. Ji, J., & Wang, X. W. (2012). Clinical implications of cancer stem cell biology in hepatocellular carcinoma. *Seminars in Oncology, 39*(4), 461–472.
106. Armas-López, L., Zúñiga, J., Arrieta, O., & Ávila-Moreno, F. (2017). The Hedgehog-GLI pathway in embryonic development and cancer: Implications for pulmonary oncology therapy. *Oncotarget, 8*(36), 60684–60703.
107. Skoda, A. M., Simovic, D., Karin, V., Kardum, V., Vranic, S., & Serman, L. (2018). The role of the Hedgehog signaling pathway in cancer: A comprehensive review. *Bosnian Journal of Basic Medical Sciences, 18*(1), 8–20.
108. Pandolfi, S., & Stecca, B. (2015). Cooperative integration between HEDGEHOG-GLI signalling and other oncogenic pathways: Implications for cancer therapy. *Expert Reviews in Molecular Medicine, 17*, e5-e.
109. Gupta, S. C., Kim, J. H., Prasad, S., & Aggarwal, B. B. (2010). Regulation of survival, proliferation, invasion, angiogenesis, and metastasis of tumor cells through modulation of inflammatory pathways by nutraceuticals. *Cancer Metastasis Reviews, 29*(3), 405–434.
110. Kasper, M., Jaks, V., Fiaschi, M., & Toftgård, R. (2009). Hedgehog signalling in breast cancer. *Carcinogenesis, 30*(6), 903–911.
111. Lauth, M., Bergström, A., Shimokawa, T., & Toftgård, R. (2007). Inhibition of GLI-mediated transcription and tumor cell growth by small-molecule antagonists. *Proceedings of the National Academy of Sciences of the United States of America., 104*(20), 8455–8460.
112. Merchant, A. A., & Matsui, W. (2010). Targeting Hedgehog--a cancer stem cell pathway. *Clinical Cancer Research, 16*(12), 3130–3140.
113. Cochrane, C. R., Szczepny, A., Watkins, D. N., & Cain, J. E. (2015). Hedgehog signaling in the maintenance of cancer stem cells. *Cancers (Basel), 7*(3), 1554–1585.
114. Malley, C. O., & Pidgeon, G. P. (2015). The mTOR pathway in obesity driven gastrointestinal cancers: Potential targets and clinical trials. *BBA Clin., 5*, 29–40.
115. Samuels, Y., & Waldman, T. (2010). Oncogenic mutations of PIK3CA in human cancers. *Current Topics in Microbiology and Immunology, 347*, 21–41.
116. Rychahou, P. G., Kang, J., Gulhati, P., Doan, H. Q., Chen, L. A., Xiao, S.-Y., et al. (2008). Akt2 overexpression plays a critical role in the establishment of colorectal cancer metastasis. *Proceedings of the National Academy of Sciences of the United States of America., 105*(51), 20315–20320.
117. Gulhati, P., Bowen, K. A., Liu, J., Stevens, P. D., Rychahou, P. G., Chen, M., et al. (2011). mTORC1 and mTORC2 regulate EMT, motility, and metastasis of colorectal cancer via RhoA and Rac1 signaling pathways. *Cancer Research, 71*(9), 3246–3256.
118. Hua, H., Kong, Q., Zhang, H., Wang, J., Luo, T., & Jiang, Y. (2019). Targeting mTOR for cancer therapy. *Journal of Hematology & Oncology, 12*(1), 71.
119. Chang, L., Graham, P. H., Hao, J., Ni, J., Bucci, J., Cozzi, P. J., et al. (2013). Acquisition of epithelial-mesenchymal transition and cancer stem cell phenotypes is associated with activation of the PI3K/Akt/mTOR pathway in prostate cancer radioresistance. *Cell Death & Disease, 4*, e875.

120. Chen, J., Shao, R., Li, F., Monteiro, M., Liu, J. P., Xu, Z. P., et al. (2015). PI3K/Akt/mTOR pathway dual inhibitor BEZ235 suppresses the stemness of colon cancer stem cells. *Clinical and Experimental Pharmacology & Physiology, 42*(12), 1317–1326.
121. Shibata, M., & Hoque, M. O. (2019). Targeting cancer stem cells: A strategy for effective eradication of cancer. *Cancers (Basel), 11*(5), 732.
122. Nishitani, S., Horie, M., Ishizaki, S., & Yano, H. (2013). Branched chain amino acid suppresses hepatocellular cancer stem cells through the activation of mammalian target of rapamycin. *PLoS One, 8*(11), e82346-e.
123. Yang, Z., Zhang, L., Ma, A., Liu, L., Li, J., Gu, J., et al. (2011). Transient mTOR inhibition facilitates continuous growth of liver tumors by modulating the maintenance of CD133+ cell populations. *PLoS One, 6*(12), e28405-e.
124. Matsui, W. H. (2016). Cancer stem cell signaling pathways. *Medicine (Baltimore), 95*(1 Suppl 1), S8–S19.
125. Schulz, A., Meyer, F., Dubrovska, A., & Borgmann, K. (2019). Cancer stem cells and radioresistance: DNA repair and beyond. *Cancers (Basel), 11*(6), 862.
126. Phi, L. T. H., Sari, I. N., Yang, Y.-G., Lee, S.-H., Jun, N., Kim, K. S., et al. (2018). Cancer stem cells (CSCs) in drug resistance and their therapeutic implications in cancer treatment. *Stem Cells International, 2018*, 5416923.
127. Wang, Q.-E. (2015). DNA damage responses in cancer stem cells: Implications for cancer therapeutic strategies. *World Journal of Biological Chemistry, 6*(3), 57–64.
128. Zhou, W., Sun, M., Li, G. H., Wu, Y. Z., Wang, Y., Jin, F., et al. (2013). Activation of the phosphorylation of ATM contributes to radioresistance of glioma stem cells. *Oncology Reports, 30*(4), 1793–1801.
129. Ahmed, S. U., Carruthers, R., Gilmour, L., Yildirim, S., Watts, C., & Chalmers, A. J. (2015). Selective inhibition of parallel DNA damage response pathways optimizes radiosensitization of glioblastoma stem-like cells. *Cancer Research, 75*(20), 4416–4428.
130. Azzam, E. I., Jay-Gerin, J.-P., & Pain, D. (2012). Ionizing radiation-induced metabolic oxidative stress and prolonged cell injury. *Cancer Letters, 327*(1–2), 48–60.
131. Diehn, M., Cho, R. W., Lobo, N. A., Kalisky, T., Dorie, M. J., Kulp, A. N., et al. (2009). Association of reactive oxygen species levels and radioresistance in cancer stem cells. *Nature, 458*(7239), 780–783.
132. Yan, Y., Zuo, X., & Wei, D. (2015). Concise review: Emerging role of CD44 in cancer stem cells: A promising biomarker and therapeutic target. *Stem Cells Translational Medicine, 4*(9), 1033–1043.
133. Ding, S., Li, C., Cheng, N., Cui, X., Xu, X., & Zhou, G. (2015). Redox regulation in cancer stem cells. *Oxidative Medicine and Cellular Longevity, 2015*, 750798.
134. Yang, N. J., & Hinner, M. J. (2015). Getting across the cell membrane: An overview for small molecules, peptides, and proteins. *Methods in Molecular Biology, 1266*, 29–53.
135. Kim, S.-S., Rait, A., Rubab, F., Rao, A. K., Kiritsy, M. C., Pirollo, K. F., et al. (2014). The clinical potential of targeted nanomedicine: Delivering to cancer stem-like cells. *Molecular Therapy, 22*(2), 278–291.
136. Abdullah, L. N., & Chow, E. K.-H. (2013). Mechanisms of chemoresistance in cancer stem cells. *Clinical and Translational Medicine, 2*(1), 3.
137. Pattabiraman, D. R., & Weinberg, R. A. (2014). Tackling the cancer stem cells - what challenges do they pose? *Nature Reviews. Drug Discovery, 13*(7), 497–512.
138. Hu, Y., & Fu, L. (2012). Targeting cancer stem cells: A new therapy to cure cancer patients. *American Journal of Cancer Research, 2*(3), 340–356.
139. Yao, S., Zhong, L., Chen, M., Zhao, Y., Li, L., Liu, L., et al. (2017). Epigallocatechin-3-gallate promotes all-trans retinoic acid-induced maturation of acute promyelocytic leukemia cells via PTEN. *International Journal of Oncology, 51*(3), 899–906.
140. Bushue, N., & Wan, Y.-J. Y. (2010). Retinoid pathway and cancer therapeutics. *Advanced Drug Delivery Reviews, 62*(13), 1285–1298.

141. Applegate, C. C., & Lane, M. A. (2015). Role of retinoids in the prevention and treatment of colorectal cancer. *World Journal of Gastrointestinal Oncology, 7*(10), 184–203.
142. Nguyen, P. H., Giraud, J., Staedel, C., Chambonnier, L., Dubus, P., Chevret, E., et al. (2016). All-trans retinoic acid targets gastric cancer stem cells and inhibits patient-derived gastric carcinoma tumor growth. *Oncogene, 35*(43), 5619–5628.
143. Jin, J., Li, X., Xing, L., Chang, Y., Wu, L., Jin, Z., et al. (2015). Addition of all-trans-retinoic acid to omeprazole and sucralfate therapy improves the prognosis of gastric dysplasia. *The Journal of International Medical Research, 43*(2), 204–216.
144. Ilson, D. H. (2018). Advances in the treatment of gastric cancer. *Current Opinion in Gastroenterology, 34*(6), 465–468.
145. Farmer, S. R. (2006). Transcriptional control of adipocyte formation. *Cell Metabolism, 4*(4), 263–273.
146. Reddy, A. T., Lakshmi, S. P., & Reddy, R. C. (2016). PPARγ as a novel therapeutic target in lung cancer. *PPAR Research, 2016*, 8972570.
147. Hatton, J. L., & Yee, L. D. (2008). Clinical use of PPARgamma ligands in cancer. *PPAR Research, 2008*, 159415.
148. Wood, W. M., Sharma, V., Bauerle, K. T., Pike, L. A., Zhou, Q., Fretwell, D. L., et al. (2011). PPARγ promotes growth and invasion of thyroid cancer cells. *PPAR Research, 2011*, 171765.
149. Mirzaei, A., Madjd, Z., Amini Kadijani, A., Alinaghi, S., & Akbari, A. (2017). Tavoosidana G. *Cancer Stem Cell's Potential Clinical Implications, 10*(1), e5897.
150. Zhao, W., Li, Y., & Zhang, X. (2017). Stemness-related markers in cancer. *Cancer Translational Medicine, 3*(3), 87–95.
151. Moding, E. J., Kastan, M. B., & Kirsch, D. G. (2013). Strategies for optimizing the response of cancer and normal tissues to radiation. *Nature Reviews. Drug Discovery, 12*(7), 526–542.
152. Plaks, V., Kong, N., & Werb, Z. (2015). The cancer stem cell niche: How essential is the niche in regulating stemness of tumor cells? *Cell Stem Cell, 16*(3), 225–238.
153. Zavras, P. D., Wang, Y., Gandhi, A., Lontos, K., & Delgoffe, G. M. (2019). Evaluating tisagenlecleucel and its potential in the treatment of relapsed or refractory diffuse large B cell lymphoma: Evidence to date. *Oncotargets and Therapy, 12*, 4543–4554.
154. Wang, Y., Chen, M., Wu, Z., Tong, C., Dai, H., Guo, Y., et al. (2018). CD133-directed CAR T cells for advanced metastasis malignancies: A phase I trial. *Oncoimmunology, 7*(7), e1440169-e.
155. Ang, W. X., Li, Z., Chi, Z., Du, S.-H., Chen, C., Tay, J. C. K., et al. (2017). Intraperitoneal immunotherapy with T cells stably and transiently expressing anti-EpCAM CAR in xenograft models of peritoneal carcinomatosis. *Oncotarget, 8*(8), 13545–13559.
156. Ning, N., Pan, Q., Zheng, F., Teitz-Tennenbaum, S., Egenti, M., Yet, J., et al. (2012). Cancer stem cell vaccination confers significant antitumor immunity. *Cancer Research, 72*(7), 1853–1864.
157. Luna, J. I., Grossenbacher, S. K., Murphy, W. J., & Canter, R. J. (2017). Targeting cancer stem cells with natural killer cell immunotherapy. *Expert Opinion on Biological Therapy, 17*(3), 313–324.
158. Codd, A. S., Kanaseki, T., Torigo, T., & Tabi, Z. (2018). Cancer stem cells as targets for immunotherapy. *Immunology, 153*(3), 304–314.
159. Oh, E., Min, B., Li, Y., Lian, C., Hong, J., Park, G.-M., et al. (2019). Cryopreserved human natural killer cells exhibit potent antitumor efficacy against orthotopic pancreatic cancer through efficient tumor-homing and cytolytic ability (running title: Cryopreserved NK Cells Exhibit Antitumor Effect). *Cancers (Basel), 11*(7), 966.
160. Hu, S., Yang, J., Shangguan, J., Eresen, A., Li, Y., Ma, Q., et al. (2019). Natural killer cell-based adoptive transfer immunotherapy for pancreatic ductal adenocarcinoma in a Kras (LSL-G12D) p53(LSL-R172H) Pdx1-Cre mouse model. *American Journal of Cancer Research, 9*(8), 1757–1765.
161. Lo Presti, E., Pizzolato, G., Gulotta, E., Cocorullo, G., Gulotta, G., Dieli, F., et al. (2017). Current advances in γδ T cell-based tumor immunotherapy. *Frontiers in Immunology, 8*, 1401.

162. Zhou, J., & Rossi, J. (2017). Aptamers as targeted therapeutics: Current potential and challenges. *Nature Reviews. Drug Discovery, 16*(3), 181–202.
163. Sakakura, C., Hagiwara, A., Nakanishi, M., Shimomura, K., Takagi, T., Yasuoka, R., et al. (2002). Differential gene expression profiles of gastric cancer cells established from primary tumour and malignant ascites. *British Journal of Cancer, 87*(10), 1153–1161.
164. Schmohl, J. U., & Vallera, D. A. (2016). CD133, selectively targeting the root of cancer. *Toxins (Basel), 8*(6), 165.
165. Glumac, P. M., & LeBeau, A. M. (2018). The role of CD133 in cancer: A concise review. *Clinical and Translational Medicine, 7*(1), 18.
166. Xiang, D., Zheng, C., Zhou, S.-F., Qiao, S., Tran, P. H.-L., Pu, C., et al. (2015). Superior performance of aptamer in tumor penetration over antibody: Implication of aptamer-based theranostics in solid tumors. *Theranostics, 5*(10), 1083–1097.
167. Zhou, G., Latchoumanin, O., Bagdesar, M., Hebbard, L., Duan, W., Liddle, C., et al. (2017). Aptamer-based therapeutic approaches to target cancer stem cells. *Theranostics, 7*(16), 3948–3961.
168. Patra, J. K., Das, G., Fraceto, L. F., Campos, E. V. R., Rodriguez-Torres, M. D. P., Acosta-Torres, L. S., et al. (2018). Nano based drug delivery systems: Recent developments and future prospects. *Journal of Nanobiotechnology, 16*(1), 71.
169. Dan, N., Setua, S., Kashyap, V. K., Khan, S., Jaggi, M., Yallapu, M. M., et al. (2018). Antibody-drug conjugates for cancer therapy: Chemistry to clinical implications. *Pharmaceuticals (Basel), 11*(2), 32.
170. Yu, B., & Liu, D. (2019). Gemtuzumab ozogamicin and novel antibody-drug conjugates in clinical trials for acute myeloid leukemia. *Biomarker Research, 7*, 24.
171. Deonarain, M. P., Kousparou, C. A., & Epenetos, A. A. (2009). Antibodies targeting cancer stem cells: A new paradigm in immunotherapy? *MAbs, 1*(1), 12–25.
172. Atanasov, A. G., Waltenberger, B., Pferschy-Wenzig, E.-M., Linder, T., Wawrosch, C., Uhrin, P., et al. (2015). Discovery and resupply of pharmacologically active plant-derived natural products: A review. *Biotechnology Advances, 33*(8), 1582–1614.
173. Falzone, L., Salomone, S., & Libra, M. (2018). Evolution of cancer pharmacological treatments at the turn of the third millennium. *Frontiers in Pharmacology, 9*, 1300.
174. Lushchak, V. I. (2012). Glutathione homeostasis and functions: Potential targets for medical interventions. *Journal of Amino Acids, 2012*, 736837.
175. Yoshikawa, M., Tsuchihashi, K., Ishimoto, T., Yae, T., Motohara, T., Sugihara, E., et al. (2013). xCT inhibition depletes CD44v-expressing tumor cells that are resistant to EGFR-targeted therapy in head and neck squamous cell carcinoma. *Cancer Research, 73*(6), 1855–1866.
176. Wada, F., Koga, H., Akiba, J., Niizeki, T., Iwamoto, H., Ikezono, Y., et al. (2018). High expression of CD44v9 and xCT in chemoresistant hepatocellular carcinoma: Potential targets by sulfasalazine. *Cancer Science, 109*(9), 2801–2810.
177. Hiyama, E., & Hiyama, K. (2007). Telomere and telomerase in stem cells. *British Journal of Cancer, 96*(7), 1020–1024.
178. Gomez, D. L. M., Armando, R. G., Cerrudo, C. S., Ghiringhelli, P. D., & Gomez, D. E. (2016). Telomerase as a cancer target. Development of new molecules. *Current Topics in Medicinal Chemistry, 16*(22), 2432–2440.
179. Djojosubroto, M. W., Chin, A. C., Go, N., Schaetzlein, S., Manns, M. P., Gryaznov, S., et al. (2005). Telomerase antagonists GRN163 and GRN163L inhibit tumor growth and increase chemosensitivity of human hepatoma. *Hepatology (Baltimore, Md), 42*(5), 1127–1136.
180. Schrank, Z., Khan, N., Osude, C., Singh, S., Miller, R. J., Merrick, C., et al. (2018). Oligonucleotides targeting telomeres and telomerase in cancer. *Molecules, 23*(9), 2267.
181. Wu, X., Zhang, J., Yang, S., Kuang, Z., Tan, G., Yang, G., et al. (2017). Telomerase antagonist imetelstat increases radiation sensitivity in esophageal squamous cell carcinoma. *Oncotarget, 8*(8), 13600–13619.

182. Xu, Y., & Goldkorn, A. (2016). Telomere and telomerase therapeutics in cancer. *Genes (Basel), 7*(6), 22.
183. Jafri, M. A., Ansari, S. A., Alqahtani, M. H., & Shay, J. W. (2016). Roles of telomeres and telomerase in cancer, and advances in telomerase-targeted therapies. *Genome Medicine, 8*(1), 69.
184. Lee, H. S., & Park, S. W. (2016). Systemic chemotherapy in advanced pancreatic cancer. *Gut Liver, 10*(3), 340–347.
185. Cozzo, A. J., Fuller, A. M., & Makowski, L. (2017). Contribution of adipose tissue to development of cancer. *Comprehensive Physiology, 8*(1), 237–282.
186. Domanska, U. M., Timmer-Bosscha, H., Nagengast, W. B., Oude Munnink, T. H., Kruizinga, R. C., Ananias, H. J. K., et al. (2012). CXCR4 inhibition with AMD3100 sensitizes prostate cancer to docetaxel chemotherapy. *Neoplasia, 14*(8), 709–718.
187. Niu, G., & Chen, X. (2010). Vascular endothelial growth factor as an anti-angiogenic target for cancer therapy. *Current Drug Targets, 11*(8), 1000–1017.
188. Williams, J. A. (2018). Using PDX for preclinical cancer drug discovery: The evolving field. *Journal of Clinical Medicine, 7*(3), 41.
189. Bregenzer, M. E., Horst, E. N., Mehta, P., Novak, C. M., Raghavan, S., Snyder, C. S., et al. (2019). Integrated cancer tissue engineering models for precision medicine. *PLoS One, 14*(5), e0216564-e.

Chapter 4
Phytochemicals Plus Checkpoint Inhibitors in GI Cancers

Krishnamurthy Nakuluri and Gowru Srivani

Abstract Malignant cancer is yet one of the overwhelming reasons for mortality and morbidity in the world. Previous literature indicates that a higher intake of fruit and vegetables is correlated with a lower incidence of various types of cancers. The predominant phytochemicals including curcumin, isothiocyanate, genistein, resveratrol, epigallocatechin gallate, and lycopene have been shown to have potential antioxidant, chemopreventive, and anticancer properties. Recent studies demonstrated numerous phytochemicals reported to have antiangiogenic, anticancer, antiproliferative, anti-metastatic, and pro-apoptotic properties. Various animal and cellular studies reveal that these phytochemicals mediate cell death and block cell cycle by numerous mechanisms. The chemopreventive, apoptotic, and anticancer properties of these phytochemicals are results from their use in monotherapy or coalition with immune checkpoint inhibitors or chemotherapeutic drugs. However, despite emerging evidence from various reports, only a few clinical trials are in progress to evaluate the therapeutic effectiveness of these phytochemicals.

Keywords Checkpoint inhibitors · Gastrointestinal cancer · Phytochemicals

Abbreviations

AKT	Protein kinase-B
AMPK	AMP-activated protein kinase
AP	Apple polysaccharides
BCL-2	B-cell lymphoma-2
COX2	Cyclooxygenase-2

K. Nakuluri (✉)
Dept. of Pediatrics, School of Medicine, University of California, San Francisco (UCSF), San Francisco, CA, USA

G. Srivani
Department of Biosciences and Biotechnology, Banasthali University, Banasthali, Rajasthan, India

G. P. Nagaraju (ed.), *Phytochemicals Targeting Tumor Microenvironment in Gastrointestinal Cancers*, https://doi.org/10.1007/978-3-030-48405-7_4

CRC	Colorectal cancer
CTLA4	Cytotoxic T-lymphocyte-associated antigen-4
EBV	Epstein-Barr virus
EGFR	Epithelial growth factor receptor
FAP	Familial adenomatous polyposis
GIT	Gastrointestinal cancer
GST	Glutathione S-transferase
HCC	Hepatocellular cancer
ICIs	Immune checkpoint inhibitors
IL-β	Interleukin-β
MAPK	Mitogen-activated protein kinase
MMR	Mismatch repair
MSI	Microsatellite instability
mTOR	Mammalian target of rapamycin
NF-κB	Nuclear factor kappa-B
NK cells	Natural killer cells
PAK1	P21-activated kinase-1
PD-1	Programmed cell death-1
PEITC	Phenethyl isothiocyanate
PGE2	Prostaglandin E2
PI3K	Phosphatidylinositol 3-kinase
ROS	Reactive oxygen species
TNF-α	Tumor necrosis factor-alpha
VEGF	Vascular endothelial growth factor

1 Introduction

Phytochemicals are the secondary plant compounds that offer helpful effects to human health and disease-preventive properties that serve a variety of functions, including deterring predators or response to tissue damage or infection. Recent studies identified that the dietary phytochemicals exert their beneficial effects on the body through a complex interplay with the host's microbiota [1, 2]. Previous studies reveal that dietary phytochemicals that are abundant in vegetables and fruits exhibit strong in vitro and in vivo chemoprotective properties [3, 4]. The dietary phytochemicals exert beneficial effects on synergy with gut microflora which assists in the reduced incidence of colorectal cancer risk [5]. Phytochemicals consist of antioxidant, antiproliferative, anticancer, and anti-inflammatory properties. The most popular phytochemicals with anticancer properties include curcumin extracted from turmeric root rhizomes, genistein obtained from soybean, lycopene from tomatoes, and resveratrol from grapes. The anticancer properties of various phytochemical compounds are the following: (a) Polyphenols act by inhibiting kinases by reducing hyperproliferation of epithelial cells, detoxifying carcinogen, inhibiting tumor cell proliferation, and inhibiting metastasis. (b) Organosulfur compounds act by inducing apoptosis, blocking cell cycle, free radical scavenging, and suppressing DNA adduct formation. (c) Alkaloids act by suppression of cancer cell metastasis, modification of cancer metabolism, and alteration of carcinogen metabolism. (d) Carotenoids are inducers of differentiation. Isothiocyanates target gastric cancer tumorigenesis at multiple levels by affecting mucosal, muscle cell layer, and *Helicobacter pylori* in the stomach [6].

Previous studies have shown that phytochemicals capable of inducing the immune system reduce oxidative damage to cells, decrease inflammation, block DNA damage, assist in DNA repair, and also help to regulate hormones. Various mechanistic insights of different phytochemical actions include inhibition of cell proliferation, differentiation, oncogene expression and suppression of cell adhesion, invasion, angiogenesis, estrogen regulation, and steroid hormone metabolism. Phytochemicals also inhibit superoxide dismutase, catalase, cyclooxygenase-2, xanthine oxidase, glutathione peroxidase, and nitric oxide synthase. The most important phytochemicals, their food sources, and beneficial effects are listed below (Table 4.1).

Various in vitro and in vivo reports have suggested that numerous phytochemicals decrease the multiplicity or incidence of induced tumors [7]. Besides these findings, numerous in vitro studies reveal that phytochemicals inhibit or downregulate many factors involved in cell signaling significant for cell proliferation

Table 4.1 The list of various categories of phytochemical compounds and their source of origin with their beneficial effects in the treatment of gastrointestinal cancers

Phytochemical (s)	Compound	Plant source	Benefits
Polyphenols	Ellagic acid, resveratrol	Green tea, grapes, berries, citrus fruits, peanuts, whole grains, and apples	Inhibits tumor formation and inflammation
Carotenoids	Lycopene, zeaxanthin, beta-carotene, lutein	Carrots, tomatoes, broccoli, apricots	Stimulate the immune response, antioxidant, and inhibit tumor growth
Terpenes	Perillyl alcohol, limonene, carnosol	Citrus fruit peel, rosemary, cherries	Antioxidant, antiproliferative, anticancer
Inositol	Phytic acid	Oats, rice, rye, soybean, corn, wheat	Antioxidant, antiproliferative, and prevents cell damage
Flavonoids	Anthocyanins, quercetin, catechins	Citrus fruits, onions, soybeans, apples	Stimulate the synthesis of detoxifying enzymes in the body and immunity
Isoflavones	Genistein, daidzein	Soybeans and soy products	Antioxidant, antiproliferative, anticancer
Indoles, glucosinolates	Isothiocyanates, sulforaphane	Broccoli, kale, cabbage, collard greens, cauliflower, and Brussels sprouts	Stimulate detoxification of carcinogens, help lower your cancer risk, and prevent tumor growth

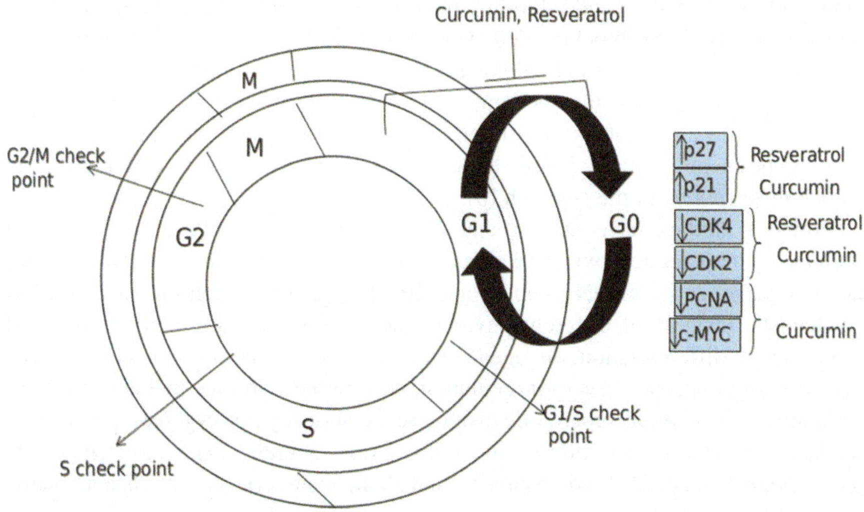

Fig. 4.1 Inhibition of several cell cycle-dependent kinases (CDK) and associated protein expression by cell cycle arrest or blocking with phytochemicals such as resveratrol and curcumin

and survival or progression of cell cycle (Fig. 4.1) and enhance signaling important for apoptosis. Phytochemicals also prevent cancer metastasis and progression but can also cause tumor cell necroptosis, apart from cell death [8, 9]. Common pathways affected by phytochemicals in these reports or studies include the tumor-promoting pathways, MAPK/ERK and PI3K/Akt, and the caspase-dependent apoptotic pathway.

Allium sativum (garlic) has previously shown to consist of several medicinal characteristics such as anticancer, antidiabetic, antimicrobial, anti-hypolipidemic, antihypertensive, and antimicrobial effects. Previous reports indicate that the intake of garlic showed a preventive effect against GI cancers [10]. Other studies reported that the consumption of garlic represses the progression of human colorectal adenoma [11]. The epidemiological reports have evidenced cancer-preventive activity of various GI cancers including colorectal, gastric, and esophageal cancers [12]. Administration of garlic enhances the cell count and activity of NK cells in patients with advanced digestive system cancer [11], since increased NK cells are correlated with antagonistic to tumor outcome, and garlic delays death due to cancer [13].

Curcumin is an alkaloid obtained from the rhizome of turmeric, which is a yellow polyphenol (diferuloylmethane). The beneficial characteristics of curcumin are accompanied by its antioxidant, cytoprotective, and anti-inflammatory features [14–16]. Extensive clinical and experimental reports have shown its curative or therapeutic efficacy to counteract various diseases such as gastrointestinal ulcers, diabetes, liver diseases, CVDs, nephropathy, arthritis, and colorectal cancer [17, 18].

Resveratrol is the most abundant phenolic compound abundant in red grapes, skin of peanuts, grapes, and other fruits, which employ its chemotherapeutic and chemopreventive reactions by regulating several biological actions. Resveratrol is recognized to induce powerful anti-inflammatory and antioxidant properties and block cell proliferation in several cancer cells [19, 20]. The ameliorative effects of resveratrol against cancer metastasis have been shown in various phases of carcinogenesis including initiation, promotion, and advancement of cancer [20]. It was shown that resveratrol also suppresses Wnt target gene expression in the usual colonic mucosa of patients with CRC [21]. Previous reports revealed that regular intake of resveratrol by patients with colorectal cancer decreases cancer cell proliferation [22]. Besides, previous reports also suggest that the administration of resveratrol mediates anticarcinogenic actions in GIT.

Viscum album is a species of mistletoe; these preparations are among the most often recommended complementary and substitute treatment for gastrointestinal cancers. *Rhus verniciflua* is a phytochemical with anti-inflammatory, antioxidant, antimicrobial, and anticancer characteristics [23, 24]. Green tea is a well-known beverage that is consumed worldwide, as it has various biological properties that include anti-inflammatory, antimicrobial, anti-arthritic, antioxidative, antiangiogenesis, and anticancer effects. The previous study reports that catechins are active components accountable for the majority of biological activities of green tea [25, 26]. A double-blind study reports that catechins from green tea were a more efficient therapeutic treatment for premalignant prostate cancer [27].

2 Phytochemicals in Colorectal Cancer

Colorectal cancer (CRC) is a member of the major gastrointestinal cancers which maintained to be a worldwide killer in the past decade. Recent reports show that CRC is the fourth most frequent cancer with an annual prevalence of 1.2 million new cases and over 6,00,000 deaths worldwide [25]. Reports showed that CRC is a good candidate for chemoprevention at the precancerous stage. Celecoxib, a cyclooxygenase-2 inhibitor, is the suggested therapy for blocking familial adenomatous polyposis (FAP) with cardiovascular adverse effects. It is believed that dietary phytochemicals are the candidates for chemoprevention. The diet rich in vegetables, fruits, spices, and grains contains helpful effects on the intestine, especially colon. Mushroom glucans, curcumin, apple polysaccharides, ginsenosides, saponins, resveratrol, and quercetin are widely studied phytochemicals to control their role in CRC prevention.

Curcumin has prominent antioxidant, anti-inflammatory, and anti-carcinogenic characteristics [28–30]. Curcumin inhibits tumor cell growth by suppressing inflammation; various in vitro reports have revealed that curcumin is utilized as a therapeutic treatment for CRC by influencing several targets. Several previous studies have revealed the molecular mechanisms indispensable for the suppression of colon cancer advancement by curcumin. The prominent targets of the signaling pathways controlled by curcumin include EGFR, Wnt/β-catenin AMPK-COX-2 [31], and MAPK. Curcumin also suppresses colon cancer cell growth by decreasing the

ERK/Egr-1/EGFR signaling and decreasing the expression of EGFR. Curcumin was also shown to block the development of chemoresistant colon cancer cells through suppression of EGFR and IGF-1R. Both survivin and IGF-1 could lead to suppression of cell death and extended survival of colon cancer cells by inhibition of the mitochondrion-mediated pathway. Besides, curcumin also reduces the levels of survivin and IGF-1 via stimulating the expression of p53 and downregulation of TNF-α levels, which results in the activation of the apoptotic signal [31]. COX-2 is a crucial player, which plays a significant role in cancer inflammation. Increased levels of COX-2 have been identified in the predominant CRC [24–28], and in a subset of adenomas. Curcumin remarkably suppressed the expression of COX-2 at mRNA and protein levels, but not COX-1. Studies report that the intake of soy is correlated with decreased occurrence of colon cancer. The soy saponin extract inhibited tumor cell growth in a dose- and time-dependent fashion. Besides, soy saponins also repress degradation of IKKBα in PMA-induced cells, whereas COX-2 and PKC expression levels are remarkably decreased.

Administration of apple polysaccharides (AP) mediates cell cycle arrest in a p53-independent way. Galectin-3 is involved in various stages of inflammation which is a prediction marker, and its altered expression is associated with cancer pathogenesis and metastasis of several types of cancers such as CRC [32, 33]. The anti-CRC efficiency of AP is ascribed to activation of death of colonic epithelial cells, and the plausible mechanism for AP to augment cell death and block carcinogenesis could be via binding of galectin-3 to its ligands [34]. Mushrooms have been known to be used as a healthy beneficial food additive for the blockage and treatment of various diseases. Reports have shown that PCNA expression reduced in colorectal adenocarcinomas of mice upon administration of mushroom glucans [35–37]. The soluble α-glucan could repress cancer cell proliferation through direct interplay with the colon cancer cells as well as by stimulation of cell death.

Resveratrol which is predominantly present in grapes inhibits IGF-1-mediated colon cancer cell proliferation by stimulating p53. Since the IGF signaling is intimately associated with obesity-induced CRC pathogenesis, resveratrol showed beneficial effects for inhibiting obesity-induced CRC [38]. Besides, it also suppresses colon cancer cell proliferation and assists cell death by inhibiting the pentose phosphate pathway and FAK, a crucial protein required for cell-ECM communication, which contributes to the anti-colon-carcinogenic effect of resveratrol in obese patients [39]. Moreover, it also employs synergistic anticancer effects on chemoresistant cancer cells by controlling the AMPK signaling. Besides, the phosphorylation level of acetyl-CoA carboxylase (ACC), a downstream target of AMPK, was upregulated by co-therapy with resveratrol as well as etoposide and enhanced phospho-ACC and pAMPK suppression of cell viability and previous reports suggest that compound C, an AMPK inhibitor, suppresses cytotoxicity [40].

3 Phytochemicals in Gastric Cancer

Gastric cancer (GC) is remarkably the seventh major frequent origin of cancer-associated mortality in the globe [40]. It is the third most principal source of cancer-associated mortality in females and males; typically the initial stages of GC are frequently clinically silent, and therefore identified in advanced stages [41–43]. GC is a solid tumor, with a complex interplay between environmental and genetic factors that attribute to the initiation and progression of cancer. The significant risk factors that confer increased risk for GC include smoking, overweight, pickles, or salty foods, and *H. pylori* infection. Exposure to chemical carcinogens or *H. pylori* infection is a source of various events that result in the spread and progression of gastric cancer [44]. Prolonged infection with *H. pylori* highly intensifies the risk of advancing GC, peptic ulcers, and mucosa-related lymphoid tissue cancers [45]. Previous studies reported that oxidative stress is a crucial player for the expansion of *H. pylori*-associated gastric carcinogenesis. Especially, *H. pylori* infection is connected with the penetration of neutrophils and macrophages into the gastric mucosa leading to the generation of various free radicals, such as ROS, superoxide, and nitric oxide that causes injury to epithelial cells and DNA damage to the vicinal cells [45, 46]. ROS-induced stress responses consequently lead to gastric mucosal injury, and ulcers finally develop into GC [47]. Therefore, agents that show strong antioxidant ability via scavenging ROS or improving antioxidant potential may be beneficial to safeguard against GC development. Previous reports revealed that *H. pylori* infection alters the expression levels of EGF, EGFR, COX2, and VEGF in gastric cancer [43, 48, 49]. COX2 expression levels were upregulated via *H. pylori* infection, elevated COX2 expression is associated with GC, and COX2 inhibition is shown to offer a notable decrease in the generation of tumors [43, 50, 51].

Curcumin was shown to consist of a broad range of biological activities including anticarcinogenic, antibacterial, anti-inflammatory, antiproliferative, antioxidant, and chemopreventive actions in multiple cancer cells [52–55]. Various reports have revealed that the antitumor action of curcumin depends on obstructing the NF-κB pathway and suppressing the IKK signaling, which phosphorylates IκB; thus it inhibits NF-κB activation and stimulates cell death [54, 56, 57]. Curcumin also suppresses the proliferation and infiltration of GC cells through the downregulation of cyclin D and suppression of PAK1 activity [58]. Besides, other studies also show that curcumin also suppresses the Akt/mTOR/p70S6 [36] signaling, stimulates ERK1/2, and mediates autophagy. It also upregulates the expression of Beclin-1-p53 which induces ROS and autophagy, consequently leading to colon cancer cell death [59–61].

Various studies have been reported that curcumin suppresses *H. pylori* infection in mice by decreasing its growth, but the process of cell growth and possible therapeutic efficacy of curcumin are yet to be demonstrated by in vitro reports using various GC cell lines [62]. Curcumin guards against chemoresistance in gastric cancer cells by decreasing NF-κB and succeeding NF-κB-induced anti-apoptotic genes in GC cell line [63]. Besides, curcumin reduces EGFR expression and the activity of PAK1, a downstream regulator of EGFR. It is also known to decrease NF-κB activity, controlled through PAK1, which mediates reduced cell proliferation by decreasing both mRNA and protein expression levels of cyclin D1 and inhibits cell cycle progression from G1 to S stage. Accordingly, curcumin also suppresses the cell proliferation and infiltration of GC cells [57].

Allicin (diallyl thiosulfinate) is an organosulfur compound noticed in garlic and has been shown to contain numerous biological activities that include anticarcinogenic, antimicrobial, and antioxidant characteristics [64, 65]. Various studies have demonstrated that it is able to prevent cell proliferation and mediates cell death in cancers including cervix, breast, colon, lung, and gastric cancer [66, 67]. It is reported that allicin also increases the level of mitochondrial cytochrome C and Bax release which plays a significant role in cell death. Besides, it is demonstrated that allicin efficiently inhibits the action of telomerase in a dose- and time-dependent way. Another report revealed that allicin induced cell cycle block at the G2/M stage and also decreased Bcl-2 expression. Allicin is correlated to chemotherapeutic agents such as AZT, and showed improved antitumor activity with lesser toxicity and side effects [66, 68].

Several recent epidemiological reports have shown an opposite relationship between red wine intake and occurrence of CVD. The cardioprotective features of red wine were ascribed to resveratrol and it has anti-inflammatory, antioxidant, and anticarcinogenic characteristics [69, 70]. It was also established that resveratrol has unique antibacterial characteristics [71] by suppressing the growth of several *H. pylori* [71, 72]. The elevated expression levels of IL-8 and enhanced generation of ROS were identified in the gastric mucosa after infection with *H. pylori*. Besides, *H. pylori*-mediated infection elevates the motility which results in morphological alterations in the co-cultured cells. Treatment with resveratrol remarkably diminished IL-8 secretion and ROS production, and distinctly suppressed morphological alterations in cells infected with *H. pylori* [59]. Hence, resveratrol is a novel therapeutic agent to combat gastric cancer.

Resveratrol also suppresses cell cycle advancement of nitrosamine-induced KATO-III and RF-1 cells through stimulating cell cycle blocking at the G0/G1 stage via suppressing kinase C-mediated mechanisms and stimulating cell death in multiple gastric cancer cell lines [73, 74]. Besides, resveratrol also inhibits cell proliferation and stimulates cell death in gastric cancer cells by generating ROS that is prevented by treating cells with SOD or catalase, resulting in suppression of resveratrol-induced cell death [75]. Resveratrol mediates cell death in esophageal cancer cells by decreasing levels of Bcl-2 and stimulating Bax [76, 77]. It can also cause cell death of transplanted cancer cells, possibly by decreased expression of Bcl-2 and increased expression of Bax by resveratrol in implanted primary GC cells in nude mice [78].

Quercetin (3,3′,4′,5,7-pentahydroxyflavone) is a flavonoid abundant in several edible and medicinal plants, and has antimicrobial, antiallergic, antioxidant, anti-inflammatory, chemopreventive, and antitumor activities [79–81]. Quercetin could inhibit the initiation, growth, metastasis, cell death, necrosis, and autophagy in tumor cells [80, 82]. Besides, quercetin also exerts pro-apoptotic gastric effects in cancer cells and inhibits the growth of cancer cell lines in all stages of the cell cycle [83]. It controls the cell cycle via the regulation of several targets such as cyclin B, P^{21}, P^{27}, and topoisomerase [80, 84, 85]. The combined use of quercetin, curcumin, and allicin could improve their beneficial effects by anticipating their synergistic properties.

The sulforaphane is an isothiocyanate, natural chemical compound which is rich in cruciferous vegetables, especially broccoli [47]. The active sulforaphane is eventually absorbed into the circulation, and it performs several functions [47]. Although sulforaphane is not itself an antioxidant, it acts as an antioxidant activity by activating Nrf2-dependent antioxidant enzymes, including glutathione S-transferase (GST), through protecting cells to counteract oxidative stress [88, 89]. Sulforaphane supports the activities of antioxidant enzymes, such as NAD(P)H NQO1 and GST when compared to other effective antioxidants in the gastric mucosa of Nrf2-deficient mice affected with *H. pylori* [47]. With these contributions sulforaphane is a more powerful antioxidant substance that arbitrates its shielding of the gastric mucosa to counteract oxidative stress. Besides, sulforaphane shows chemoprotective properties that are corroborated with its in vitro antibacterial activity [47]. In a previous clinical report of *H. pylori*-infected patients, the group that had broccoli for 8 weeks appears to have reduced levels of markers of *H. pylori* colonization and markers of gastric inflammation in contrast to the placebo group [86]. Mice treated with broccoli rich in sulforaphane showed reduced gastric bacterial colonization and decreased expression of TNF-α and IL-1β in the gastric mucosa, giving rise to the progression of inflammation and impediment of high salt-mediated gastric corpus atrophy [87]. Surprisingly, the antibacterial and anti-inflammatory actions of sulforaphane were not detected in mice with *Nrf2* gene knockout, indicating that sulforaphane acts its effect through *Nrf2* [87].

4 Phytochemicals in Esophageal Cancer

Esophageal cancer is the eighth most prevalent cancer and is the sixth most frequent element of cancer-associated mortality [88]. Owing to the absence of symptoms, patients are hardly aware of their condition until the final stage of cancer [89]. Despite emerging technology in current cancer therapy, including chemotherapy, radiation treatment, and esophagogastric resection, patients with esophageal cancer are not generally cured of cancer [90]. Reports for the previous years evidenced that Americans and Europeans suffering from esophageal adenocarcinoma have comparatively low survival rates, up to 10–15% and 10%, respectively [91]. Furthermore, it is proposed that the esophageal cancers are resistant to systematic therapies and, thus, substitute approaches for the novel therapies of esophageal adenocarcinoma are necessary.

The predominant risk factors for the causation of esophageal cancer include tobacco smoking, drinking of alcoholic beverages [92], lower intake of fruits and vegetables [94], and intake of salt-cured, salt-pickled, and moldy foods [93]. Hence, avoiding cigarette smoking, reducing alcohol consumption, greater fruit and vegetable intake, and consuming foods consisting of nitrosamines and nitrosamine precursors are crucial for impeding esophageal cancer. Besides such lifestyle modifications, recognizing foods or food components that can assist to impede, suppress, and/or delay the manifestation of cancer is crucial [94, 95]. Previous reports have shown the valuable effects of phytochemicals, including curcumin, isothiocyanates, and resveratrol, against esophageal cancer. Despite the fact that basic mechanisms are not yet studied, such phytochemicals are known to counteract disease progression by triggering discrete proteins.

Previous reports revealed that isothiocyanates, especially PEITC, have been shown to protect against esophageal cancer by suppressing tumor prevalence and multiplicity [96]. Various studies demonstrated that PEITC inhibits N-nitrosobenzylmethylamine-mediated esophageal carcinogenesis which shows that PEITC represses the action of cytochrome P450 and also impedes DNA methylation [94, 96, 97]. The antioxidant activity of curcumin attributes to counteract against esophageal tumorigenesis by augmenting the action and/or expression of antioxidant enzymes, such as SOD, and diminishing COX-2. A recent report demonstrated that curcumin reversed the inhibition of SOD-1 and activation of *COX-2* expression ensuing upon usage with bile acid in HET-1A cell line [98]. Besides, curcumin employs its anticancer action with its anti-inflammatory properties by regulating the expression of NF-κB, which is involved in cancer initiation, promotion, and tumor progression. It is shown that NF-κB activity is correlated with increased cell proliferation, invasion, angiogenesis, cancer metastasis, inhibition of cell death, and chemoresistance in several classes of cancers [56, 99, 100]. Numerous studies revealed that curcumin suppresses NF-κB activity in esophageal cancer and also safeguards against bile acid-induced increased NF-κB activity in an esophageal cell line [101–103]. Recent studies reveal that curcumin also induces cell death and blocks the cell cycle by obstructing Notch signaling. Recently it was found that Notch signaling increased in esophageal cancer, which plays a crucial role in apoptosis, cancer cell proliferation, cancer stem cell maintenance, and renewal and which acts as a therapeutic target. Polyphenols especially epigallocatechin gallate are the abundant and active components among tea polyphenols, which show anticarcinogenic effects by inhibition of MAPK, phosphorylation of EGFR, and activator protein-1 and cell transformation [104–106].

Type of cancer	Phytochemical	Targets/mechanisms	Chemopreventive action	Ref
Gastric cancer	Curcumin	Activation of programmed cell death genes *Bcl-2* and *Bcl-xL*	Chemoresistance	[63]
		Downregulation of NF-κB		[63]
		Downregulation of EGFR-PAK1	Inhibition of cell proliferation and invasion	[58]
	Resveratrol	Suppression of cell cycle progression	Inhibition of PKC	[74, 107]
		Suppression of cell death	Decreased cyclin D1 expression	[107]
	Sulforaphane	Induction of Nrf2	Protection against oxidative stress	[108–110]
		Augmentation of GST and glutathione levels	Antibacterial activity	[108, 110, 111]
		A decrease in gastric bacterial colonization	Antibacterial activity	
Colon cancer	Resveratrol	IGF-1, p53	Anti-proliferation	[38]
		PPP-FAK signaling	Apoptosis	[112]
		AMPK	Apoptosis growth inhibition	[40]
Esophageal cancer	Isothiocyanate	Suppression of DNA methylation	Suppression of DNA damage	[97]
		Suppression of cytochrome P450 enzyme activity	Suppression of tumorigenesis	[93, 113]
		Suppression of phosphorylated ERK1/2, c-Jun, and COX-2 expressions	Anti-inflammation	[114]
		Decreased COX-2 expression and PGE_2 production		[115]
		Suppression of EGFR phosphorylation	Growth inhibition	[116]
		Activation of cell cycle arrest	Inhibition of cyclin D1	[34]

5 Immune Checkpoint Inhibitors

The immune system protects from disease, eliminating bacteria and viruses, especially T cells that stimulate the immune response. The surface proteins on T cells activate the immune response and various other proteins that turn it off by activating checkpoints. Various drugs that prevent checkpoint proteins are known as checkpoint inhibitors. These checkpoint inhibitors block the expression of proteins on tumor cells from pushing the stop button, which in turn activates T cells and is able to target the tumor cells. Various cancer cells express elevated levels of checkpoint proteins, which can switch off T-cell signals. Thus, the tumor cells drive a stop button on the immune system, and T lymphocytes cannot recognize and kill cancer cells. The ICIs that prevent/block checkpoint proteins include (a) PD-1: nivolumab (Opdivo) and pembrolizumab (Keytruda), (b) PD-L1: atezolizumab (also known as MPDL3280A), and (c) CTLA-4: ipilimumab (Yervoy).

Checkpoint inhibitors are used for the immunotherapy of various types of cancers, which prevent proteins that stop the immune system from invading the cancer cells. Checkpoint inhibitors are considered as immunotherapy, a kind of monoclonal antibody or targeted therapy. The first approved anticancer checkpoint inhibitor was ipilimumab, which blocks CTLA4. The currently approved immune checkpoint inhibitor target molecules include-CTLA4, PD-1, and PD-L1. The recent compelling data reveals that ICIs are effective in GI cancers and previous reports have shown that ipilimumab and anti-PD-L1 antibody (ICIs) show improved survival rates in cancer patients [117, 118]. Several clinical reports revealed significant efficacy of ICIs in the treatment of various tumors in the end stages of cancer patients. Currently, the objective of immunotherapy is to improve the immune system and assist to counteract various cancers, but it was not a huge success due to immune checkpoints. These checkpoints act as brakes in the immune system, besides also being repressed by tumor cells, and assist the tumor cells in their growth and cancer metastasis. ICIs liberate these breaks and stimulate the activity of the immune system to combat cancers. ICIs act by repressing the immune checkpoint, which increases the binding of APCs and cytotoxic T cells. This is accompanied by proliferation and enhanced activity of T cells against cancers. The major targets of ICIs are PD-1, PD-L1, and CTLA-4. Cancer immunotherapy is an emerging era in the therapy of cancers and recent reports revealed its efficacy in the treatment of end-stage cancers [119].

6 Gastrointestinal (GI) Cancers

The gastrointestinal (GI) cancers account for four million deaths every year, which are responsible for 40% of deaths of all cancer-associated morbidity and mortality. The most prevalent GI cancers include pancreatic cancer, gastric cancer, esophageal cancer, hepatocellular carcinoma (HCC), colorectal cancers (CRC), and gastric that are most fatal cancers. Immunotherapy has been demonstrated to be successful in several gastrointestinal cancers, but attentive individual patient-specific treatment is required to improve the treatment efficacy. The drugs that inhibit or block checkpoints are known as immune checkpoint inhibitors (Table 4.2). The ICIs play a profound role as anticancer agents, especially in GI cancers. The ICIs have been playing an emerging role in the recent few years and various clinical trials have already attempted to test the effectiveness in several malignant cancers. Recent data suggest that ICIs are shown to be emerging therapeutic drug candidates for treating GI malignancies and the most effective option. Ipilimumab, which is an ICI, has

Table 4.2 The clinical trials undergone by using immune checkpoint inhibitors for the therapeutic treatment of various gastrointestinal cancers

Type of cancer	Agent	Mechanism of action	Clinical trial NCT. No.	Clinical status
Hepatocellular cancer	Pembrolizumab (MK-3475)	Humanized mAb against PD-1 and PD-2 that encounters T cells Downregulates T-cell receptor signaling	NCT02702401 NCT02702414	III and II
	Nivolumab Sorafenib	Inhibits PD-1 Targeted the CheckMate 459: Checkpoint pathway	NCT02576559	III
	Combinational therapy of galunisertib and nivolumab	Downregulates the SMAD2, targets the PD1 that stimulates the T cells	NCT02423343	I and II
Colorectal cancer	Pembrolizumab (MK-3475) dMMR/MSI-H	Act as immune checkpoint inhibitor, targets the CTLA-4 (cytotoxic T-lymphocyte antigen-4)	NCT02563002 NCT02460198	II and III
Esophageal cancer	Pembrolizumab (third-line therapy)	PD-1 inhibitor	NCT02559687	II
	Pembrolizumab vs. docetaxel, paclitaxel/ irinotecan	Act as immune checkpoint inhibitors (CTLA-4, PD-1)	NCT02564263	III
	Nivolumab	PD-1 inhibitor	NCT02569242	III
Stomach cancer	Pembrolizumab combination with cisplatin, 5-FU placebo, 5-FU	Act as immune checkpoint inhibitors (CTLA-4 and CD-152, PD-1)	NCT02494583	III
	Nivolumab (ONO-4538)	Immune checkpoint inhibitor, acts against the EGFR and blocks binding of the TGF-α and EGF to EGFR	NCT02267343	III
	Nivolumab Ipilimumab Oxaliplatin Fluoropyrimidine	PD-L1 inhibitor	NCT02872116	III

shown to improve survival rate upon treatment in end-stage cancer. Till now, immunotherapy is shown to magnify the immune system, thereby helping to counteract against cancers. Cancer cells can get deserted from the immune system by suppressing tumor-explicit T cells. The major cytotoxic T-cell immune checkpoint receptors result in T-cell downregulation and functional suppression: PD-1 and CTLA-4. ICIs act by repressing the immune checkpoint, which improves the attachment of antigen-presenting cells and cytotoxic T cells. ICIs act as brakes on the immune surveillance and intensify the activity of the immune system. Some of the targets of ICIs include PD-1, PD-L1, and CTLA-4.

Various types of cancers including gastrointestinal (GI) cancers express PD-L1 on their tumor cells, which are stimulated by PD-1 receptors on T cells. The association of PD-1 with PD-L1 assists cancer cell immune escape by downregulating T-cell activation [120, 121]. ICIs have been intended to block PD-1- or CTLA-4-conciliated inhibitory signals and improve antitumor immunity [120]. Immunotherapy with ICIs exhibited remarkable clinical benefits in the treatment of some solid and hematologic malignancies [122]. The ICIs which suppress PD-1/PD-L1 interplay have been a principal alternative for treating GI cancer patients. Both PD-L1 and PD-L2 receptors are present on tumor cells which bind to PD-1 and impair the T-cell stimulation consequently suppressing the immune system. ICIs which act on both PD-L1 and PD-L2 repress this interaction and release brakes of the immune system promoting stimulation and proliferation of cytotoxic T cells and assisting in eliminating cancer cells. Both PD-L1 and PD-L2 are expressed on various cells such as multiple myeloma, breast, colon, bladder, renal cell, and lung cancer. A recent report reveals that 43.9% of esophageal squamous cell carcinoma patients had PD-L1 or PD-L2 expression and in gastric carcinoma patients PD-L1 expression was 42.2% [123, 124]. Previous reports have shown compelling evidence with respect to the expression levels of both PD-L1 and PD-L2 in esophageal and gastric cancers [119].

7 Colorectal Cancer

CRC is the most prevalent, lethal cancer accounting for 8% of deaths, and the third most common cancer in males and the second in females in the world [125, 126]. Besides chemotherapy as well as surgical resection, recent therapeutic treatment options include VEGF- and EGFR-targeted agents that have been used for treating CRC, but these targeted treatments have enhanced metastatic patient survival [127]. CRC is categorized into three types: (a) sporadic CRC, (b) familial CRC, and (c) hereditary CRC. 70–75% of sporadic CRC is connected with lifestyle such as smoking, alcohol, diet, and obesity. Familial CRC and hereditary CRC are correlated with germline mutation which accounts for 20% and 5%, respectively [128]. Previous reports reveal that ICIs are beneficial for only a small group of patients with colorectal cancer.

A preliminary clinical trial revealed the effect of pembrolizumab on patients with metastatic CRC that manifested greater response rates in mismatch repair (MMR)-impaired tumors, while MMR-efficient cancers exhibited no therapeutic effect at all [119]. The MMR proteins act as safeguards during cell replication, while they rectify any type of error due to deletion and insertion by DNA polymerase and reduce the frequency of mutation during cell replication. Mutations in MMR proteins cause defective DNA replication which leads to microsatellite instability (MSI). Previous clinical trial data also reveal that ICIs in patients with CRC with MSI are promising [119]. The germline mutations in MMR genes such as MSH6, MLH1, and MSH2 cause an autosomal dominant disorder, Lynch syndrome [129]. These germline mutations significantly play a significant role in the manifestation of CRC in Lynch syndrome patients with MSI [130]. The higher number of mutations is associated with the greater number of neoantigen and stimulates an immune response, which leads to increased $CD4^+$ T cells, lytic enzymes, $CD8^+$ T cells, and upregulation of costimulatory molecules for APCs in the tumor microenvironment [131–135]. As a result, with the more immunogenic type of CRC and greater density of tumor-infiltrating lymphocytes, the frequency for the progress of ICIs in CRC therapy is larger. Recent numerous clinical trials revealed the productive effect of pembrolizumab in CRC patients (Table 4.2) [136–138].

8 Gastric Cancer

The Cancer Genome Atlas has categorized gastric cancer by molecular subtype: (a) microsatellite unstable, (b) Epstein-Barr virus (EBV) positive, (c) genetically stable, and (d) chromosomal instability tumors [139]. In this subtype, EBV-linked tumors are correlated with increased levels of PD-L1/2 expression, and suitable for therapeutic directing PD-1 and its ligands [139]. Besides, microsatellite-unstable cancers possess increased mutations, which are accompanied by a greater response to ICIs in other tumors [140]. With these possible suggestions for the use of ICIs in gastric cancer, several clinical trials are already established. The first results of the phase 1b KEYNOTE-012 clinical report assess the effectiveness and safety of ICI (pembrolizumab) in gastric cancer patients. Pembrolizumab was evaluated along with 5-fluorouracil and cisplatin (FP) for the therapy of end-stage gastric cancer [141]. As per recent initial safety data from KEYNOTE-059, pembrolizumab was used for FP patients with end-stage gastric cancer. The KEYNOTE-061 trial is performed to determine pembrolizumab versus paclitaxel after the failure of selected platinum and fluoropyrimidine therapy for patients with advanced gastric cancer and KEYNOTE-062 study is to assess pembrolizumab in combination with 5-fluorouracil and cisplatin as a selected treatment in end-stage gastric cancer patients. In CheckMate-032 trial nivolumab along with ipilimumab was evaluated in patients with advanced-stage gastric cancer (Table 4.2).

9 Esophageal Cancer

Few recent data reveal that ICIs also act as blockades in esophageal cancer, which has been shown in the results of phase KEYNOTE-028. KEYNOTE-028 trial assessed pembrolizumab in patients with PD-L1-positive final-stage esophageal cancer. Recent clinical reports of nivolumab as a relief therapy and adjuvant treatment are also under development for advanced esophageal carcinoma [122].

10 Hepatocellular Cancer

Hepatocellular cancer is a dangerous tumor, most often connected with liver disease which causes it more lethal and crucial to treat. Previous reports have shown that treatment with tremelimumab has antitumor activity in advanced hepatocellular carcinoma (HCC) patients, with a 17% response rate and stable disease of 76% [142]. Besides, nivolumab was also used to treat cancer patients with sorafenib-refractory or sorafenib-intolerant HCC in any case in which hepatitis status has shown 23% response rate.

11 Conclusion

Phytochemicals have always been a predominant source for the identification of novel therapeutics for various human diseases. Hence, these could be a good unique drug candidate for the improvement of anticancer therapy. Regular consumption of fruits and vegetables might counteract cancer. Among the various phytochemicals that have been reported for anticancer, only a few clinical trials were in progress to assess the therapeutic efficacy of these phytochemicals. The prominent phytochemicals including *Allium sativum*, camptothecin, resveratrol, *Rhus verniciflua*, curcumin, green tea, *Panax ginseng*, and *Viscum album* had the adequate results of clinical evidence for reinforcing their anticancer effects. It is believed that herbal preparations consisting of several phytochemicals exert enhanced effectiveness than taking the same phytochemical independently. The mix of the anticancer phytochemicals exhibits greater effectiveness and produces more active therapeutic agents for cancer. The consumption of isothiocyanates is epidemiologically correlated with reduced risk of gastric cancers. The chemopreventive actions of several phytochemicals have been well demonstrated including curcumin, mushroom glucans, ginsenosides, soy saponins, resveratrol, and quercetin on various cancers and the probable mechanisms have been well studied. Therefore, supportive therapeutics are used besides the present chemotherapy drugs such as phytochemicals to counteract several types of cancer. These phytochemicals have shown beneficial and synergistic effects as these are absolutely safe and generally target several cell signaling pathways.

The ICIs are also leading novel emerging immunotherapy for treating advanced stages of cancer. Immunotherapy was recently demonstrated to be more powerful in several GI cancers; nevertheless, cautious patient selection is necessary to enhance treatment efficacy. Numerous clinical trials have been enlivened by recent success in some other types of cancers, and have also attempted to assess the potency of ICIs in

GI cancers. Recent reports proposed that it might be impressive in a few patients with GI cancers. The immune-repressive mechanisms and microenvironment neighboring GI cancers are still ambiguous correlated with other cancers. To enhance the efficacy of ICIs in GI cancers, we should study a deeper consideration of the tumor-immune system and microenvironment. Besides, it is necessary to establish appropriate biomarkers that anticipate the effectiveness of this type of immunotherapy. Nevertheless, further studies are required to acknowledge the role of PD-L1 expression and these plausible biomarkers in determining the response to ICIs in GI cancers. Current approaches for treating cancers are varying among multimodality combination therapy strategies. Initially, traditional chemotherapy can be used along with ICIs to treat patients with GI cancers. The current chemotherapeutic agents impair tumor cells and generally deliver RNA, intracellular peptides, and proteins which may turn into effective tumor-linked antigens to magnify the potency of ICIs. Based on the immune-modulating effects of VEGF to suppress the T-cell infiltration and dendritic cells into tumors, ICIs are perhaps used along with VEGF inhibitors.

References

1. Eid, H., Wright, M., Anil Kumar, N., Qawasmeh, A., Hassan, S., Mocan, A., Nabavi, S., Rastrelli, L., Atanasov, A., & Haddad, P. (2017). Significance of microbiota in obesity and metabolic diseases and the modulatory potential by medicinal plant and food ingredients. *Frontiers in Pharmacology, 8*, 387. https://doi.org/10.3389/fphar.2017.00387.
2. Espín, J. C., González-Sarrías, A., & Tomás-Barberán, F. A. (2017). The gut microbiota: A key factor in the therapeutic effects of (poly)phenols. *Biochemical Pharmacology, 139*, 82–93.
3. Rajamanickam, S., & Agarwal, R. (2008). Natural products and colon cancer: Current status and future prospects. *Drug Development Research, 69*(7), 460–471.
4. Tammariello, A. E., & Milner, J. A. (2010). Mouse models for unraveling the importance of diet in colon cancer prevention. *The Journal of Nutritional Biochemistry, 21*(2), 77–88.
5. Ricciardiello, L., Bazzoli, F., & Fogliano, V. (2011). Phytochemicals and colorectal cancer prevention—Myth or reality? *Nature Reviews Gastroenterology & Hepatology, 8*(10), 592–596.
6. Øverby, A., Zhao, C.-M., & Chen, D. (2014). Plant phytochemicals: Potential anticancer agents against gastric cancer. *Current Opinion in Pharmacology, 19*, 6–10.
7. Maru, G. B., Hudlikar, R. R., Kumar, G., Gandhi, K., & Mahimkar, M. B. (2016). Understanding the molecular mechanisms of cancer prevention by dietary phytochemicals: From experimental models to clinical trials. *World Journal of Biological Chemistry, 7*(1), 88.
8. Khorsandi, L., Orazizadeh, M., Niazvand, F., Abbaspour, M., Mansouri, E., & Khodadadi, A. (2017). Quercetin induces apoptosis and necroptosis in MCF-7 breast cancer cells. *Bratislavske lekarske listy, 118*(2), 123–128.
9. Lin, W., & Tongyi, S. (2014). Role of Bax/Bcl-2 family members in green tea polyphenol induced necroptosis of p53-deficient Hep3B cells. *Tumor Biology, 35*(8), 8065–8075.
10. Fleischauer, A. T., Poole, C., & Arab, L. (2000). Garlic consumption and cancer prevention: Meta-analyses of colorectal and stomach cancers. *The American Journal of Clinical Nutrition, 72*(4), 1047–1052.
11. Tanaka, S., Haruma, K., Yoshihara, M., Kajiyama, G., Kira, K., Amagase, H., & Chayama, K. (2006). Aged garlic extract has potential suppressive effect on colorectal adenomas in humans. *The Journal of Nutrition, 136*(3), 821S–826S.

12. Nicastro, H. L., Ross, S. A., & Milner, J. A. (2015). Garlic and onions: Their cancer prevention properties. *Cancer Prevention Research (Philadelphia, Pa.), 8*(3), 181–189.
13. Coca, S., Perez-Piqueras, J., Martinez, D., Colmenarejo, A., Saez, M. A., Vallejo, C., Martos, J. A., & Moreno, M. (1997). The prognostic significance of intratumoral natural killer cells in patients with colorectal carcinoma. *Cancer: Interdisciplinary International Journal of the American Cancer Society, 79*(12), 2320–2328.
14. Alinejad, B., Ghorbani, A., & Sadeghnia, H. R. (2013). Effects of combinations of curcumin, linalool, rutin, safranal, and thymoquinone on glucose/serum deprivation-induced cell death. *Avicenna Journal of Phytomedicine, 3*(4), 321–328.
15. Yamazaki, E., Mizuoka, K., Masuda, G., & Nakae, T. (1988). Study of bacterial infection in the antimicrobial susceptibility against various clinical isolates. II. Analysis based on the source of clinical specimens. *Kansenshogaku zasshi The Journal of the Japanese Association for Infectious Diseases, 62*(9), 772.
16. Noorafshan, A., & Ashkani-Esfahani, S. (2013). A review of therapeutic effects of curcumin. *Current Pharmaceutical Design, 19*(11), 2032–2046.
17. Temraz, S., Mukherji, D., & Shamseddine, A. (2013). Potential targets for colorectal cancer prevention. *International Journal of Molecular Sciences, 14*(9), 17279–17303.
18. Hosseini, A., & Ghorbani, A. (2015). Cancer therapy with phytochemicals: Evidence from clinical studies. *Avicenna Journal of Phytomedicine, 5*(2), 84.
19. Athar, M., Back, J. H., Tang, X., Kim, K. H., Kopelovich, L., Bickers, D. R., & Kim, A. L. (2007). Resveratrol: A review of preclinical studies for human cancer prevention. *Toxicology and Applied Pharmacology, 224*(3), 274–283.
20. Smoliga, J. M., Baur, J. A., & Hausenblas, H. A. (2011). Resveratrol and health – a comprehensive review of human clinical trials. *Molecular Nutrition & Food Research, 55* (8), 1129–1141.
21. Nguyen, A. V., Martinez, M., Stamos, M. J., Moyer, M. P., Planutis, K., Hope, C., & Holcombe, R. F. (2009). Results of a phase I pilot clinical trial examining the effect of plant-derived resveratrol and grape powder on Wnt pathway target gene expression in colonic mucosa and colon cancer. *Cancer Management and Research, 1*, 25–37.
22. Patel, K. R., Brown, V. A., Jones, D. J. L., Britton, R. G., Hemingway, D., Miller, A. S., West, K. P., Booth, T. D., Perloff, M., Crowell, J. A., et al. (2010). Clinical pharmacology of resveratrol and its metabolites in colorectal cancer patients. *Cancer Research, 70*(19), 7392–7399.
23. Kim, J. H., Park, C. Y., & Lee, S. J. (2006). Effects of sun ginseng on subjective quality of life in cancer patients: A double-blind, placebo-controlled pilot trial. *Journal of Clinical Pharmacy and Therapeutics, 31*(4), 331–334.
24. Lee, S., Jung, H., Eo, W., Lee, S., Kim, S., & Shim, B. (2010). Rhus verniciflua Stokes extract as a potential option for treatment of metastatic renal cell carcinoma: Report of two cases. *Annals of Oncology, 21*(6), 1383–1385.
25. Bettuzzi, S., Brausi, M., Rizzi, F., Castagnetti, G., Peracchia, G., & Corti, A. (2006). Chemoprevention of human prostate cancer by oral administration of green tea catechins in volunteers with high-grade prostate intraepithelial neoplasia: A preliminary report from a one-year proof-of-principle study. *Cancer Research, 66*(2), 1234–1240.
26. Chacko, S. M., Thambi, P. T., Kuttan, R., & Nishigaki, I. (2010). Beneficial effects of green tea: A literature review. *Chinese Medicine, 5*, 13–13.
27. Jemal, A., Bray, F., Center, M. M., Ferlay, J., Ward, E., & Forman, D. (2011). Global cancer statistics. *CA: a Cancer Journal for Clinicians, 61*(2), 69–90.
28. Esatbeyoglu, T., Huebbe, P., Ernst, I. M. A., Chin, D., Wagner, A. E., & Rimbach, G. (2012). Curcumin—from molecule to biological function. *Angewandte Chemie International Edition, 51*(22), 5308–5332.
29. Goel, A., & Aggarwal, B. B. (2010). Curcumin, the golden spice from Indian saffron, is a chemosensitizer and radiosensitizer for tumors and chemoprotector and radioprotector for normal organs. *Nutrition and Cancer, 62*(7), 919–930.

30. Lee, K. W., Bode, A. M., & Dong, Z. (2011). Molecular targets of phytochemicals for cancer prevention. *Nature Reviews Cancer, 11*(3), 211–218.
31. Lee, Y. K., Park, S. Y., Kim, Y. M., & Park, O. J. (2009). Regulatory effect of the AMPK–COX-2 signaling pathway in curcumin-induced apoptosis in HT-29 colon cancer cells. *Annals of the New York Academy of Sciences, 1171*(1), 489–494.
32. Tsuboi, K., Shimura, T., Masuda, N., Ide, M., Tsutsumi, S., Yamaguchi, S., Asao, T., & Kuwano, H. (2007). Galectin-3 expression in colorectal cancer: Relation to invasion and metastasis. *Anticancer Research, 27*(4B), 2289–2296.
33. Endo, K., Kohnoe, S., Tsujita, E., Watanabe, A., Nakashima, H., Baba, H., & Maehara, Y. (2005). Galectin-3 expression is a potent prognostic marker in colorectal cancer. *Anticancer Research, 25*(4), 3117–3121.
34. Li, Y., Liu, L., Niu, Y., Feng, J., Sun, Y., Kong, X., Chen, Y., Chen, X., Gan, H., & Cao, S. (2012). Modified apple polysaccharide prevents against tumorigenesis in a mouse model of colitis-associated colon cancer: Role of galectin-3 and apoptosis in cancer prevention. *European Journal of Nutrition, 51*(1), 107–117.
35. Lavi, I., Friesem, D., Geresh, S., Hadar, Y., & Schwartz, B. (2006). An aqueous polysaccharide extract from the edible mushroom Pleurotus ostreatus induces anti-proliferative and pro-apoptotic effects on HT-29 colon cancer cells. *Cancer Letters, 244*(1), 61–70.
36. Xie, J., Wang, C., Wicks, S., Yin, J., Kong, J., Li, J., Li, Y., & Yuan, C. (2006). Ganoderma lucidum extract inhibits proliferation of SW 480 human colorectal cancer cells. *Experimental Oncology*.
37. Lavi, I., Nimri, L., Levinson, D., Peri, I., Hadar, Y., & Schwartz, B. (2012). Glucans from the edible mushroom Pleurotus pulmonarius inhibit colitis-associated colon carcinogenesis in mice. *Journal of Gastroenterology, 47*(5), 504–518.
38. LeRoith, D., & Roberts, C. T. (2003). The insulin-like growth factor system and cancer. *Cancer Letters, 195*(2), 127–137.
39. Vanamala, J., Radhakrishnan, S., Reddivari, L., Bhat, V. B., & Ptitsyn, A. (2011). Resveratrol suppresses human colon cancer cell proliferation and induces apoptosis via targeting the pentose phosphate and the talin-FAK signaling pathways - a proteomic approach. *Proteome Science, 9*(1), 49–49.
40. Hwang, J.-T., Kwak, D. W., Lin, S. K., Kim, H. M., Kim, Y. M., & Park, O. J. (2007). Resveratrol induces apoptosis in chemoresistant cancer cells via modulation of AMPK signaling pathway. *Annals of the New York Academy of Sciences, 1095*(1), 441–448.
41. Wadhwa, R., Song, S., Lee, J.-S., Yao, Y., Wei, Q., & Ajani, J. A. (2013). Gastric cancer - molecular and clinical dimensions. *Nature Reviews. Clinical Oncology, 10*(11), 643–655.
42. McLean, M. H., & El-Omar, E. M. (2014). Genetics of gastric cancer. *Nature Reviews Gastroenterology & Hepatology, 11*(11), 664–674.
43. Romano, M., Ricci, V., & Zarrilli, R. (2006). Mechanisms of disease: Helicobacter pylori-related gastric carcinogenesis—Implications for chemoprevention. *Nature Clinical Practice Gastroenterology & Hepatology, 3*(11), 622–632.
44. Williams, P. (1999). Review article: The pharmacology of rabeprazole. *Alimentary Pharmacology & Therapeutics, 13*(s3), 3–10.
45. Wroblewski, L. E., Peek, R. M., Jr., & Wilson, K. T. (2010). Helicobacter pylori and gastric cancer: Factors that modulate disease risk. *Clinical Microbiology Reviews, 23*(4), 713–739.
46. S-Y, L. E. E., SHIN, Y. W., & K-B, H. A. H. M. (2008). Phytoceuticals: Mighty but ignored weapons against helicobacter pylori infection. *Journal of Digestive Diseases, 9*(3), 129–139.
47. Yanaka, A. (2011). Sulforaphane enhances protection and repair of gastric mucosa against oxidative stress in vitro, and demonstrates anti-inflammatory effects on Helicobacter pylori-infected gastric mucosae in mice and human subjects. *Current Pharmaceutical Design, 17* (16), 1532–1540.
48. Yan, F., Cao, H., Chaturvedi, R., Krishna, U., Hobbs, S. S., Dempsey, P. J., Peek, R. M., Jr., Cover, T. L., Washington, M. K., Wilson, K. T., et al. (2009). Epidermal growth factor

receptor activation protects gastric epithelial cells from Helicobacter pylori-induced apoptosis. *Gastroenterology, 136*(4), 1297–e1293.
49. Boughan, P. K., Argent, R. H., Body-Malapel, M., Park, J.-H., Ewings, K. E., Bowie, A. G., Ong, S. J., Cook, S. J., Sorensen, O. E., & Manzo, B. A. (2006). Nucleotide-binding oligomerization domain-1 and epidermal growth factor receptor critical regulators of β-defensins during helicobacter pylori infection. *Journal of Biological Chemistry, 281*(17), 11637–11648.
50. Wong, B. C. Y., & Zhang, L. (2012). Ma J-l, Pan K-f, Li J-y, Shen L, Liu W-d, Feng G-s, Zhang X-d, Li J *et al*: Effects of selective COX-2 inhibitor and <em>Helicobacter pylori</em> eradication on precancerous gastric lesions. *Gut, 61*(6), 812–818.
51. Wu, C.-Y., Wang, C.-J., Tseng, C.-C., Chen, H.-P., Wu, M.-S., Lin, J.-T., Inoue, H., & Chen, G.-H. (2005). Helicobacter pylori promote gastric cancer cells invasion through a NF-kappaB and COX-2-mediated pathway. *World Journal of Gastroenterology, 11*(21), 3197–3203.
52. Koosirirat, C., Linpisarn, S., Changsom, D., Chawansuntati, K., & Wipasa, J. (2010). Investigation of the anti-inflammatory effect of Curcuma longa in Helicobacter pylori-infected patients. *International Immunopharmacology, 10*(7), 815–818.
53. Y-m, P., Zheng, J.-b., & Y-b, Z. (2013). Li J: Characterization of a novel curcumin analog P1 as potent inhibitor of the NF-κB signaling pathway with distinct mechanisms. *Acta Pharmacologica Sinica, 34*(7), 939–950.
54. Shehzad, A., Wahid, F., & Lee, Y. S. (2010). Curcumin in cancer chemoprevention: Molecular targets, pharmacokinetics, bioavailability, and clinical trials. *Archiv der Pharmazie, 343*(9), 489–499.
55. Duvoix, A., Blasius, R., Delhalle, S., Schnekenburger, M., Morceau, F., Henry, E., Dicato, M., & Diederich, M. (2005). Chemopreventive and therapeutic effects of curcumin. *Cancer Letters, 223*(2), 181–190.
56. Kunnumakkara, A. B., Guha, S., Krishnan, S., Diagaradjane, P., Gelovani, J., & Aggarwal, B. B. (2007). Curcumin potentiates antitumor activity of gemcitabine in an orthotopic model of pancreatic cancer through suppression of proliferation, angiogenesis, and inhibition of nuclear factor-κB-regulated gene products. *Cancer Research, 67*(8), 3853–3861.
57. Foryst-Ludwig, A., Neumann, M., Schneider-Brachert, W., & Naumann, M. (2004). Curcumin blocks NF-κB and the motogenic response in helicobacter pylori-infected epithelial cells. *Biochemical and Biophysical Research Communications, 316*(4), 1065–1072.
58. Cai, X.-Z., Wang, J., Xiao-Dong, L., Wang, G.-L., Liu, F.-N., Cheng, M.-S., & Li, F. (2009). Curcumin suppresses proliferation and invasion in human gastric cancer cells by downregulation of PAK1 activity and cyclin D1 expression. *Cancer Biology & Therapy, 8*(14), 1360–1368.
59. Zaidi, S. F. H., Ahmed, K., Yamamoto, T., Kondo, T., Usmanghani, K., Kadowaki, M., & Sugiyama, T. (2009). Effect of resveratrol on Helicobacter pylori-induced interleukin-8 secretion, reactive oxygen species generation and morphological changes in human gastric epithelial cells. *Biological and Pharmaceutical Bulletin, 32*(11), 1931–1935.
60. Lee, Y. J., Kim, N.-Y., Suh, Y.-A., & Lee, C. (2011). Involvement of ROS in curcumin-induced autophagic cell death. *Korean J Physiology Pharmacology, 15*(1), 1–7.
61. Singletary, K., & Milner, J. (2008). Diet, autophagy, and cancer: A review. *Cancer Epidemiology and Prevention Biomarkers, 17*(7), 1596–1610.
62. De, R., Kundu, P., Swarnakar, S., Ramamurthy, T., Chowdhury, A., Nair, G. B., & Mukhopadhyay, A. K. (2009). Antimicrobial activity of curcumin against Helicobacter pylori isolates from India and during infections in mice. *Antimicrobial Agents and Chemotherapy, 53*(4), 1592–1597.
63. Yu, L.-L., Wu, J.-G., Dai, N., Yu, H.-G., & Si, J.-M. (2011). Curcumin reverses chemoresistance of human gastric cancer cells by downregulating the NF-κB transcription factor. *Oncology Reports, 26*(5), 1197–1203.

64. Cha, J. H., Choi, Y. J., Cha, S. H., Choi, C. H., & Cho, W. H. (2012). Allicin inhibits cell growth and induces apoptosis in U87MG human glioblastoma cells through an ERK-dependent pathway. *Oncology Reports, 28*(1), 41–48.
65. Z-M, Z., Zhong, N., Gao, H.-Q., Zhang, S.-Z., Yuan, W., Hua, X., Xing, M., Hou, H.-S., Lin, X.-Y., & Qing, S. (2006). Inducing apoptosis and upregulation of Bax and Fas ligand expression by allicin in hepatocellular carcinoma in Balb/c nude mice. *Chinese Medical Journal, 119*(5), 422–426.
66. Tao, M., Gao, L., Pan, J., & Wang, X. (2013). Study on the inhibitory effect of allicin on human gastric cancer cell line SGC-7901 and its mechanism. *African Journal of Traditional, Complementary, and Alternative Medicines, 11*(1), 176–179.
67. Park, S.-Y., Cho, S.-J., Kwon, H.-C., Lee, K.-R., Rhee, D.-K., & Pyo, S. (2005). Caspase-independent cell death by allicin in human epithelial carcinoma cells: Involvement of PKA. *Cancer Letters, 224*(1), 123–132.
68. Sun, L., & Wang, X. (2003). Effects of allicin on both telomerase activity and apoptosis in gastric cancer SGC-7901 cells. *World Journal of Gastroenterology, 9*(9), 1930–1934.
69. Catalgol, B., Batirel, S., Taga, Y., & Ozer, N. K. (2012). Resveratrol: French paradox revisited. *Frontiers in Pharmacology, 3*, 141–141.
70. Hung, L.-M., Chen, J.-K., Huang, S.-S., Lee, R.-S., & Su, M.-J. (2000). Cardioprotective effect of resveratrol, a natural antioxidant derived from grapes. *Cardiovascular Research, 47* (3), 549–555.
71. Mahady, G. B., Pendland, S. L., & Chadwick, L. R. (2003). Resveratrol and red wine extracts inhibit the growth of CagA+ strains of helicobacter pylori in vitro. *The American Journal of Gastroenterology, 98*(6), 1440–1441.
72. Mahady, G. B., & Pendland, S. L. (2000). Resveratrol inhibits the growth of Helicobacter pylori in vitro. *The American Journal of Gastroenterology, 95*(7), 1849.
73. Atten, M. J., Attar, B. M., Milson, T., & Holian, O. (2001). Resveratrol-induced inactivation of human gastric adenocarcinoma cells through a protein kinase C-mediated mechanism 11 Abbreviations: COX-1, cyclooxygenase-1; COX-2, cyclooxygenase-2; PKC, protein kinase C; ERK1/ERK2, mitogen-activated protein kinases; NA, nitrosamine(s); TCA, trichloroacetic acid; and PMSF, phenylmethylsulfonyl fluoride. *Biochemical Pharmacology, 62*(10), 1123–1132.
74. Atten, M. J., Godoy-Romero, E., Attar, B. M., Milson, T., Zopel, M., & Holian, O. (2005). Resveratrol regulates cellular PKC α and δ to inhibit growth and induce apoptosis in gastric cancer cells. *Investigational New Drugs, 23*(2), 111–119.
75. Aquilano, K., Baldelli, S., & Rotilio, G. (2009). Ciriolo MR: Trans-resveratrol inhibits H2O2-induced adenocarcinoma gastric cells proliferation via inactivation of MEK1/2-ERK1/2-c-Jun signalling axis. *Biochemical Pharmacology, 77*(3), 337–347.
76. Wang, L., Liu, L., Shi, Y., Cao, H., Chaturvedi, R., Calcutt, M. W., Hu, T., Ren, X., Wilson, K. T., Polk, D. B., et al. (2012). Berberine induces caspase-independent cell death in colon tumor cells through activation of apoptosis-inducing factor. *PLoS One, 7*(5), e36418–e36418.
77. Zhou, H.-B., Yan, Y., Sun, Y.-N., & Zhu, J.-R. (2003). Resveratrol induces apoptosis in human esophageal carcinoma cells. *World Journal of Gastroenterology, 9*(3), 408–411.
78. Zhou, H.-B., Chen, J.-J., Wang, W.-X., Cai, J.-T., & Du, Q. (2005). Anticancer activity of resveratrol on implanted human primary gastric carcinoma cells in nude mice. *World Journal of Gastroenterology, 11*(2), 280–284.
79. Chen, C., Zhou, J., & Ji, C. (2010). Quercetin: A potential drug to reverse multidrug resistance. *Life Sciences, 87*(11), 333–338.
80. Dajas, F. (2012). Life or death: Neuroprotective and anticancer effects of quercetin. *Journal of Ethnopharmacology, 143*(2), 383–396.
81. Zhang, L., Kong, Y., Wu, D., Zhang, H., Wu, J., Chen, J., Ding, J., Hu, L., Jiang, H., & Shen, X. (2008). Three flavonoids targeting the beta-hydroxyacyl-acyl carrier protein dehydratase from Helicobacter pylori: Crystal structure characterization with enzymatic inhibition assay. *Protein Science, 17*(11), 1971–1978.

82. Bi, Y., Shen, C., Li, C., Liu, Y., Gao, D., Shi, C., Peng, F., Liu, Z., Zhao, B., & Zheng, Z. (2016). Inhibition of autophagy induced by quercetin at a late stage enhances cytotoxic effects on glioma cells. *Tumor Biology, 37*(3), 3549–3560.
83. Borska, S., Chmielewska, M., Wysocka, T., Drag-Zalesinska, M., Zabel, M., & Dziegiel, P. (2012). In vitro effect of quercetin on human gastric carcinoma: Targeting cancer cells death and MDR. *Food and Chemical Toxicology, 50*(9), 3375–3383.
84. Gibellini, L., Pinti, M., Nasi, M., Montagna, J. P., De Biasi, S., Roat, E., Bertoncelli, L., Cooper, E. L., & Cossarizza, A. (2011). Quercetin and cancer chemoprevention. *Evidence-based Complementary and Alternative Medicine, 2011*, 591356–591356.
85. Jeong, J.-H., An, J. Y., Kwon, Y. T., Rhee, J. G., & Lee, Y. J. (2009). Effects of low dose quercetin: Cancer cell-specific inhibition of cell cycle progression. *Journal of Cellular Biochemistry, 106*(1), 73–82.
86. HUISSEN, C. H., & KUIJPERS, E. W. (1991). Quick cytochemical staining of blood and bone marrow cells in a microwave oven. *Clinical & Laboratory Haematology, 13*(2), 197–205.
87. Yanaka, A., Fahey, J. W., Fukumoto, A., Nakayama, M., Inoue, S., Zhang, S., Tauchi, M., Suzuki, H., Hyodo, I., & Yamamoto, M. (2009). Dietary sulforaphane-rich broccoli sprouts reduce colonization and attenuate gastritis in Helicobacter pylori-infected mice and humans. *Cancer Prevention Research, 2*(4), 353–360.
88. Parkin, D. M., Bray, F., Ferlay, J., & Pisani, P. (2005). Global cancer statistics, 2002. *CA: a Cancer Journal for Clinicians, 55*(2), 74–108.
89. Jemal, A., Siegel, R., Ward, E., Murray, T., Xu, J., & Thun, M. J. (2007). Cancer statistics, 2007. *CA: a Cancer Journal for Clinicians, 57*(1), 43–66.
90. Subramaniam, D., Ponnurangam, S., Ramamoorthy, P., Standing, D., Battafarano, R. J., Anant, S., & Sharma, P. (2012). Curcumin induces cell death in esophageal cancer cells through modulating Notch signaling. *PLoS One, 7*(2), e30590–e30590.
91. Sant, M., Aareleid, T., Berrino, F., Bielska Lasota, M., Carli, P., Faivre, J., Grosclaude, P., Hedelin, G., Matsuda, T., & Møller, H. (2003). EUROCARE-3: Survival of cancer patients diagnosed 1990–94—Results and commentary. *Annals of Oncology, 14*(suppl_5), v61–v118.
92. Wynder, E. L., & Bross, I. J. (1961). A study of etiological factors in cancer of the esophagus. *Cancer, 14*(2), 389–413.
93. Stoner, G. D., Kresty, L. A., Carlton, P. S., Siglin, J. C., & Morse, M. A. (1999). Isothiocyanates and freeze-dried strawberries as inhibitors of esophageal cancer. *Toxicological Sciences: An Official Journal of the Society of Toxicology, 52*(suppl_1), 95–100.
94. Stoner, G. D., & Gupta, A. (2001). Etiology and chemoprevention of esophageal squamous cell carcinoma. *Carcinogenesis, 22*(11), 1737–1746.
95. Engel, L. S., Chow, W. H., Vaughan, T. L., Gammon, M. D., Risch, H. A., Stanford, J. L., Schoenberg, J. B., Mayne, S. T., Dubrow, R., & Rotterdam, H. (2003). Population attributable risks of esophageal and gastric cancers. *Journal of the National Cancer Institute, 95*(18), 1404–1413.
96. Wilkinson, J. T., Morse, M. A., Kresty, L. A., & Stoner, G. D. (1995). Effect of alkyl chain length on inhibition of N-nitrosomethylbenzylamine-induced esophageal tumorigenesis and DNA methylation by isothiocyanates. *Carcinogenesis, 16*(5), 1011–1015.
97. Morse, M. A., Lu, J., Gopalakrishnan, R., Peterson, L. A., Wani, G., & Stoner, G. D. (1997). Mechanism of enhancement of esophageal tumorigenesis by 6-phenylhexyl isothiocyanate. *Cancer Letters, 112*(1), 119–125.
98. Bower, M. R., Aiyer, H. S., Li, Y., & Martin, R. C. G. (2010). Chemoprotective effects of curcumin in esophageal epithelial cells exposed to bile acids. *World Journal of Gastroenterology, 16*(33), 4152–4158.
99. Arlt, A., Gehrz, A., Müerköster, S., Vorndamm, J., Kruse, M.-L., Fölsch, U. R., & Schäfer, H. (2003). Role of NF-κB and Akt/PI3K in the resistance of pancreatic carcinoma cell lines against gemcitabine-induced cell death. *Oncogene, 22*(21), 3243.

100. Rayet, B., & Gelinas, C. (1999). Aberrant rel/nfkb genes and activity in human cancer. *Oncogene, 18*(49), 6938.
101. Hartojo, W., Silvers, A. L., Thomas, D. G., Seder, C. W., Lin, L., Rao, H., Wang, Z., Greenson, J. K., Giordano, T. J., Orringer, M. B., et al. (2010). Curcumin promotes apoptosis, increases chemosensitivity, and inhibits nuclear factor kappaB in esophageal adenocarcinoma. *Translational Oncology, 3*(2), 99–108.
102. Tian F, Song M, Xu P, Liu H, Xue L: Curcumin promotes apoptosis of esophageal squamous carcinoma cell lines through inhibition of NF-kappaB signaling pathway. *Ai zheng= Aizheng=* Chinese Journal of Cancer 2008, 27(6):566–570.
103. Rawat, N., Alhamdani, A., McAdam, E., Cronin, J., Eltahir, Z., Lewis, P., Griffiths, P., Baxter, J. N., & Jenkins, G. J. (2012). Curcumin abrogates bile-induced NF-κB activity and DNA damage in vitro and suppresses NF-κB activity whilst promoting apoptosis in vivo, suggesting chemopreventative potential in Barrett's oesophagus. *Clinical and Translational Oncology, 14* (4), 302–311.
104. Chung, J. Y., Huang, C., Meng, X., Dong, Z., & Yang, C. S. (1999). Inhibition of activator protein 1 activity and cell growth by purified green tea and black tea polyphenols in H-<em>ras</em>–transformed cells. *Structure-Activity Relationship and Mechanisms Involved, 59*(18), 4610–4617.
105. Chung, J. Y., Park, J. O., Phyu, H., Dong, Z., & Yang, C. S. (2001). Mechanisms of inhibition of the Ras-MAP kinase signaling pathway in 30.7 b Ras 12 cells by tea polyphenols (−)-epigallocatechin-3-gallate and theaflavin-3, 3′-digallate. *The FASEB Journal, 15*(11), 2022–2024.
106. Dong, Z., Ma, W.-Y., Huang, C., & Yang, C. S. (1997). Inhibition of tumor promoter-induced activator protein 1 activation and cell transformation by tea polyphenols,(−)-epigallocatechin gallate, and theaflavins. *Cancer Research, 57*(19), 4414–4419.
107. Atten, M. J., Attar, B. M., Milson, T., & Holian, O. (2001). Resveratrol-induced inactivation of human gastric adenocarcinoma cells through a protein kinase C-mediated mechanism. *Biochemical Pharmacology, 62*(10), 1423–1432.
108. Ramos-Gomez, M., Kwak, M.-K., Dolan, P. M., Itoh, K., Yamamoto, M., Talalay, P., & Kensler, T. W. (2001). Sensitivity to carcinogenesis is increased and chemoprotective efficacy of enzyme inducers is lost in nrf2 transcription factor deficient mice. *Proceedings of the National Academy of Sciences, 98*(6), 3410–3415.
109. Friedman, K. J., Highsmith, W., Jr., & Silverman, L. (1991). Detecting multiple cystic fibrosis mutations by polymerase chain reaction-mediated site-directed mutagenesis. *Clinical Chemistry, 37*(5), 753–755.
110. Fahey, J. W., Haristoy, X., Dolan, P. M., Kensler, T. W., Scholtus, I., Stephenson, K. K., Talalay, P., & Lozniewski, A. (2002). Sulforaphane inhibits extracellular, intracellular, and antibiotic-resistant strains of Helicobacter pylori and prevents benzo [a] pyrene-induced stomach tumors. *Proceedings of the National Academy of Sciences, 99*(11), 7610–7615.
111. Fahey, J. W., Zhang, Y., & Talalay, P. (1997). Broccoli sprouts: An exceptionally rich source of inducers of enzymes that protect against chemical carcinogens. *Proceedings of the National Academy of Sciences, 94*(19), 10367–10372.
112. Vanamala, J., Radhakrishnan, S., Reddivari, L., Bhat, V. B., & Ptitsyn, A. (2011). Resveratrol suppresses human colon cancer cell proliferation and induces apoptosis via targeting the pentose phosphate and the talin-FAK signaling pathways - a proteomic approach. *Proteome Science, 9*(1), 49.
113. Stoner, G. D., & Morse, M. A. (1997). Isothiocyanates and plant polyphenols as inhibitors of lung and esophageal cancer. *Cancer Letters, 114*(1–2), 113–119.
114. Ye, F., Zhang, G.-H., Guan, B.-X., & Xu, X.-C. (2012). Suppression of esophageal cancer cell growth using curcumin,(−)-epigallocatechin-3-gallate and lovastatin. *World journal of gastroenterology: WJG, 18*(2), 126.
115. Li, Z. G., Shimada, Y., Sato, F., Maeda, M., Itami, A., Kaganoi, J., Komoto, I., Kawabe, A., & Imamura, M. (2002). Inhibitory effects of epigallocatechin-3-gallate on N-

nitrosomethylbenzylamine-induced esophageal tumorigenesis in F344 rats. *International Journal of Oncology, 21*(6), 1275–1283.
116. Hou, Z., Sang, S., You, H., Lee, M.-J., Hong, J., Chin, K.-V., & Yang, C. S. (2005). Mechanism of action of (−)-epigallocatechin-3-gallate: Auto-oxidation-dependent inactivation of epidermal growth factor receptor and direct effects on growth inhibition in human esophageal cancer KYSE 150 cells. *Cancer Research, 65*(17), 8049–8056.
117. Brahmer, J. R., Tykodi, S. S., Chow, L. Q. M., Hwu, W.-J., Topalian, S. L., Hwu, P., Drake, C. G., Camacho, L. H., Kauh, J., Odunsi, K., et al. (2012). Safety and activity of anti-PD-L1 antibody in patients with advanced cancer. *The New England Journal of Medicine, 366*(26), 2455–2465.
118. Hodi, F. S., O'Day, S. J., McDermott, D. F., Weber, R. W., Sosman, J. A., Haanen, J. B., Gonzalez, R., Robert, C., Schadendorf, D., Hassel, J. C., et al. (2010). Improved survival with ipilimumab in patients with metastatic melanoma. *The New England Journal of Medicine, 363* (8), 711–723.
119. Jindal, V. (2018). Immune checkpoint inhibitors in gastrointestinal malignancies. *Journal of Gastrointestinal Oncology, 9*(2), 390–403.
120. Pardoll, D. M. (2012). The blockade of immune checkpoints in cancer immunotherapy. *Nature Reviews. Cancer, 12*(4), 252–264.
121. Korman, A. J., Peggs, K. S., & Allison, J. P. (2006). Checkpoint blockade in cancer immunotherapy. In *Advances in Immunology* (Vol. 90, pp. 297–339). Cambridge: Academic Press.
122. Kim, B. J., Jang, H. J., Kim, H. S., & Kim, J. H. (2017). Current status of immune checkpoint inhibitors in gastrointestinal cancers. *Journal of Cancer, 8*(8), 1460–1465.
123. Wu, C., Zhu, Y., Jiang, J., Zhao, J., Zhang, X.-G., & Xu, N. (2006). Immunohistochemical localization of programmed death-1 ligand-1 (PD-L1) in gastric carcinoma and its clinical significance. *Acta Histochemica, 108*(1), 19–24.
124. Ohigashi, Y., Sho, M., Yamada, Y., Tsurui, Y., Hamada, K., Ikeda, N., Mizuno, T., Yoriki, R., Kashizuka, H., & Yane, K. (2005). Clinical significance of programmed death-1 ligand-1 and programmed death-1 ligand-2 expression in human esophageal cancer. *Clinical Cancer Research, 11*(8), 2947–2953.
125. Siegel, R. L., Miller, K. D., & Jemal, A. (2017). Cancer statistics, 2017. *CA: a Cancer Journal for Clinicians, 67*(1), 7–30.
126. Torre, L. A., Bray, F., Siegel, R. L., Ferlay, J., Lortet-Tieulent, J., & Jemal, A. (2015). Global cancer statistics, 2012. *CA: a Cancer Journal for Clinicians, 65*(2), 87–108.
127. Bilgin, B., Sendur, M. A. N., Bülent Akıncı, M., Şener Dede, D., & Yalçın, B. (2017). Targeting the PD-1 pathway: A new hope for gastrointestinal cancers. *Current Medical Research and Opinion, 33*(4), 749–759.
128. Gippini, A. P., Rodríguez, I. L., Torre, A. C., & Barrio, E. G. (1990). Alcohol withdrawal syndrome at the internal medicine department of a general hospital; epidemiology and hospital costs. *Anales de medicina interna (Madrid, Spain: 1984), 1990*, 171–173.
129. Kastrinos, F., Ojha, R. P., Leenen, C., Alvero, C., Mercado, R. C., Balmaña, J., Valenzuela, I., Balaguer, F., Green, R., Lindor, N. M., et al. (2015). Comparison of prediction models for lynch syndrome among individuals with colorectal cancer. *Journal of the National Cancer Institute, 108*(2), djv308.
130. Hemminki, A., Peltomäki, P., Mecklin, J.-P., Järvinen, H., Salovaara, R., Nyström-Lahti, M., de la Chapelle, A., & Aaltonen, L. A. (1994). Loss of the wild type MLH1 gene is a feature of hereditary nonpolyposis colorectal cancer. *Nature Genetics, 8*(4), 405–410.
131. Saeterdal, I., Bjørheim, J., Lislerud, K., Gjertsen, M. K., Bukholm, I. K., Olsen, O. C., Nesland, J. M., Eriksen, J. A., Møller, M., Lindblom, A., et al. (2001). Frameshift-mutation-derived peptides as tumor-specific antigens in inherited and spontaneous colorectal cancer. *Proceedings of the National Academy of Sciences of the United States of America, 98*(23), 13255–13260.

132. Phillips, S. M., Banerjea, A., Feakins, R., Li, S. R., Bustin, S. A., & Dorudi, S. (2004). Tumour-infiltrating lymphocytes in colorectal cancer with microsatellite instability are activated and cytotoxic. *BJS (British Journal of Surgery), 91*(4), 469–475.
133. Quinn, E., Hawkins, N., Yip, Y. L., Suter, C., & Ward, R. (2003). CD103+ intraepithelial lymphocytes—A unique population in microsatellite unstable sporadic colorectal cancer. *European Journal of Cancer, 39*(4), 469–475.
134. Galon, J., Costes, A., Sanchez-Cabo, F., Kirilovsky, A., Mlecnik, B., Lagorce-Pagès, C., Tosolini, M., Camus, M., Berger, A., Wind, P., et al. (2006). Type, density, and location of immune cells within human colorectal tumors predict clinical outcome. *Science, 313*(5795), 1960–1964.
135. Schumacher, T. N., & Schreiber, R. D. (2015). Neoantigens in cancer immunotherapy. *Science, 348*(6230), 69–74.
136. Plimack, E. R., Bellmunt, J., Gupta, S., Berger, R., Chow, L. Q., Juco, J., Lunceford, J., Saraf, S., Perini, R. F., & O'Donnell, P. H. (2017). Safety and activity of pembrolizumab in patients with locally advanced or metastatic urothelial cancer (KEYNOTE-012): A non-randomised, open-label, phase 1b study. *The Lancet Oncology, 18*(2), 212–220.
137. Nanda, R., Chow, L. Q. M., Dees, E. C., Berger, R., Gupta, S., Geva, R., Pusztai, L., Pathiraja, K., Aktan, G., Cheng, J. D., et al. (2016). Pembrolizumab in patients with advanced triple-negative breast cancer: Phase Ib KEYNOTE-012 study. *Journal of Clinical Oncology, 34*(21), 2460–2467.
138. Diaz, L. A., Marabelle, A., Delord, J.-P., Shapira-Frommer, R., Geva, R., Peled, N., Kim, T. W., Andre, T., Van Cutsem, E., & Guimbaud, R. (2017). Pembrolizumab therapy for microsatellite instability high (MSI-H) colorectal cancer (CRC) and non-CRC. *American Society of Clinical Oncology.*
139. Network, C. G. A. R. (2014). Comprehensive molecular characterization of gastric adenocarcinoma. *Nature, 513*(7517), 202–209.
140. Le, D. T., Uram, J. N., Wang, H., Bartlett, B. R., Kemberling, H., Eyring, A. D., Skora, A. D., Luber, B. S., Azad, N. S., Laheru, D., et al. (2015). PD-1 blockade in tumors with mismatch-repair deficiency. *The New England Journal of Medicine, 372*(26), 2509–2520.
141. Muro, K., Chung, H. C., Shankaran, V., Geva, R., Catenacci, D., Gupta, S., Eder, J. P., Golan, T., Le, D. T., & Burtness, B. (2016). Pembrolizumab for patients with PD-L1-positive advanced gastric cancer (KEYNOTE-012): A multicentre, open-label, phase 1b trial. *The Lancet Oncology, 17*(6), 717–726.
142. Sangro, B., Gomez-Martin, C., de la Mata, M., Iñarrairaegui, M., Garralda, E., Barrera, P., Riezu-Boj, J. I., Larrea, E., Alfaro, C., Sarobe, P., et al. (2013). A clinical trial of CTLA-4 blockade with tremelimumab in patients with hepatocellular carcinoma and chronic hepatitis C. *Journal of Hepatology, 59*(1), 81–88.

Chapter 5
Crucial Role of Curcumin in Gut Microbiota Associated with GI Cancers

Santoshi Muppala and Siva Krishna Prasad Konduru

Abstract The widespread cause of cancer occurs due to alterations in genetic and environmental components; in addition to this, gut microbiota plays a profound role in causing cancer incidence. Human body consists of significant number of microorganisms having a potential impact on human health. Gut is ubiquitously enriched with microbiota which has a critical role in the CRC advancement. Changes in the metabolite agility by microbiome and their structural impact on adjacent epithelial cells will be detrimental to drive cancer progression. Research on animal models showed reduced tumorigenesis when suspended in germ-free environment. This clearly depicts the importance of the microbes or its products in driving the inflammation and cancer progression. Curcumin, also known as *Curcuma longa*, is the most active constituent of the ground rhizome of the *Curcuma longa* plant, which has been demonstrated to have anti-inflammatory, antioxidative, and antiproliferative properties.

Current literature shows the importance of curcumin influence on gut microbiota in the regulation of immune mediated inflammatory processes. This book chapter highlights direct relationship of curcumin in gut microbiota with genetic and environmental factors resulting in GI cancer progression. Taken together, gut microbiota is the key player of GI progression. There is an urgent need of using curcumin as one of the phytochemicals controlling the reign of gut microbiota that can definitely be helpful in reducing the risk of developing GI cancers and will have a better therapeutic role in patient treatment outcomes.

Keywords Curcumin · Gut microbiome · Inflammation · Cancer

S. Muppala (✉)
Department of Cardiovascular and Metabolic Sciences, Lerner Research Institute, Cleveland Clinic, Cleveland, OH, USA
e-mail: muppals@ccf.org

S. K. P. Konduru
Sangre Grande Hospital, Eastern Regional Health Authority, Sangre Grande, Trinidad and Tobago

G. P. Nagaraju (ed.), *Phytochemicals Targeting Tumor Microenvironment in Gastrointestinal Cancers*, https://doi.org/10.1007/978-3-030-48405-7_5

Abbreviations

GI	Gastrointestinal
OC	Esophageal cancer
CRC	Colorectal cancer
PC	Pancreatic cancer
LC	Liver cancer
MAPK	Mitogen-activated protein kinase pathway

1 Introduction

The microbial population in the gut is associated to many human diseases including cancer. The beneficial effect of curcumin on tumorigenesis was associated with the maintenance of a more diverse colonic microbial ecology. Existing literature states that the effects of curcumin/polyphenols are associated to changes in the gut microbiota. Thus, novel role of curcumin provides insights into metabolic regulation of GI cancers which may lead to effective therapy.

Microbiota-harboring intestine has the ability to progress cancer. Diet is one of the key determinants of the microbial population, so dietary interventions are an important part of the treatment. The maintenance of the gut microbiota called homeostasis significantly contributes to the status of resident microorganisms [1]. Phytochemicals have the tendency to modulate antimicrobial activity. Curcumin as one of the phytochemical candidates has the ability to regulate gut microbiota by its antimicrobial activity [2].

Studies on healthy adults show that there are multiple changes in the urine composition by consuming the curcumin extract [3]. The incidence of occurrence of cancer, esp. CRC, one of the most aggressive GI cancers, is mostly related to lifestyle. Existing studies demonstrate that dietary phenolics regulate different markers and signaling pathways [4]. In addition to curcumin, other dietary ingredients such as resveratrol and fatty acids are thoroughly used for the treatment and impediment of cancer, especially as they alter the crucial pathways that regulate metastasis, tumor growth, and invasion [5].

It is a known fact that different microorganisms adapt to gut microbiome for living in the intestine. When there is a disturbance in the gut microbiome, there is reduced number of microbial diversity which can trigger the immune system repression and thereby result in many types of diseases including cancer in human bodies. Therefore, gut microbiome is highly important in engaging cancer therapy, esp. with different GI cancers [6]. An interesting study on CRC reports that the leading cause of death is the increasing incidence of colorectal cancer which occurs due to the dysbiosis of the gut microbiome [7].

The great advantage of the phytochemicals, e.g., curcumin, is that they have a wide spectrum of antimicrobial activities. Thus far, ingestion of phytochemicals can have antimicrobial activity by regulating gut microbiota [2]. Recent evidence suggests that curcumin is one of the biologically active components of *Curcuma longa* that have received a lot of attention for the clinical improvement of many GI cancers including esophageal, prostate, and colorectal cancer. Much more efforts need to be addressed to define the effects of curcumin on cancer regulation [8].

Curcumin is known to possess many properties including anticancer, antiviral, antioxidant, and anti-inflammatory which makes it an ideal candidate for therapies of many diseases including cancer. The major drawback is its poor bioavailability [9]. Curcumin, one of the polyphenols, has a long history of using as a spice compound in the diet. It possesses a broad spectrum of antimicrobial activity but it possesses very poor bioavailability. Henceforth, it does not reinforce clinical application. Existing studies indicate that oral ingestion of curcumin results in the accumulation in the intestine being able to regulate the gut microbiota. There are more challenges on curcumin being used as a pharmacological compound and more importantly how this natural compound acts to combat cancer [10].

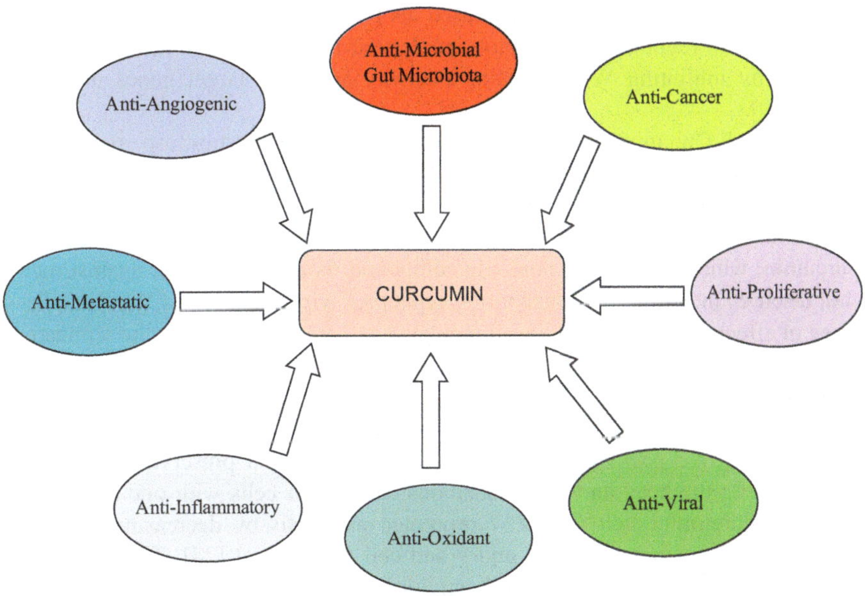

2 Crucial Roles of Curcumin

Anti-microbial: Curcumin has extensive antimicrobial effects and is safer at high concentrations. Combinations of curcumin and antibiotics work efficiently in treating the multidrug-resistant bacteria [11]. Curcumin has a wide range of antimicrobial activities. Antimicrobial photodynamic therapy is one of the best approaches to treat chronic wound infections based on curcumin-silica nanoparticles for the treatment of chronic wounds [12]. Curcumin gel shows beneficial effect on the improvement of chronic periodontitis and has clinical significance as a successful drug delivery agent [13].

Anti-cancer: Curcumin along with cyclodextrin-graphene oxide core (Cur@CD-GO)-coated nanofibers (NFs) appears to be a better therapeutic approach than single-drug loading. These NFs show potential anticancer properties which are more reliable and sustainable [14]. Current literature states that curcumin having anticarcinogenic properties can be an effective natural anticancer therapeutic agent [15]. Existing studies indicate that the novel complex of curcumin along with cyclodextrin polymer has demonstrated significant antitumor benefits against human cancers [16].

Anti-proliferative: Curcumin has been extensively used along with adjuvants or nanoparticles to improve its bioavailability and has been demonstrated to increase its antiproliferative properties [17]. Curcumin in combination with small molecule called tolfenamic acid showed significant antiproliferative properties in the inhibition of NF-kappaB activity and increased apoptosis in colorectal cancer cell lines [18]. Curcumin regulates pro-apoptotic molecular mechanism and has a significant potential by inhibiting Wnt signaling pathway and their target genes in gastric cancer [19].

Anti-viral: Curcumin is known to possess antiviral properties, esp. synthesis of nanocurcumin with better physical and chemical properties. This formulation was very beneficial in the treatment against dengue virus [20]. Curcumin has significant applications as a safe antiviral compound in the field of biomedical research. Curcumin, which is a highly nontoxic compound, is able to combat against many viral diseases including influenza virus, hepatitis C virus, and HIV [21]. Boundless range of effects of curcumin are well regulated and are able to inhibit the replication of herpesvirus which is associated with Kaposi's sarcoma, particularly hindered cell invasion [22].

Anti-oxidant: Curcumin has both antimicrobial and antioxidant properties and is used as an active packaging ingredient for high-potential preservation purposes [23]. Treating the head-and-neck squamous cell cancer cells with one of the analogues of curcumin such as WZ37 promoted apoptosis by decreasing oxidative pathways such as mitochondrial injury and cell cycle arrest [24]. There has been increasing evidence on the biological activities of curcumin as an antioxidant; study on pancreatitis mice model showed significant inhibition of acute pancreatitis inflammation [25]. It has extremely powerful antioxidant properties and can be a reducer of oxidative stress.

Anti-inflammatory: There is increasing evidence on the role of curcumin as an anti-inflammatory agent and a neuroprotective against many cancers and also neurological diseases like Alzheimer's and Parkinson's disease [26]. Existing studies on curcumin showed significant reduction in the LPS-induced inflammation in microglia through the regulation of NF-kappaB pathway [27]. Another study has shown curcumin analogue C66 to inhibit inflammation in LPS-induced lung injury by inhibiting JNK pathway; thereby curcumin may benefit as a prospective beneficial agent for acute lung injury [28].

Anti-metastatic: Curcumin is known to possess antimetastatic activity in many cancers. Curcumin along with the aminonaphthoquinone derivatives is known to suppress breast cancer metastasis significantly [29]. An analogue of curcumin named as pentagamavunon-1 (PGV-1) is highly potential in the inhibition of metastasis of breast cancer cell lines [30]. Existing data on the treatment of metastatic cancers has reported polyphenols including curcumin as one of the chemoprotective and preventative agents despite its poor solubility and bioavailability which can be enhanced using nanoparticle formulations [31].

Anti-angiogenic: Curcumin serves as a supplementary antiangiogenic compound which has been well documented on studies related to cancer treatments [32]. Numerous reports indicate that curcumin has potential antiangiogenic and wound-healing effects [33]. Curcumin is known to exhibit antiangiogenic properties by inhibiting the pathway connected with MAPK besides inhibiting cell migration and tube formation [34]. Moreover, curcumin possesses tumor-suppressor properties by inhibiting angiogenesis mediated by insulin growth factor-1 receptor [35].

3 Curcumin as a Therapeutic Remedial of GI Cancers

Esophageal cancer: Esophageal cancer is one of the most commonly occurring cancers and the sixth most common among the death-causing cancers worldwide. Curcumin has been widely used for the inhibition of inflammation associated with the advancement of cancer. Many pro-oncogenic pathways are being targeted with the application of curcumin [36]. Current clinical studies on curcumin show that it has a protective role in the healing of ulcers of the gastrointestinal tract [37]. Another study showed that curcumin inhibited apoptosis of squamous cell carcinoma through inducing cell growth arrest by targeting STAT3 signaling pathway [38].

Liver cancer: With liver cancer being the fifth most common death-causing cancers around the world, lot of attention has been focused on curcumin as a therapeutic aid for the treatment of liver cancer; especially, studies on curcumin-associated nanoparticles have shown their potential to inhibit the growth of liver cancer cells [39]. NF-kappaB is one of the targeting pathways of curcumin to inhibit the steatosis associated with the liver as outlined in a study on the prevention of nonalcoholic fatty liver disease (NAFLD) [40]. Curcumin inhibits hepatocellular carcinoma cell migration, invasion, and proliferation and thereby has a very important medicinal value for the prevention of liver cancer [41].

Colorectal cancer: Colorectal cancer is the second most occurring among the types of cancers. Existing reports indicate that curcumin is one of the most reliable therapeutic tools for the prevention of CRC, because its contribution is highly significant in the inhibition of inflammatory signaling pathways [42]. Some derivatives of curcumin, namely calebin A, blocked NF-kappa B pathway; thereby CRC cell line invasion, proliferation, and metastasis were significantly repressed

[43]. Many curcumin analogues along with the fusion with nanoparticles which are known to be anti-inflammatory are found to be very effective in the treatment of colitis-related colorectal cancer [44].

Pancreatic cancer: Pancreatic cancer is the fourth leading cause of cancer deaths around the world. Nanoparticle-associated curcumin is shown to be relevant for its inhibitory effects on tumor microenvironment, esp. by downregulating IL-10 expression [45]. Current studies report that curcumin plays one of the major roles in the inhibition of mitogen-activated protein kinase (MAPK) pathway which is a crucial regulator of inflammatory pathway [46]. Existing literature supports the role of curcumin in the effective treatment of acute pancreatitis and ongoing clinical trial advancements correspond and are supportive to the therapeutic response of curcumin [47].

4 Highlights

- This book chapter highlights the underlying effects of curcumin on regulating gut microbiota associated with GI progression.
- It reveals the role of curcumin and gut microbiota in the regulation of different types of GI cancers.
- The antimicrobial and antimetastatic role of curcumin in connection to GI is discussed.
- It ponders on how gut microbiota is strongly connected in manipulating tumor microenvironment and renders response to therapeutics, esp. curcumin.

5 Conclusions

Further research needs are to be focused on the development of the nanotherapeutics in combination with curcumin and should be effective in case of bioavailability and biodegradability. Curcumin analogues and formulations seem to be very crucial in the ongoing clinical trial advancements in the treatments of different types of GI cancers. Using curcumin as a natural therapy in addition to the chemotherapy will be more beneficial to reduce cytotoxicity and prognosis of a patient's life. Existing scientific literature reinforces the strategy that the effective sources of curcumin are powerful chemotherapeutic and cancer preventative tools for GI carcinogenesis.

References

1. Dudek-Wicher, R. K., Junka, A., & Bartoszewicz, M. (2018). The influence of antibiotics and dietary components on gut microbiota. *Przegląd Gastroenterologiczny, 13*, 85–92.

2. Lakes, J. E., Richards, C. I., & Flythe, M. D. (2019). Inhibition of Bacteroidetes and Firmicutes by select phytochemicals. *Anaerobe, 61*, 102145.
3. Peron, G., Sut, S., Dal Ben, S., Voinovich, D., & Dall'Acqua, S. (2020). Untargeted UPLC-MS metabolomics reveals multiple changes of urine composition in healthy adult volunteers after consumption of Curcuma longa L. extract. *Food Research International, 127*, 108730.
4. Nunez-Sanchez, M. A., Gonzalez-Sarrias, A., Romo-Vaquero, M., Garcia-Villalba, R., Selma, M. V., Tomas-Barberan, F. A., Garcia-Conesa, M. T., & Espin, J. C. (2015). Dietary phenolics against colorectal cancer--from promising preclinical results to poor translation into clinical trials: Pitfalls and future needs. *Molecular Nutrition & Food Research, 59*, 1274–1291.
5. Riaz Rajoka, M. S., Jin, M., Haobin, Z., Li, Q., Shao, D., Huang, Q., & Shi, J. (2018). Impact of dietary compounds on cancer-related gut microbiota and microRNA. *Applied Microbiology and Biotechnology, 102*, 4291–4303.
6. Ichikawa, M., Sujino, T., & Kanai, T. (2019). The relationship between gut microbiome, immune system, and Cancer. *Gan to Kagaku Ryoho, 46*, 1807–1813.
7. Sanyaolu, L. N., Oakley, N. J., Nurmatov, U., Dolwani, S., & Ahmed, H. (2019). Antibiotic exposure and the risk of colorectal adenoma and carcinoma: A systematic review and meta-analysis of observational studies. *Colorectal Disease*.
8. Peterson, C. T., Vaughn, A. R., Sharma, V., Chopra, D., Mills, P. J., Peterson, S. N., & Sivamani, R. K. (2018). Effects of turmeric and curcumin dietary supplementation on human gut microbiota: A double-blind, randomized, placebo-controlled pilot study. *Journal of Evidence-Based Integrative Medicine, 23*, 2515690X18790725.
9. Lopresti, B. I. B. A. L. (2018). The problem of curcumin and its bioavailability: Could its gastrointestinal influence contribute to its overall health-enhancing effects? *Advances in Nutrition, 9*, 41–50.
10. Shen, L., & Ji, H. F. (2019). Bidirectional interactions between dietary curcumin and gut microbiota. *Critical Reviews in Food Science and Nutrition, 59*, 2896–2902.
11. Yasbolaghi Sharahi, J., Aliakbar Ahovan, Z., Taghizadeh Maleki, D., Riahi Rad, Z., Riahi Rad, Z., Goudarzi, M., Shariati, A., Bostanghadiri, N., Abbasi, E., & Hashemi, A. (2020). In vitro antibacterial activity of curcumin-meropenem combination against extensively drug-resistant (XDR) bacteria isolated from burn wound infections. *Avicenna Journal of Phytomedicine, 10*, 3–10.
12. Mirzahosseinipour, M., Khorsandi, K., Hosseinzadeh, R., Ghazaeian, M., & Shahidi, F. K. (2019). Antimicrobial photodynamic and wound healing activity of curcumin encapsulated in silica nanoparticles. *Photodiagnosis and Photodynamic Therapy*, 101639.
13. Nagasri, M., Madhulatha, M., Musalaiah, S. V., Kumar, P. A., Krishna, C. H., & Kumar, P. M. (2015). Efficacy of curcumin as an adjunct to scaling and root planning in chronic periodontitis patients: A clinical and microbiological study. *Journal of Pharmacy & Bioallied Sciences, 7*, S554–S558.
14. Sattari, S., Tehrani, A. D., Adeli, M., Soleimani, K., & Rashidipour, M. (2019). Fabrication of new generation of co-delivery systems based on graphene-g-cyclodextrin/chitosan nanofiber. *International Journal of Biological Macromolecules*.
15. Wang, X. J., Chen, J. Y., Fu, L. Q., & Yan, M. J. (2020). Recent advances in natural therapeutic approaches for the treatment of cancer. *Journal of Chemotherapy*, 1–13.
16. Chen, J., Cao, X., Qin, X., Liu, H., Chen, S., Zhong, S., & Li, Y. (2019). Proteomic analysis of the molecular mechanism of curcumin/beta-cyclodextrin polymer inclusion complex inhibiting HepG2 cells growth. *Journal of Food Biochemistry*, e13119.
17. Alkhader, E., Roberts, C. J., Rosli, R., Yuen, K. H., Seow, E. K., Lee, Y. Z., & Billa, N. (2018). Pharmacokinetic and anti-colon cancer properties of curcumin-containing chitosan-pectinate composite nanoparticles. *Journal of Biomaterials Science. Polymer Edition, 29*, 2281–2298.
18. Sankpal, U. T., Nagaraju, G. P., Gottipolu, S. R., Hurtado, M., Jordan, C. G., Simecka, J. W., Shoji, M., El-Rayes, B., & Basha, R. (2016). Combination of tolfenamic acid and curcumin induces colon cancer cell growth inhibition through modulating specific transcription factors and reactive oxygen species. *Oncotarget, 7*, 3186–3200.

19. Zheng, R., Deng, Q., Liu, Y., & Zhao, P. (2017). Curcumin inhibits gastric carcinoma cell growth and induces apoptosis by suppressing the Wnt/beta-catenin signaling pathway. *Medical Science Monitor, 23*, 163–171.
20. Nabila, N., Suada, N. K., Denis, D., Yohan, B., Adi, A. C., Veterini, A. S., Anindya, A. L., Sasmono, R. T., & Rachmawati, H. (2019). Antiviral action of curcumin encapsulated in nanoemulsion against four serotypes of dengue virus. *Pharmaceutical Nanotechnology.*
21. Praditya, D., Kirchhoff, L., Bruning, J., Rachmawati, H., Steinmann, J., & Steinmann, E. (2019). Anti-infective properties of the golden spice curcumin. *Frontiers in Microbiology, 10*, 912.
22. Li, H., Zhong, C., Wang, Q., Chen, W., & Yuan, Y. (2019). Curcumin is an APE1 redox inhibitor and exhibits an antiviral activity against KSHV replication and pathogenesis. *Antiviral Research, 167*, 98–103.
23. Roy, S., & Rhim, J. W. (2019). Preparation of antimicrobial and antioxidant gelatin/curcumin composite films for active food packaging application. *Colloids and Surfaces. B, Biointerfaces, 188*, 110761.
24. Zhang, Z., Lin, R., Liu, Z., Yan, T., Xia, Y., Zhao, L., Lin, F., Zhang, X., Li, C., & Wang, Y. (2019). Curcumin analog, WZ37, promotes G2/M arrest and apoptosis of HNSCC cells through Akt/mTOR inhibition. *Toxicology In Vitro, 65*, 104754.
25. Siriviriyakul, P., Chingchit, T., Klaikeaw, N., Chayanupatkul, M., & Werawatganon, D. (2019). Effects of curcumin on oxidative stress, inflammation and apoptosis in L-arginine induced acute pancreatitis in mice. *Heliyon, 5*, e02222.
26. Forouzanfar, F., Read, M. I., Barreto, G. E., & Sahebkar, A. (2019). Neuroprotective effects of curcumin alleviates lipopolysaccharide (LPS)-activated neuroinflammation via modulation of miR-199b-5p/IκB kinase β (IKKβ)/nuclear factor kappa B (NF-κB) pathway in microglia through autophagy modulation. *IUBMB Life.*
27. Gao, F., Shen, J., Zhao, L., Hao, Q., & Yang, Y. (2019). Curcumin alleviates lipopolysaccharide (LPS)-activated neuroinflammation via modulation of miR-199b-5p/IkappaB kinase beta (IKKbeta)/nuclear factor kappa B (NF-kappaB) pathway in microglia. *Medical Science Monitor, 25*, 9801–9810.
28. Xiao, Z., Xu, F., Zhu, X., Bai, B., Guo, L., Liang, G., Shan, X., Zhang, Y., Zhao, Y., & Zhang, B. (2019). Inhibition of JNK phosphorylation by curcumin analog C66 protects LPS-induced acute lung injury. *Drug Design, Development and Therapy, 13*, 4161–4171.
29. Pereira, M. C., Mohammed, R., VAN Otterlo, W. A. L., DE Koning, C. B., & Davids, H. (2020). In vitro analysis of the combinatory effects of novel aminonaphthoquinone derivatives and curcumin on breast cancer progression. *Anticancer Research, 40*, 229–238.
30. Meiyanto, E., Putri, H., Arum Larasati, Y., Yudi Utomo, R., Istighfari Jenie, R., Ikawati, M., Lestari, B., Yoneda-Kato, N., Nakamae, I., Kawaichi, M., & Kato, J. Y. (2019). Antiproliferative and anti-metastatic potential of Curcumin analogue, pentagamavunon-1 (PGV-1), toward highly metastatic breast cancer cells in correlation with ROS generation. *Advanced Pharmaceutical Bulletin, 9*, 445–452.
31. Heenatigala Palliyage, G., Singh, S., Ashby, C. R., Jr., Tiwari, A. K., & Chauhan, H. (2019). Pharmaceutical topical delivery of poorly soluble polyphenols: Potential role in prevention and treatment of melanoma. *AAPS PharmSciTech, 20*, 250.
32. Xiang, D. B., Zhang, K. Q., Zeng, Y. L., Yan, Q. Z., Shi, Z., Tuo, Q. H., Lin, L. M., Xia, B. H., Wu, P., & Liao, D. F. (2020). Curcumin: From a controversial "panacea" to effective antineoplastic products. *Medicine (Baltimore), 99*, e18467.
33. Yang, B. Y., Hu, C. H., Huang, W. C., Ho, C. Y., Yao, C. H., & Huang, C. H. (2019). Effects of bilayer nanofibrous scaffolds containing curcumin/lithospermi radix extract on wound healing in streptozotocin-induced diabetic rats. *Polymers (Basel)*, 11.
34. Hosseini, A., Rasmi, Y., Rahbarghazi, R., Aramwit, P., Daeihassani, B., & Saboory, E. (2019). Curcumin modulates the angiogenic potential of human endothelial cells via FAK/P-38 MAPK signaling pathway. *Gene, 688*, 7–12.

35. Chen, Y., Zhong, W., Chen, B., Yang, C., Zhou, S., & Liu, J. (2018). Effect of curcumin on vascular endothelial growth factor in hypoxic HepG2 cells via the insulin-like growth factor 1 receptor signaling pathway. *Experimental and Therapeutic Medicine, 15*, 2922–2928.
36. Komal, K., Chaudhary, S., Yadav, P., Parmanik, R., & Singh, M. (2019). The therapeutic and preventive efficacy of curcumin and its derivatives in esophageal cancer. *Asian Pacific Journal of Cancer Prevention, 20*, 1329–1337.
37. Kwiecien, S., Magierowski, M., Majka, J., Ptak-Belowska, A., Wojcik, D., Sliwowski, Z., Magierowska, K., & Brzozowski, T. (2019). Curcumin: A potent protectant against esophageal and gastric disorders. *International Journal of Molecular Sciences, 20*.
38. Liu, Y., Wang, X., Zeng, S., Zhang, X., Zhao, J., Zhang, X., Chen, X., Yang, W., Yang, Y., Dong, Z., Zhu, J., Xu, X., & Tian, F. (2018). The natural polyphenol curcumin induces apoptosis by suppressing STAT3 signaling in esophageal squamous cell carcinoma. *Journal of Experimental & Clinical Cancer Research, 37*, 303.
39. Chen, X. P., Li, Y., Zhang, Y., & Li, G. W. (2019). Formulation, characterization and evaluation of curcumin-loaded PLGA-TPGS nanoparticles for liver cancer treatment. *Drug Design, Development and Therapy, 13*, 3569–3578.
40. Feng, D., Zou, J., Su, D., Mai, H., Zhang, S., Li, P., & Zheng, X. (2019). Curcumin prevents high-fat diet-induced hepatic steatosis in ApoE(−/−) mice by improving intestinal barrier function and reducing endotoxin and liver TLR4/NF-kappaB inflammation. *Nutrition & Metabolism (London), 16*, 79.
41. Zhao, Z., Malhotra, A., & Seng, W. Y. (2019). Curcumin modulates hepatocellular carcinoma by reducing UNC119 expression. *Journal of Environmental Pathology, Toxicology and Oncology, 38*, 195–203.
42. Wu, R., Wang, L., Yin, R., Hudlikar, R., Li, S., Kuo, H. D., Peter, R., Sargsyan, D., Guo, Y., Liu, X., & Kong, A. T. (2020). Epigenetics/epigenomics and prevention by curcumin of early stages of inflammatory-driven colon cancer. *Molecular Carcinogenesis, 59*, 227–236.
43. Buhrmann, C., Popper, B., Kunnumakkara, A. B., Aggarwal, B. B., & Shakibaei, M. (2019). Evidence that calebin A, a component of Curcuma longa, suppresses NF-B mediated proliferation, invasion and metastasis of human colorectal cancer induced by TNF-beta (lymphotoxin). *Nutrients, 11*.
44. Han, W., Xie, B., Li, Y., Shi, L., Wan, J., Chen, X., & Wang, H. (2019). Orally deliverable nanotherapeutics for the synergistic treatment of colitis-associated colorectal cancer. *Theranostics, 9*, 7458–7473.
45. Madamsetty, V. S., Pal, K., Keshavan, S., Caulfield, T. R., Dutta, S. K., Wang, E., Fadeel, B., & Mukhopadhyay, D. (2019). Development of multi-drug loaded PEGylated nanodiamonds to inhibit tumor growth and metastasis in genetically engineered mouse models of pancreatic cancer. *Nanoscale, 11*, 22006–22018.
46. Wang, Y., Bu, C., Wu, K., Wang, R., & Wang, J. (2019). Curcumin protects the pancreas from acute pancreatitis via the mitogen-activated protein kinase signaling pathway. *Molecular Medicine Reports, 20*, 3027–3034.
47. Tarasiuk, A., & Fichna, J. (2019). Effectiveness and therapeutic value of phytochemicals in acute pancreatitis: A review. *Pancreatology, 19*, 481–487.

Chapter 6
Cellular and Molecular Mechanisms of Garlic Compounds in Common GI Cancers

Rama Rao Malla

Abstract The major gastrointestinal (GI) tract cancers are stomach, colorectal, pancreas, and liver cancers, which are foremost prevalent cancers worldwide, accounting for more deaths than any other cancers of human body. The GI tract cancers affect both men and women with preventable lifestyle risk factors including diet. Garlic is a globally used food ingredient with innumerable medicinal benefits due to the presence of sulfur-containing natural constituents such as alliin, methiin, DAS, DADS, DATS, SAC, and SAMC. They reduce GI cancer growth by inhibiting proliferation through disruption of microtubule-mediated cytoskeleton formation, inhibiting different cyclin/cyclin-dependent kinases in a phase-specific manner, and inducing apoptosis through mitochondrial dependent and independent pathways. The garlic compounds inhibit angiogenesis in GI cancers by downregulating VEGF, AKT/ERK, and NO signaling in tumor-induced endothelial cells. They also inhibit metastasis by inhibiting NF-κB and MMP2/9 signaling pathways. They exhibit antitumor by increasing the activity of NK cells, by secreting cytokine and chemokines, and by enhancing phagocytic activity of macrophages. Therefore, the consumption of garlic compounds may provide some kind of preventive mechanism against GI cancers through modulation of immune system.

Keywords Apoptosis · Gastrointestinal tract cancers · Garlic compounds · Proliferation and metastasis

Abbreviations

AGE	Aged garlic extract
AMC	Allyl mercaptan
COX2	Cyclooxygenase-2
CYP	Cytochrome P450

R. R. Malla (✉)
Cancer Biology Lab, Department of Biochemistry and Bioinformatics, Institute of Science, GITAM (Deemed to be University), Visakhapatnam, India

G. P. Nagaraju (ed.), *Phytochemicals Targeting Tumor Microenvironment in Gastrointestinal Cancers*, https://doi.org/10.1007/978-3-030-48405-7_6

DADS	Diallyl disulfide
DAS	Diallyl sulfide
DATS	Diallyl trisulfide
DNMT1	DNA methyltransferase 1
DVLS-2	Disheveled-2
EMT	Epithelial-mesenchymal transition
FGF-2	Fibroblast growth factor-2
FN	Fibronectin
GSAC	γ-Glutamyl-S-allyl-L-cysteines
HDAC	Histone deacetylase
HIF	Hypoxia-inducible factor
HMG-CoA	β-Hydroxy β-methylglutaryl-CoA
HUVAC	Human umbilical vein endothelial cells
IFN-gamma	Interferon-gamma
IL-2	Interleukin 2
JNK1	c-Jun N-terminal kinases
LEF-1	Lymphoid enhancer factor
MAP kinase	Mitogen-activated protein kinase
MCP-1	Monocyte chemoattractant protein-1
MDM2	Mouse double minute 2 homolog
MDR1	Multidrug resistance protein 1
MMP-2	Matrix metalloproteinase-2
MRP1	Multidrug resistance-associated protein 1
MSI	Microsatellite instability
NK cells	Natural killer cells
NO	Nitric oxide
Nrf-2	Nuclear factor erythroid 2-related factor 2
OSC	Organosulfur compound
PARP	Poly (ADP-ribose) polymerase
PCD	Programmed cell death
ROS	Reactive oxygen species
SAC	S-allyl cysteine
SAMC	S-allyl mercaptocysteine
SPRC	S-propargyl-L-cysteine
STAT-3	Signal transducer and activator of transcription 3
TAMs	Tumor-associated macrophages
TGF-alpha	Transforming growth factor-alpha
TIMP	Tissue inhibitor of metallopeptidase
TNF-alpha	Tumor necrosis factor-alpha
VEGF	Vascular endothelial growth factor
VEGFR-2	Vascular endothelial growth factor receptor-2
VHL	von Hippel-Lindau

1 Introduction

Gastrointestinal tract (GI) cancers are a group of malignancies of GI tract and accessory organs. The etiological causes of GI cancers are primarily preventable lifestyle habits including diet, exercise, alcohol and tobacco, and sanitation. Globally, GI tract cancers are one of the foremost prevalent cancers, diagnosed in more than four million new cases every year, and affect both men and women. The major GI cancers including stomach, colorectal, pancreas, and liver cancers account for more deaths than any other cancers of human body [1]. Worldwide, these cancers are foremost medical and economic burden to patients in both developed and developing countries. Genomic biomarkers have been recognized as valid genetic tools for diagnosis as well as treatment of GI tract cancers [2]. Microsatellite instability (MSI) is recognized as a most promising marker for prognosis and prediction of GI cancers [3, 4]. Also, genotyping of tumors [5] and RAS/BRAF [6], PI3K/Akt [7], Wnt/ß-catenin, and STAT-3 are recognized as important markers of GI tract cancers [8, 9]. Further, genome and epigenome-based biomarkers for GI tract cancers were discovered using high-throughput technology. *RAS/BRAF mutant* genes are predicted as prognostic markers in colon cancer. However, MSI has been demonstrated as a most promising marker for colon cancer. Yu and Cheung proposed MSI as a prognostic biomarker of adenocarcinoma of pancreas [10]. Even though extensive efforts are devoted to develop novel drugs and diagnostic markers, the prognosis of advanced GI cancers is very poor. Large body of experimental as well as epidemiological studies has provided ample evidence to support associations of prevention and reduction of cancer risk with intake of essential cooking ingredients. Garlic is one of the commonly used ingredients of dishes and an extensively used natural remedy in folk medicines. The immunomodulatory and antioxidant activities of garlic are related to anticancer activity against several cancers [11].

2 Health Benefits of Garlic

Garlic has health benefits mainly by sulfur-containing organic compounds as well as their derivatives. The medicinal claims of garlic are treatment of leprosy, diarrhea, constipation, and infections. Garlic can be used as expectorant, antispasmodic, antiseptic, and antihypertensive agent. Further, garlic can be used as bactericidal [12], antibiotic [13], and antifungal [14] agent. Additionally, garlic can reduce chronic bronchitis [15], infections of upper respiratory tract [16], as well as influenza [17, 18]. It can also diminish sugar levels in blood [19] and risk of heart diseases [20, 21]. The most compelling studies reported significant correlation between reduction of risks of GI tract cancers and intake of garlic [22–25].

3 Biologically Active Compounds of Garlic

Garlic is a globally used spice with innumerable medicinal benefits. The most important sulfur-containing natural constituents of fresh garlic are S-ally-L-cysteine sulfoxide (alliin), S-methylcysteine sulfoxide (methiin), γ-glutamyl-S-allyl-L-cysteines (GSAC), and S-allylcysteine. Allicin is a typical garlic compound with pungent smell formed from alliin by allinase during crushing or cutting of garlic [12, 13, 26]. It is highly unstable and rapidly converted to diallyl sulfide (DAS), diallyl disulfide (DADS), diallyl trisulfide (DATS), as well as diallyl tetrasulfide. Allicin, ajoene, allyl propyl disulfide (APDS), DAS, DADS, DATS, S-allyl cysteine (SAC), and S-allyl mercaptocysteine (SAMC) are prominent biologically active compounds of garlic [27]. The prominent organosulfur compounds of garlic and their biological activities of garlic compounds are depicted in Table 6.1.

3.1 Inhibition of Tumor Growth

Organosulfur garlic compounds inhibit proliferation of different human cancer cells [28] including prostate [29], skin [30], colorectal [31], lung [32], neuroblastoma [33], and melanoma [34] cancers. SAMC inhibits growth of colorectal cancer [35] by disruption of microtubules, which are required for the formation of cytoskeleton, and mitotic spindle, which is required for cell division [36]. DADS suppresses H-ras oncogene-containing tumor growth in xenograft model through decreasing the activity of HMG-CoA reductase and by inhibiting binding of p21 to membrane without affecting farnesyl transferase activity [37].

3.2 Inhibition of Cell Cycle

Cell cycle involves simulation of growth, replication, and division, controlled by checkpoints through diverse signal transduction pathways [38, 39]. The checkpoints witness the completion of events in each phase of cell cycle during genomic instability and DNA damage [38, 39]. Most commonly used anticancer agents primarily target cell cycle and interfere with different phases depending on cells, mode of action, as well as target. Garlic-derived compounds can suppress colon cancer cell proliferation by arresting cell cycle [40] through decreasing Cdk1/cyclin B1 activity, disrupting Cdk1 and cyclin B1 complex, and decreasing Cdc25C expression [41]. DATS mediates cell cycle arrest in G2/M phase due to oligosulfide chain (OSC) length [41–44]. In PC-3 cells, DATS mediates cell cycle arrest by increasing phosphorylation of Cdk1 at Tyr 15, inhibiting Cdc25C activity of Cdk1/cyclin B1 complex, increasing phosphorylation at inhibitory site (Ser216), as well as downregulating Cdc25C protein level [45]. It also induces mitotic arrest by altering tubulin network and chromatin condensation as well as by increasing histone H3

Table 6.1 Summary of anticancer activity of allyl sulfides against GI tract cancers

Garlic compound	Mechanism of action of garlic compounds			
	Gastric cancer	Colon cancer	Liver cancer	Pancreatic cancer
DADS	• Inhibits migration and invasiveness • Inhibits MMP-2 and -9 activity • Represses claudin proteins • Induces apoptosis • Decreases Bcl-2 expression • Enhances Fas and Bax expression • Increases caspase-3 activity	• Inhibits proliferation • Enhances apoptosis • Targets ECM proteins • Reduces metastasis • Targets MMP-2, −7, and -9 • Modulates PI3K, Ras, MAP kinases, ERK1/2, JNK1/2, pathways • Enhances early apoptosis • Enhances genomic DNA degradation • Induces cell cycle arrest • Enhances ROS levels • Increases cyclin B1 activity	• Affects proliferation and viability • Induces apoptosis • Activates MAPK pathway • Enhances intracellular ROS • Induces dysregulation of mitochondrial membrane potential • Triggers DNA damage • Induces G2/M cell cycle arrest • Increases mitochondrial apoptotic pathway	• Invasion and migration ability • Protects against cerulein-induced acute pancreatitis
Allicin	• Induces apoptosis • Activates caspase-3 • Activates p38 MAP kinase signaling pathway • Induces mitochondrial dependent apoptosis • Enhances Fas/Fas ligand-dependent apoptosis	• Induces cytotoxicity • Promotes apoptosis • Increases Nrf2 expression	• Induces genotoxicity • Inhibits CYP enzymes • Induces phase II enzymes • Sensitizes HCC cells to 5-FU-induced apoptosis • Ameliorates tamoxifen-induced liver injury • Induces p53-mediated autophagy	• Effectively induces apoptosis • Induces caspase-3 expression • Causes DNA fragmentation • Inhibits cell cycle • Induces p21 (Waf1/Cip1) cyclin-dependent kinase inhibitor expression • Enhances ROS generation
SAMC	• Inhibits tumor growth • Induces apoptosis • Modulates	• In combination with rapamycin, induces apoptosis • Upregulates Bax/Bcl-2 ratio	• Inhibits metastasis • Targets Ki-67 and PCNA • Induces cell cycle arrest at S/G2	–

(continued)

Table 6.1 (continued)

Garlic compound	Mechanism of action of garlic compounds			
	Gastric cancer	Colon cancer	Liver cancer	Pancreatic cancer
	MAPK and PI3K/Akt signaling pathways • Induces depolymerization of microtubule • Activates JNK-1	• Inhibits autophagic activity • Promotes MAPK inhibitor-induced apoptosis	transition • Induces apoptosis • Downregulates Bcl-xL and Bcl-2 proteins • Activates caspase-3 and -9 • Downregulates Cdc25c, Cdc2, and cyclin B1	
DAS	• Protects from MNNG-induced damages • Inhibits cytochrome P450 2E1	• Exhibits chemopreventive activity by increasing G2/M arrest • Increases STAT1-mediated PCD • Upregulates NF-kB expression • Increases caspase-3 activity • Suppresses ERK-2 activity • Promotes expression of drug-resistant gene MDR1 • Promotes expression of MRP3 gene	• Prevents initiation of estrogen-induced cancer • Protects against N-nitrosodiethylamine-induced tumorigenesis • Modulates testosterone-induced oxidative stress • Displays antigenotoxic activity • Prevents hepatocarcinogenesis	–
DATS	• Enhances chemosensitivity by attenuating NF-kB activity	• Enhances MRP1 expression • Inhibits NF-κB pathway • Hamper COX-2 pathway	• Enhances caspase-3-dependent apoptosis • Reduces viability of J5 liver cancer cells • Enhances G2/M phase arrest	• Enhances caspase-3-dependent apoptosis • Reduces viability of J5 liver cancer cells • Inhibits cell proliferation • Induces caspase-3 activity

phosphorylation at serine 10 in PC cells [42]. DATS also arrests cell division at prometaphase of PC-3 cells by activating Chk1 and by accumulating APC/C and cyclin A B1 along with hyperphosphorylation of securin [43]. DADS and SAMC also induce mitotic attest in PC-3 cells [43]. DATS mediates cell cycle arrest through generation of ROS in a JNK-dependent pathway [Ref]. In colorectal cancer cells, DATS induces mitotic arrest in mitotic cells by disrupting the network of microtubules as well as inhibiting the formation of spindle via oxidation-dependent tubulin β (cysteine-12 and -354) modifications [46]. The summary of the mechanism of DATS-mediated G2M arrest of cell cycle is depicted in Fig. 6.1.

Ajoene causes cells cycle arrest at G2/M phase by disrupting microtubule network and inhibiting tubulin polymerization [47]. DADS also mediates cell cycle arrest at S phase [48]. The synthetic derivative of DATS, allitridi, arrests cell cycle in G1 phase by decreasing cyclin D1 level and increasing p27 protein level in gastric cancer cells [49]. The arrest of cell cycle progression by garlic compounds can be mediated by histone modifications. The garlic compound-dependent histone acetylation affects cancer cell proliferation by regulating gene expression. For instance, DADS enhances H4 and H3 histone acetylation, but inhibits deacetylases [50]. Allicin, SAMC, and SAC inhibit colon cancer growth by increasing acetylation of histones [51]. The DADS induces cell cycle of colorectal cancer cells in G2/M phase by inhibiting hyperacetylation of histones H3 and H4, and histone deacetylase, and upregulating p21 levels [52]. DADS also affects cell cycle by decreasing tumor cells at the G1 and S phases with concomitant increasing of G2/M phase [40]. DADS is known to reduce proliferation of cells by inducting cell cycle arrest through inhibition of p34cdc2 kinase [41]. It also inhibits growth of implanted H-ras-dependent tumors by preventing the interaction of p21H-ras with cell membrane in nude mice [37]. The summary of garlic compound-mediated cell cycle arrest is presented in Fig. 6.1.

3.3 Apoptosis

Apoptosis/programmed cell death (PCD) with conserved and tight regulation is essential for normal development of embryo as well as maintenance of tissue homeostasis. Deregulation of apoptosis is the basis for various pathological states of cancer. Hence, apoptosis is an effective target for cancer treatment as well as prevention [53, 54]. The garlic compounds majorly mediate intrinsic or mitochondrial dependent apoptosis by promoting dissipation of mitochondrial membrane potential ($\Delta\Psi m$) along with release of apoptotic mediators into cytosol [55, 56]. The ultimate fate of the mitochondrial dependent apoptosis depends on the levels of anti-apoptotic (Bcl-2 and Bcl-xL) as well as pro-apoptotic (Bax and Bak) proteins of Bcl-2 family [57].

Garlic-derived compounds trigger PCD by modulating Bcl-2 protein levels. For instance, DAS and DADS increase Bax/Bcl-2 ratio in lung cancer cells [58, 59]. DADS treatment also upregulates Bax level with concomitant

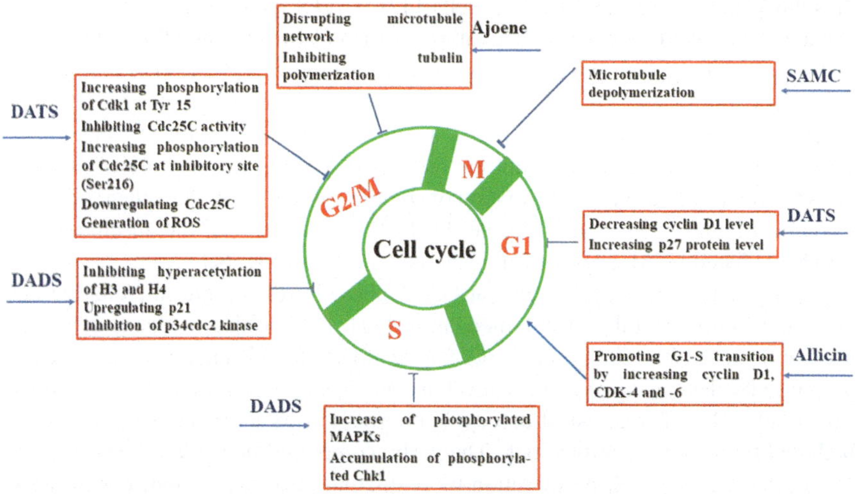

Fig. 6.1 Mechanism of garlic compounds on cell cycle. DATS induces cell arrest at G2M phase by increasing phosphorylation of Cdk1 at Tyr 15, inhibiting Cdc25C activity, increasing phosphorylation of Cdc25C at inhibitory site (Ser216), downregulating Cdc25C and generation of ROS, and inducing cell cycle arrest at G1 phase by decreasing cyclin D1 and increasing p27 protein levels. DADS causes cell cycle arrest at G2M phase by inhibiting hyperacetylation of H3 and H4, upregulating p21, and inhibiting p34cdc2 kinase and S phase by increasing phosphorylated MAPKs and accumulating phosphorylated Chk1. SAMC inhibits cell cycle at M phase by inducing depolymerization of microtubules. Allicin promotes G1-S transition by increasing cyclin D1, CDK-4, and -6. Ajoene induces G2M cell arrest by disrupting microtubule network and inhibiting tubulin polymerization

downregulation of Bcl-xL [60]. DAS and DADS increase apoptosis by enhancing p53 and Bax expression and decreasing Bcl-2 expression [59]. DADS and DATS induce apoptosis by changing the morphology as well as by causing fragmentation of DNA [31, 32]. DADS induces DNA fragmentation by increasing intracellular Ca^{2+} and activating Ca^{2+}-dependent endonucleases.

DATS is more potent in inducing apoptosis compared to other oil-soluble garlic compounds [61]. It induces apoptosis by decreasing expression and JNK-dependent hyperphosphorylation of Bcl-2, which decreases Bcl-2:Bax association and promotes intrinsic apoptotic pathway [61]. DATS also enhances PCD by increasing the expression of Bax as well as Bak [62]. DATS stimulates apoptosis mainly by controlling Akt-mediated Bad pathway [63]. Akt enhances sequestration of Bad in cytosol by phosphorylation and consequently reduces interaction of Bad with Bcl-2 protein. In fact, DATS reduces Akt-dependent phosphorylated Bad (Ser155 and Ser136) levels, thereby diminishing Bad and 14-3-3β interaction [63]. It is experimentally demonstrated that ROS is an intermediary of garlic-induced apoptotic cell death mechanisms. DADS induces cell death by generating ROS [64] via activation of JNK [65]. OSC induces apoptosis by increasing intracellular calcium. They induce release of intracellular Ca^{2+} along with hydrogen peroxide level and activate caspase-3 [31, 32, 66, 67]. DAS and DADS can activate calpain by increasing calcium levels [58]. The Z ajoene promotes apoptosis by caspase-dependent cleavage of Bcl-2 via generation of ROS [68]. SAMC can also induce apoptosis by triggering activation of caspase cascade [36]. The mechanism of garlic compound-induced apoptosis is summarized in Fig. 6.2.

4 Antimetastatic Activity

Angiogenesis is indispensable for tumor growth beyond 1 mm in diameter [69]. Recent reports demonstrated that garlic-derived compounds inhibit tumor-induced angiogenesis and metastasis in cellular and animal models (Fig. 6.3). AGE inhibits proliferation and invasiveness of the endothelial cells by increasing cell adhesion to collagen and fibronectin [70]. AGE reduces endothelial cell-mediated formation of capillary tubes [70]. Even DATS is more efficacious in reducing the viability of HUVEC by increasing active caspase-3 and cleaving PARP as well as apoptosis [71]. DATS mediates reduction of capillary tube formation as well as migration of HUVEC by suppressing the secretion of VEGF, downregulating the expression of VEGFR-2, and inactivating Akt and activating ERK ½ [71]. Alliin also reduces VEGF- and FGF-2-mediated angiogenesis [72]. DADS and DAS reduce MMP-2 and -9 expression [73]. Alliin inhibits FGF2- and VEGF-mediated angiogenesis by upregulating p53 expression and by enhancing the release of NO [72]. Ajoene inhibits metastasis by disrupting the vimentin network [74]. DAS is another OCS of garlic that increases circulatory antiangiogenic factors and IL-2 and TIMP in C57BL/6 mice implanted with B16F-10 melanoma cells [75]. It can also inhibit differentiation [73] and angiogenic features of HUVAC cells by inactivating Akt and downregulating VEGF and VEGF-R2 [71].

Taylor et al. [92] reported that ajoene significantly inhibited lung metastasis of cancer cells. Likewise, SAMC reduced the lung metastasis without effect on local metastasis [93]. DATS inhibited hypoxia-dependent hematogenous metastasis by reducing HIF-1α mRNA expression [76]. DADS suppresses cancer metastasis by SRC/Ras/ERK signaling-dependent upregulation of miR-34a [77]. It can also inhibit invasiveness and cancer metastasis by repressing tight-junction protein claudin and by inactivating invasive proteins MMP-2 and -9 [78]. DADS reduces gastric cancer cell motility and invasion by upregulating the expression of TIMP-1 and -2 [79]. DADS reduces FN-induced metastasis by reducing the activity of gelatinases. It suppresses FN-mediated EMT by enhancing the expression of E-cadherin and cytokeratin-18 and by reducing the expression of N-cadherin and vimentin as well as snail, slug, and twist. It inhibits DVLS-2 and LEF-1 by preventing β-catenin translocation into nucleus and by phosphorylation-dependent inhibition of glycogen synthase kinase-3β [80]. DADS suppresses metastasis by modulating MMP/TIMP ratio through blocking NF-κB and PI3K/AKT pathways [81]. DATS diminishes cancer progression and experimental metastasis by targeting metastasis-related

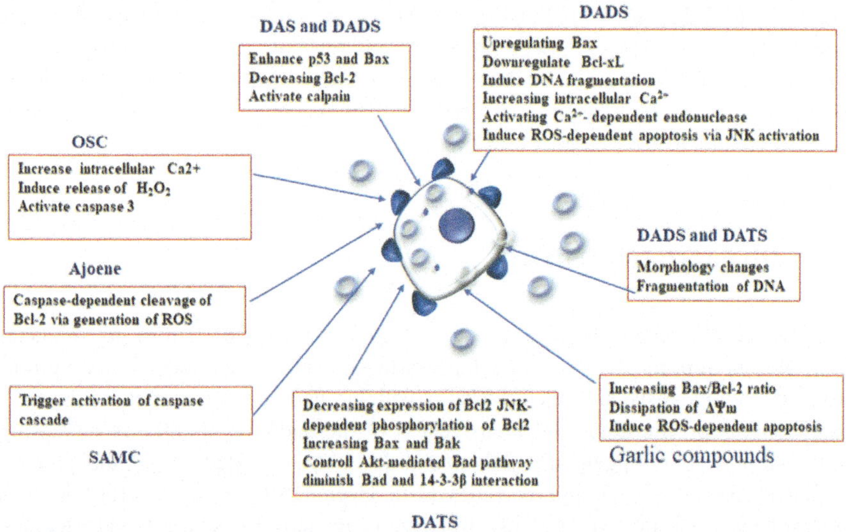

Fig. 6.2 Mechanisms of garlic compound-induced apoptosis. DAS and DADS enhance p53 and Bax, decrease Bcl-2 expression, and activate calpain. DADS upregulates Bax, downregulates Bcl-xL, induces DNA fragmentation, increases intracellular Ca^{2+}, activates Ca^{2+}-dependent endonuclease, and induces ROS-dependent apoptosis via JNK activation; DADS and DATS alter morphology and induce DNA fragmentation. DATS decreases the expression of Bcl2- and JNK-dependent phosphorylation of Bcl2, increases Bax and Bak, controls Akt-mediated Bad pathway, and diminishes Bad and 14-3-3β interaction. SAMC can trigger activation of caspase cascade. Ajoene enhances caspase-dependent cleavage of Bcl-2 via generation of ROS. Oligosulfur compounds (OSC) increase intracellular Ca^{2+}, induce release of H_2O_2, and activate caspase-3

genes, and NF-κB and MMP2/9 genes mediated by thioredoxin system [82]. DATS suppresses colon cancer stem cells by targeting colon spheres and stem cell markers via Wnt/β-catenin pathway [83].

5 Epigenetic Regulation

DADS inhibits cell cycle, induces apoptosis and autophagy, inhibits angiogenesis, and enhances ROS generation in cancer cells by modulating histone deacetylase (HDAC) [84]. It can reduce the metastasis of breast cancer cells by post-transcriptionally attenuating HIF-1α via von Hippel-Lindau (VHL)-dependent degradation [76]. Garlic can regulate gene expression by inhibiting histone deacetylase-mediated histone acetylation [85]. SAC inhibits proliferation of ovarian cancer cells by DNMT1-dependent methylation of DNA [86]. DATS increases the sensitivity of gastric cancer cells to docetaxel by diminishing NF-κB activity through epigenetic upregulation of metallothionein 2A [87]. These studies demonstrated that garlic compounds regulate gene expression through epigenetic mechanism.

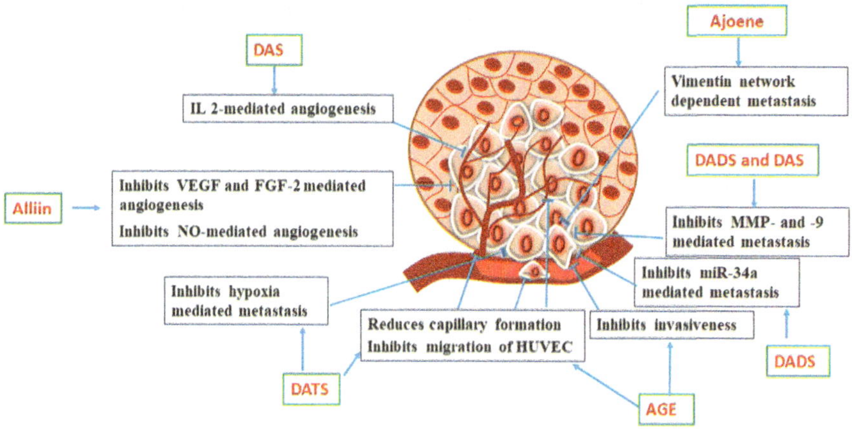

Fig. 6.3 Effect of garlic compounds on metastasis. DAS inhibits IL-2-mediated angiogenesis. DATS inhibits hypoxia-mediated metastasis, and reduces capillary formation and migration of HUVEC. AGE inhibits invasiveness of cancer cells and capillary formation of endothelial cells. DADS inhibits miR-34a-mediated metastasis. DADS and DAS inhibit MMP- and -9-mediated metastasis. Ajoene inhibits vimentin network-dependent metastasis. Alliin inhibits VEGF- and FGF-2-mediated and NO-mediated angiogenesis

6 Antitumor Immunity

AGE (500 mg/day) increases the activity of natural killer (NK) cells in advanced hepatic cancer patients [88]. ABGE-treated gastric cancer cells exhibit antitumor and immunomodulatory activity [89] by secreting IL-2, TNF-alpha, and IFN-gamma, by increasing the activity of NK cells and by enhancing the phagocytic activity of macrophages [90]. Garlic compounds prevent cancer by modulating immune response [91]. DADS inhibits cancer metastasis through modulation of tumor-associated macrophages (TAMs) via suppression of TNFα-mediated release of MCP-1 [92]. These studies support the anticancer activity of garlic compounds through immunomodulation.

The organic sulfuric compounds present in the garlic inhibit major GI tract cancers through different mechanisms. They exhibit stronger antitumor activity against GI malignancies by inhibiting the expression of oncogenes controlling tumor cell proliferation, cell cycle regulation, apoptosis, metastasis, and antitumor immunity (Table 6.1).

7 Antitumor Mechanisms in Gastric Cancer

DADS induces inhibition of migration and invasiveness by enhancing tightness of the tight junctions, and transepithelial electrical resistance [79]. It inhibits MMP-2 and -9 activities along with repression of claudin proteins (claudin-2, -3, and -4). DADS decreases gastric cancer cell growth by inducing apoptosis via decreased Bcl-2 expression-enhanced Fas, and Bax expression, as well as increased activity of casp-3 [93]. Allicin induces apoptosis by activating caspase-3 via p38 MAP kinase signaling pathway [94]. SAMC inhibits human gastric cancer growth in xenografts by inducing apoptosis through modulating MAPK and PI3K/Akt signaling pathways [95]. SAMC can induce apoptosis by depolymerizing microtubule and activating JNK-1 [36]. Allicin induces both mitochondrial dependent intrinsic and Fas/Fas ligand-dependent extrinsic apoptosis pathways in gastric cancers [96]. Garlic oil inhibits proliferation of gastric cancer cells by targeting the expression of cyclin E and autocrine and paracrine loops of TGF-α [97]. Further, combination of garlic oil and resveratrol prompts apoptosis synergistically in gastric cancer cells by increasing Fas and Bax and decreasing Bcl-2 expression [98]. SAMC inhibits gastric cancer cell growth by causing dose-dependent reduction of proliferation and induction of DNA fragmentation and caspase-3 activity via Bax and p53. It inhibits implanted gastric tumors in nude mice by regulating Bcl-2 and Bax expression [99].

8 Antitumor Mechanisms in Colorectal Cancer

Organosulfur garlic compounds are also reported to target metastasis. DADS reduces colorectal cancer growth by inhibiting proliferation and enhancing apoptosis via targeting extracellular matrix proteins [100]. For instance DAS, DADS, and DATS reduce metastasis by targeting MMP-2, -7, and -9 via modulating PI3K, Ras, MAP kinases, ERK1/2, and JNK1/2 pathways [101]. DADS reduces development of colorectal tumors along with dietary factors such as short-chain fatty acids/polysaccharides by reducing cell proliferation, enhancing early apoptosis, activating caspase-3 and -9, and enhancing genomic DNA degradation as well as cell cycle arrest [102].

Allicin induces cytotoxicity and apoptosis via increased expression of Nrf2 transcription factor. DADS inhibits proliferation of colon cancer cells by enhancing ROS-dependent G2/M arrest of cell cycle via increased activity of cyclin B1 and apoptosis by activating p53 [103]. Allyl sulfides modulate the activity of histone deacetylases. Allyl mercaptan (AM) is most potent in inhibiting the activity of histone deacetylase compared to its precursors, DADS and SAMC [104]. AM induces G1-phase arrest by increasing the p21 expression in colorectal cancer cells [105]. DAS exhibits chemopreventive activity by increasing G2/M arrest and STAT1-mediated PCD as well as upregulating NF-kB and caspase-3 and suppressing ERK-2 activity [106]. DADS treatment significantly raises the intracellular Ca^{2+} by enhancing Ca^{2+} influx.

DAS, DADS, and DATS promote the expression of drug-resistant gene multidrug resistant 1 (MDR1) while DAS and DADS promote the expression of MRP3 gene, whereas DATS alone enhances the expression of MRP1 in colorectal cancer cells. However, DADS and DATS induce the expression of MDR1 and MRP1 genes, DADS promotes MRP3 gene while DADS and DATS increase MRP4 and MRP6 genes in in vivo xenograft model [107]. DATS inhibits NF-κB and COX-2 pathways [107]. These observations suggest the antimetastatic proliferation of colon cancer cells by targeting potentials of organosulfur garlic compounds.

9 Antitumor Mechanisms in Liver Cancer

SAC inhibits metastasis of liver cancer cells by targeting Ki-67 and PCNA and inducing cell cycle arrest at S/G2 transition [108]. It also induces apoptosis by downregulating Bcl-xL and Bcl-2 proteins and activating caspase-3 and -9. Moreover, SAC enhances S-phase cell arrest by downregulating Cdc25c, Cdc2, and cyclin B1. DATS showed significantly high anticancer activity against HepG2 cells in caspase-3-dependent apoptosis compared to DAS and DADS [109]. Similarly, DATS reduces viability of J5 liver cancer cells by enhancing the arrest of cells at G2/M phase. DATS-treated group displays significant number of G2/M arrest cells compared to DADS- and DAS-treated groups with increased Cdk7 and cyclin B1 protein levels due to difference in the allyl groups [110]. Water-soluble garlic extracts induced significantly marked effects on HepG2 cells compared to oil-soluble extracts [111]. They induce p53/p21-mediated G2/M arrest of cells and JNK-dependent apoptosis [112]. DADS affects proliferation and viability of hepatic cells by inducing apoptosis through activation of MAPK pathway [112]. Allicin, DAS, DADS, SAC, and AM induce genotoxicity by inhibiting CYP enzymes and inducting phase II enzymes [113]. SAC along with cisplatin inhibits tumor progression and metastasis of liver cancer cells in orthotopic xenograft [113]. Garlic oil reduces N-nitrosodiethylamine (NDEA)-induced liver cancer by decreasing Bcl-2, Bcl-xl, and β-arrestin-2 as well as increasing Bax and caspase-3 [114]. DMBA-induced liver carcinogenesis was prevented by DAS [115, 116].

10 Antitumor Mechanisms in Pancreatic Cancer

DATS reduces the viability of pancreatic carcinoma cells by enhancing G2/M phase and apoptotic cells via increasing Fas, p21, p53, and cyclin B1 expression and decreasing Akt, cyclin D1, MDM2, and Bcl-2 expression [117]. It also increases cleaved caspase 3 and PARP as well as Bim-s and Bim-L isoforms in apoptotic pancreatic cells [117]. S-propargyl-L-cysteine (SPRC) reduces pancreatic cancer growth by inhibiting proliferation and promoting G2/M cell arrest and JNK-dependent apoptosis by enhancing its phosphorylation and by reducing its ubiquitin-dependent degradation [118]. Garlicin at higher concentration inhibits pancreatic tumor growth, while at lower concentration reduces cancer cell invasion and migration via targeting PI3K/AKT signaling pathway [119]. Allicin enhances apoptosis in pancreatic cancer cells by increasing caspase-3 activity, DNA fragmentation, and cell cycle arrest also inducing the expression of p21 (Waf1/Cip1), generation of ROS, and depletion of GSH [120]. Garlic oil shows remarkable inhibition of pancreatic cancer cell proliferation by accumulating cells at G2M phase and presenting significant level of apoptosis [121].

11 Conclusion

In recent past, there has been an increase in research on the impact of garlic and its derivatives in the treatment of various cancers especially GI and associated cancers. The sulfur-containing garlic compounds target multiple cellular mechanisms including proliferation, cell cycle, apoptosis, metastasis, and angiogenesis, which infer their anticancer activities. Garlic compounds also regulate gene expression through modulation of genes controlling epigenetic mechanisms. Further, limited studies demonstrated the antitumor immunity especially aged garlic extract. Additional information on cellular and molecular mechanisms of garlic compounds is required to understand their cancer-preventive mechanism in clinical studies.

Acknowledgments This review was supported by DST-EMR (EMR/2016/002694, dt. 21st August 2017) (RRM) and CSIR (NO. 37(1683)/17/EMR-II, dt. 5th May 2017) (RRM), New Delhi, India.

Conflict of interest: The authors declared that there is no conflict of interest.

References

1. Bjelakovic, G., Nikolova, D., Simonetti, R. G., & Gluud, C. (2008). Antioxidant supplements for preventing gastrointestinal cancers. *Cochrane Database of Systematic Reviews*, (3).
2. Badreddine, R., & Wang, K. K. (2008). Biomarkers in gastrointestinal cancers. *The American Journal of Gastroenterology, 103*(8), 2106–2110.
3. Gupta, R., Sinha, S., & Paul, R. N. (2018). The impact of microsatellite stability status in colorectal cancer. *Current Problems in Cancer, 42*(6), 548–559.
4. Fornasarig, M., Magris, R., & De Re, V. (2018). Molecular and pathological features of gastric cancer in lynch syndrome and familial adenomatous polyposis., *19*(6).
5. Wong, N., Taniere, P., Walsh, S., Wallace, A., Nonaka, D., Jones, T., & Gonzalez, D. (2019). Gastrointestinal stromal tumor with multiple primary tyrosine kinase mutations-clinicopathologic and molecular characterization. *Applied Immunohistochemistry & Molecular Morphology: AIMM, 27*(6), 461–465.

6. Sawada, K., Nakamura, Y., Yamanaka, T., Kuboki, Y., Yamaguchi, D., Yuki, S., Yoshino, T., Komatsu, Y., Sakamoto, N., Okamoto, W., & Fujii, S. (2018). Prognostic and predictive value of HER2 amplification in patients with metastatic colorectal cancer. *Clinical Colorectal Cancer, 17*(3), 198–205.
7. Yin, J., Ji, Z., Hong, Y., Song, Z., Hu, N., Zhuang, M., Bian, B., Liu, Y., & Wu, F. (2018). Sh-MARCH8 inhibits tumorigenesis via PI3K pathway in gastric cancer. *Cellular Physiology and Biochemistry : International Journal of Experimental Cellular Physiology, Biochemistry, and Pharmacology, 49*(1), 306–321.
8. Zhan, T., Rindtorff, N., & Boutros, M. (2017). Wnt signaling in cancer., *36*(11), 1461–1473.
9. Zhang, G. J., Li, L. F., Yang, G. D., Xia, S. S., Wang, R., Leng, Z. W., Liu, Z. L., Tian, H. P., He, Y., Meng, C. Y., Liu, D. Z., Hou, S. L., Tang, X. G., & Zhou, T. (2017). MiR-92a promotes stem cell-like properties by activating Wnt/beta-catenin signaling in colorectal cancer. *Oncotarget, 8*(60), 101760–101770.
10. Sharma, K. L., & Bhatia, V. (2018). Gastrointestinal cancers: Molecular genetics and biomarkers., *2018*, 4513860.
11. Guo, Z., Gong, J., Li, Y., Gu, L., Cao, L., Wang, Z., Zhu, W., & Li, J. (2016). Mucosal microRNAs expression profiles before and after exclusive enteral nutrition therapy in adult patients with Crohn's disease. *Nutrients, 8*(8).
12. Cavallito, C. J., & Bailey, J. H. (1944). Allicin, the antibacterial principle of Allium sativum. I. Isolation, physical properties and antibacterial action. *Journal of the American Chemical Society, 66*(11), 1950–1951.
13. Stoll, A., & Seebeck, E. (1951). Chemical investigations on alliin, the specific principle of garlic. *Advances in Enzymology and Related Subjects of Biochemistry, 11*, 377–400.
14. Moore, G. S., & Atkins, R. D. (1977). The fungicidal and fungistatic effects of an aqueous garlic extract on medically important yeast-like fungi. *Mycologia, 69*(2), 341–348.
15. Gitt, A. K., Winter, U. J., Fritsch, J., Pothoff, G., Sedlak, M., Ehmanns, S., Ostmann, H., & Hilger, H. H. (1994). Comparison of four different methods for respiratory determination of the anaerobic threshold in normal people, and heart- and lung patients. *Zeitschrift fur Kardiologie, 83*(Suppl 3), 37–42.
16. Lissiman, E., Bhasale, A. L., & Cohen, M. (2014). Garlic for the common cold. *The Cochrane Database of Systematic Reviews, 11*, Cd006206.
17. Rasool, A., Khan, M. U., Ali, M. A., Anjum, A. A., Ahmed, I., Aslam, A., Mustafa, G., Masood, S., Ali, M. A., & Nawaz, M. (2017). Anti-avian influenza virus H9N2 activity of aqueous extracts of Zingiber officinalis (ginger) and Allium sativum (garlic) in chick embryos. *Pakistan Journal of Pharmaceutical Sciences, 30*(4), 1341–1344.
18. Tsai, Y., Cole, L. L., Davis, L. E., Lockwood, S. J., Simmons, V., & Wild, G. C. (1985). Antiviral properties of garlic: In vitro effects on influenza B. *Herpes Simplex and Coxsackie Viruses, Planta Medica, 51*(5), 460–461.
19. Sheela, C., Kumud, K., & Augusti, K. (1995). Anti-diabetic effects of onion and garlic sulfoxide amino acids in rats. *Planta Medica, 61*(04), 356–357.
20. Orekhov, A. N., & Grünwald, J. (1997). Effects of garlic on atherosclerosis. *Nutrition, 13* (7–8), 656–663.
21. Milner, J. (1999). Functional foods and health promotion. *The Journal of Nutrition, 129*(7), 1395S–1397S.
22. Fleischauer, A. T., & Arab, L. (2001). Garlic and cancer: A critical review of the epidemiologic literature. *The Journal of Nutrition, 131*(3), 1032S–1040S.
23. Fleischauer, A. T., Poole, C., & Arab, L. (2000). Garlic consumption and cancer prevention: Meta-analyses of colorectal and stomach cancers. *The American Journal of Clinical Nutrition, 72*(4), 1047–1052.
24. Sumiyoshi, H., & Wargovich, M. J. (1990). Chemoprevention of 1,2-dimethylhydrazine-induced colon cancer in mice by naturally occurring organosulfur compounds. *Cancer Research, 50*(16), 5084–5087.

25. Wargovich, M. J. (1987). Diallyl sulfide, a flavor component of garlic (Allium sativum), inhibits dimethylhydrazine-induced colon cancer. *Carcinogenesis, 8*(3), 487–489.
26. Shenoy, N. R., & Choughuley, A. S. (1992). Inhibitory effect of diet related sulphydryl compounds on the formation of carcinogenic nitrosamines. *Cancer Letters, 65*(3), 227–232.
27. Agarwal, K. C. (1996). Therapeutic actions of garlic constituents. *Medicinal Research Reviews, 16*(1), 111–124.
28. Sundaram, S. G., & Milner, J. A. (1993). Impact of organosulfur compounds in garlic on canine mammary tumor cells in culture. *Cancer Letters, 74*(1–2), 85–90.
29. Pinto, J. T., Qiao, C., Xing, J., Rivlin, R. S., Protomastro, M. L., Weissler, M. L., Tao, Y., Thaler, H., & Heston, W. D. (1997). Effects of garlic thioallyl derivatives on growth, glutathione concentration, and polyamine formation of human prostate carcinoma cells in culture. *The American Journal of Clinical Nutrition, 66*(2), 398–405.
30. Wang, H. C., Pao, J., Lin, S. Y., & Sheen, L. Y. (2012). Molecular mechanisms of garlic-derived allyl sulfides in the inhibition of skin cancer progression. *Annals of the New York Academy of Sciences, 1271*, 44–52.
31. Sundaram, S. G., & Milner, J. A. (1996). Diallyl disulfide induces apoptosis of human colon tumor cells. *Carcinogenesis, 17*(4), 669–673.
32. Sakamoto, K., Lawson, L. D., & Milner, J. A. (1997). Allyl sulfides from garlic suppress the in vitro proliferation of human A549 lung tumor cells. *Nutrition and Cancer, 29*(2), 152–156.
33. Karmakar, S., Choudhury, S. R., Banik, N. L., & Ray, S. K. (2011). Molecular mechanisms of anti-cancer action of garlic compounds in neuroblastoma. *Anti-Cancer Agents in Medicinal Chemistry, 11*(4), 398–407.
34. Pratheeshkumar, P., Thejass, P., & Kutan, G. (2010). Diallyl disulfide induces caspase-dependent apoptosis via mitochondria-mediated intrinsic pathway in B16F-10 melanoma cells by up-regulating p53, caspase-3 and down-regulating pro-inflammatory cytokines and nuclear factor-kappabeta-mediated Bcl-2 activation. *Journal of Environmental Pathology, Toxicology and Oncology : Official Organ of the International Society for Environmental Toxicology and Cancer, 29*(2), 113–125.
35. Liang, D., Qin, Y., Zhao, W., Zhai, X., Guo, Z., Wang, R., Tong, L., Lin, L., Chen, H., Wong, Y. C., & Zhong, Z. (2011). S-allylmercaptocysteine effectively inhibits the proliferation of colorectal cancer cells under in vitro and in vivo conditions. *Cancer Letters, 310*(1), 69–76.
36. Xiao, D., Pinto, J. T., Soh, J. W., Deguchi, A., Gundersen, G. G., Palazzo, A. F., Yoon, J. T., Shirin, H., & Weinstein, I. B. (2003). Induction of apoptosis by the garlic-derived compound S-allylmercaptocysteine (SAMC) is associated with microtubule depolymerization and c-Jun NH(2)-terminal kinase 1 activation. *Cancer Research, 63*(20), 6825–6837.
37. Singh, S. V., Mohan, R. R., Agarwal, R., Benson, P. J., Hu, X., Rudy, M. A., Xia, H., Katoh, A., Srivastava, S. K., Mukhtar, H., Gupta, V., & Zaren, H. A. (1996). Novel anti-carcinogenic activity of an organosulfide from garlic: Inhibition of H-RAS oncogene transformed tumor growth in vivo by diallyl disulfide is associated with inhibition of p21H-RAS processing. *Biochemical and Biophysical Research Communications, 225*(2), 660–665.
38. Molinari, M. (2000). Cell cycle checkpoints and their inactivation in human cancer. *Cell Proliferation, 33*(5), 261–274.
39. Murray, A. W. (2004). Recycling the cell cycle: Cyclins revisited. *Cell, 116*(2), 221–234.
40. Knowles, L. M., & Milner, J. A. (1998). Depressed p34cdc2 kinase activity and G2/M phase arrest induced by diallyl disulfide in HCT-15 cells. *Nutrition and Cancer, 30*(3), 169–174.
41. Knowles, L. M., & Milner, J. A. (2000). Diallyl disulfide inhibits p34(cdc2) kinase activity through changes in complex formation and phosphorylation. *Carcinogenesis, 21*(6), 1129–1134.
42. Herman-Antosiewicz, A., & Singh, S. V. (2005). Checkpoint kinase 1 regulates diallyl trisulfide-induced mitotic arrest in human prostate cancer cells. *The Journal of Biological Chemistry, 280*(31), 28519–28528.
43. Herman-Antosiewicz, A., Stan, S. D., Hahm, E. R., Xiao, D., & Singh, S. V. (2007). Activation of a novel ataxia-telangiectasia mutated and Rad3 related/checkpoint kinase

1-dependent prometaphase checkpoint in cancer cells by diallyl trisulfide, a promising cancer chemopreventive constituent of processed garlic. *Molecular Cancer Therapeutics, 6*(4), 1249–1261.

44. Antosiewicz, J., Herman-Antosiewicz, A., Marynowski, S. W., & Singh, S. V. (2006). C-Jun NH(2)-terminal kinase signaling axis regulates diallyl trisulfide-induced generation of reactive oxygen species and cell cycle arrest in human prostate cancer cells. *Cancer Research, 66*(10), 5379–5386.
45. Xiao, D., Herman-Antosiewicz, A., Antosiewicz, J., Xiao, H., Brisson, M., Lazo, J. S., & Singh, S. V. (2005). Diallyl trisulfide-induced G(2)-M phase cell cycle arrest in human prostate cancer cells is caused by reactive oxygen species-dependent destruction and hyperphosphorylation of Cdc 25 C. *Oncogene, 24*(41), 6256–6268.
46. Hosono, T., Fukao, T., Ogihara, J., Ito, Y., Shiba, H., Seki, T., & Ariga, T. (2005). Diallyl trisulfide suppresses the proliferation and induces apoptosis of human colon cancer cells through oxidative modification of beta-tubulin. *The Journal of Biological Chemistry, 280* (50), 41487–41493.
47. Li, M., Ciu, J. R., Ye, Y., Min, J. M., Zhang, L. H., Wang, K., Gares, M., Cros, J., Wright, M., & Leung-Tack, J. (2002). Antitumor activity of Z-ajoene, a natural compound purified from garlic: Antimitotic and microtubule-interaction properties. *Carcinogenesis, 23*(4), 573–579.
48. Zhang, Y. W., Wen, J., Xiao, J. B., Talbot, S. G., Li, G. C., & Xu, M. (2006). Induction of apoptosis and transient increase of phosphorylated MAPKs by diallyl disulfide treatment in human nasopharyngeal carcinoma CNE2 cells. *Archives of Pharmacal Research, 29*(12), 1125–1131.
49. Lan, H., & Lu, Y. Y. (2003). Effect of allitridi on cyclin D1 and p27(Kip1) protein expression in gastric carcinoma BGC823 cells. *Ai zheng = Aizheng = Chinese Journal of Cancer, 22*(12), 1268–1271.
50. Lea, M. A., Randolph, V. M., & Patel, M. (1999). Increased acetylation of histones induced by diallyl disulfide and structurally related molecules. *International Journal of Oncology, 15*(2), 347–352.
51. Lea, M. A., Rasheed, M., Randolph, V. M., Khan, F., Shareef, A., & desBordes, C. (2002). Induction of histone acetylation and inhibition of growth of mouse erythroleukemia cells by S-allylmercaptocysteine. *Nutrition and Cancer, 43*(1), 90–102.
52. Druesne, N., Pagniez, A., Mayeur, C., Thomas, M., Cherbuy, C., Duee, P. H., Martel, P., & Chaumontet, C. (2004). Repetitive treatments of colon HT-29 cells with diallyl disulfide induce a prolonged hyperacetylation of histone H3 K14. *Annals of the New York Academy of Sciences, 1030*, 612–621.
53. Kaufmann, S. H., & Gores, G. J. (2000). Apoptosis in cancer: Cause and cure. *BioEssays : News and Reviews in Molecular, Cellular and Developmental Biology, 22*(11), 1007–1017.
54. Ghobrial, I. M., Witzig, T. E., & Adjei, A. A. (2005). Targeting apoptosis pathways in cancer therapy. *CA: a Cancer Journal for Clinicians, 55*(3), 178–194.
55. Hengartner, M. O. (2000). The biochemistry of apoptosis. *Nature, 407*(6805), 770–776.
56. Thornberry, N. A., & Lazebnik, Y. (1998). Caspases: Enemies within. *Science (New York, N. Y.), 281*(5381), 1312–1316.
57. Chao, D. T., & Korsmeyer, S. J. (1998). BCL-2 family: Regulators of cell death. *Annual Review of Immunology, 16*, 395–419.
58. Karmakar, S., Banik, N. L., Patel, S. J., & Ray, S. K. (2007). Garlic compounds induced calpain and intrinsic caspase cascade for apoptosis in human malignant neuroblastoma SH-SY5Y cells. *Apoptosis : An International Journal On Programmed Cell Death, 12*(4), 671–684.
59. Hong, Y. S., Ham, Y. A., Choi, J. H., & Kim, J. (2000). Effects of allyl sulfur compounds and garlic extract on the expression of Bcl-2, Bax, and p53 in non-small cell lung cancer cell lines. *Experimental & Molecular Medicine, 32*(3), 127–134.

60. Nakagawa, H., Tsuta, K., Kiuchi, K., Senzaki, H., Tanaka, K., Hioki, K., & Tsubura, A. (2001). Growth inhibitory effects of diallyl disulfide on human breast cancer cell lines. *Carcinogenesis, 22*(6), 891–897.
61. Xiao, D., Choi, S., Johnson, D. E., Vogel, V. G., Johnson, C. S., Trump, D. L., Lee, Y. J., & Singh, S. V. (2004). Diallyl trisulfide-induced apoptosis in human prostate cancer cells involves c-Jun N-terminal kinase and extracellular-signal regulated kinase-mediated phosphorylation of Bcl-2. *Oncogene, 23*(33), 5594–5606.
62. Kim, Y. A., Xiao, D., Xiao, H., Powolny, A. A., Lew, K. L., Reilly, M. L., Zeng, Y., Wang, Z., & Singh, S. V. (2007). Mitochondria-mediated apoptosis by diallyl trisulfide in human prostate cancer cells is associated with generation of reactive oxygen species and regulated by Bax/Bak. *Molecular Cancer Therapeutics, 6*(5), 1599–1609.
63. Xiao, D., & Singh, S. V. (2006). Diallyl trisulfide, a constituent of processed garlic, inactivates Akt to trigger mitochondrial translocation of BAD and caspase-mediated apoptosis in human prostate cancer cells. *Carcinogenesis, 27*(3), 533–540.
64. Kwon, K. B., Yoo, S. J., Ryu, D. G., Yang, J. Y., Rho, H. W., Kim, J. S., Park, J. W., Kim, H. R., & Park, B. H. (2002). Induction of apoptosis by diallyl disulfide through activation of caspase-3 in human leukemia HL-60 cells. *Biochemical Pharmacology, 63*(1), 41–47.
65. Filomeni, G., Aquilano, K., Rotilio, G., & Ciriolo, M. R. (2003). Reactive oxygen species-dependent c-Jun NH2-terminal kinase/c-Jun signaling cascade mediates neuroblastoma cell death induced by diallyl disulfide. *Cancer Research, 63*(18), 5940–5949.
66. Sundaram, S. G., & Milner, J. A. (1996). Diallyl disulfide inhibits the proliferation of human tumor cells in culture. *Biochimica et Biophysica Acta, 1315*(1), 15–20.
67. Park, E. K., Kwon, K. B., Park, K. I., Park, B. H., & Jhee, E. C. (2002). Role of Ca(2+) in diallyl disulfide-induced apoptotic cell death of HCT-15 cells. *Experimental & Molecular Medicine, 34*(3), 250–257.
68. Li, M., Min, J. M., Cui, J. R., Zhang, L. H., Wang, K., Valette, A., Davrinche, C., Wright, M., & Leung-Tack, J. (2002). Z-ajoene induces apoptosis of HL-60 cells: Involvement of Bcl-2 cleavage. *Nutrition and Cancer, 42*(2), 241–247.
69. Folkman, J. (2003). Fundamental concepts of the angiogenic process. *Current Molecular Medicine, 3*(7), 643–651.
70. Matsuura, N., Miyamae, Y., Yamane, K., Nagao, Y., Hamada, Y., Kawaguchi, N., Katsuki, T., Hirata, K., Sumi, S., & Ishikawa, H. (2006). Aged garlic extract inhibits angiogenesis and proliferation of colorectal carcinoma cells. *The Journal of Nutrition, 136*(3 Suppl), 842s–846s.
71. Xiao, D., Li, M., Herman-Antosiewicz, A., Antosiewicz, J., Xiao, H., Lew, K. L., Zeng, Y., Marynowski, S. W., & Singh, S. V. (2006). Diallyl trisulfide inhibits angiogenic features of human umbilical vein endothelial cells by causing Akt inactivation and down-regulation of VEGF and VEGF-R2. *Nutrition and Cancer, 55*(1), 94–107.
72. Mousa, A. S., & Mousa, S. A. (2005). Anti-angiogenesis efficacy of the garlic ingredient alliin and antioxidants: Role of nitric oxide and p53. *Nutrition and Cancer, 53*(1), 104–110.
73. Thejass, P., & Kuttan, G. (2007). Inhibition of angiogenic differentiation of human umbilical vein endothelial cells by diallyl disulfide (DADS). *Life Sciences, 80*(6), 515–521.
74. Kaschula, C. H., Tuveri, R., Ngarande, E., Dzobo, K., Barnett, C., Kusza, D. A., Graham, L. M., Katz, A. A., Rafudeen, M. S., Parker, M. I., Hunter, R., & Schafer, G. (2019). The garlic compound ajoene covalently binds vimentin, disrupts the vimentin network and exerts anti-metastatic activity in cancer cells. *BMC Cancer, 19*(1), 248.
75. Thejass, P., & Kuttan, G. (2007). Antiangiogenic activity of diallyl sulfide (DAS). *International Immunopharmacology, 7*(3), 295–305.
76. Wei, Z., Shan, Y., Tao, L., Liu, Y., Zhu, Z., Liu, Z., Wu, Y., Chen, W., Wang, A., & Lu, Y. (2017). Diallyl trisulfides, a natural histone deacetylase inhibitor, attenuate HIF-1alpha synthesis, and decreases breast cancer metastasis. *Molecular Carcinogenesis, 56*(10), 2317–2331.

77. Xiao, X., Chen, B., Liu, X., Liu, P., Zheng, G., Ye, F., Tang, H., & Xie, X. (2014). Diallyl disulfide suppresses SRC/Ras/ERK signaling-mediated proliferation and metastasis in human breast cancer by up-regulating miR-34a. *PLoS One, 9*(11), e112720.
78. Shin, D. Y., Kim, G. Y., Kim, J. I., Yoon, M. K., Kwon, T. K., Lee, S. J., Choi, Y. W., Kang, H. S., Yoo, Y. H., & Choi, Y. H. (2010). Anti-invasive activity of diallyl disulfide through tightening of tight junctions and inhibition of matrix metalloproteinase activities in LNCaP prostate cancer cells. *Toxicology In Vitro : An International Journal Published in Association with BIBRA, 24*(6), 1569–1576.
79. Park, H. S., Kim, G. Y., Choi, I. W., Kim, N. D., Hwang, H. J., Choi, Y. W., & Choi, Y. H. (2011). Inhibition of matrix metalloproteinase activities and tightening of tight junctions by diallyl disulfide in AGS human gastric carcinoma cells. *Journal of Food Science, 76*(4), T105–T111.
80. Das, B., & Sinha, D. (2019). Diallyl disulphide suppresses the canonical Wnt signaling pathway and reverses the fibronectin-induced epithelial mesenchymal transition of A549 lung cancer cells. *Food & Function, 10*(1), 191–202.
81. Yin, X., Feng, C., Han, L., Ma, Y., Jiao, Y., Wang, J., Jia, L., Jing, F., Gao, X., Zhang, Y., & Zhang, J. (2018). Diallyl disulfide inhibits the metastasis of type esophageal gastric junction adenocarcinoma cells via NF-kappaB and PI3K/AKT signaling pathways in vitro. *Oncology Reports, 39*(2), 784–794.
82. Liu, Y., Zhao, Y., Wei, Z., Tao, L., Sheng, X., Wang, S., Chen, J., Ruan, J., Liu, Z., Cao, Y., Shan, Y., Wang, A., Chen, W., & Lu, Y. (2018). Targeting thioredoxin system with an organosulfur compound, diallyl trisulfide (DATS), attenuates progression and metastasis of triple-negative breast cancer (TNBC). *Cellular Physiology and Biochemistry : International Journal of Experimental Cellular Physiology, Biochemistry, and Pharmacology, 50*(5), 1945–1963.
83. Zhang, Q., Li, X. T., Chen, Y., Chen, J. Q., Zhu, J. Y., Meng, Y., Wang, X. Q., Li, Y., Geng, S. S., Xie, C. F., Wu, J. S., & Zhong, C. Y. (2018). Wnt/beta-catenin signaling mediates the suppressive effects of diallyl trisulfide on colorectal cancer stem cells., *81*(6), 969–977.
84. Singh, A. K., Bishayee, A., Pandey, A. K. (2018). Targeting histone deacetylases with natural and synthetic agents: An emerging anticancer strategy. *Nutrients, 10*(6), 731.
85. Druesne-Pecollo, N., & Latino-Martel, P. (2011). Modulation of histone acetylation by garlic sulfur compounds. *Anti-Cancer Agents in Medicinal Chemistry, 11*(3), 254–259.
86. Xu, Y., Su, D., Zhu, L., Zhang, S., Ma, S., Wu, K., Yuan, Q., & Lin, N. (2018). S-allylcysteine suppresses ovarian cancer cell proliferation by DNA methylation through DNMT1. *Journal of Ovarian Research, 11*(1), 39.
87. Pan, Y., Lin, S., Xing, R., Zhu, M., Lin, B., Cui, J., Li, W., Gao, J., Shen, L., Zhao, Y., Guo, M., Wang, J. M., Huang, J., & Lu, Y. (2016). Epigenetic upregulation of metallothionein 2a by diallyl trisulfide enhances chemosensitivity of human gastric cancer cells to docetaxel through attenuating NF-kappaB activation. *Antioxidants & Redox Signaling, 24*(15), 839–854.
88. Ishikawa, H., Saeki, T., Otani, T., Suzuki, T., Shimozuma, K., Nishino, H., Fukuda, S., & Morimoto, K. (2006). Aged garlic extract prevents a decline of NK cell number and activity in patients with advanced cancer. *The Journal of Nutrition, 136*(3 Suppl), 816s–820s.
89. Wang, X., Jiao, F., Wang, Q. W., Wang, J., Yang, K., Hu, R. R., Liu, H. C., Wang, H. Y., & Wang, Y. S. (2012). Aged black garlic extract induces inhibition of gastric cancer cell growth in vitro and in vivo. *Molecular Medicine Reports, 5*(1), 66–72.
90. Kyo, E., Uda, N., Suzuki, A., Kakimoto, M., Ushijima, M., Kasuga, S., & Itakura, Y. (1998). Immunomodulation and antitumor activities of aged garlic extract. *Phytomedicine : International Journal of Phytotherapy and Phytopharmacology, 5*(4), 259–267.
91. Schafer, G., & Kaschula, C. H. (2014). The immunomodulation and anti-inflammatory effects of garlic organosulfur compounds in cancer chemoprevention. *Anti-Cancer Agents in Medicinal Chemistry, 14*(2), 233–240.

92. Bauer, D., Mazzio, E., Soliman, K. F., Taka, E., Oriaku, E., Womble, T., & Darling-Reed, S. (2014). Diallyl disulfide inhibits TNFalpha-induced CCL2 release by MDA-MB-231 cells. *Anticancer Research, 34*(6), 2763–2770.
93. Lee, J. E., Lee, R. A., Kim, K. H., & Lee, J. H. (2011). Induction of apoptosis with diallyl disulfide in AGS gastric cancer cell line. *Journal of the Korean Surgical Society, 81*(2), 85–95.
94. Zhang, X., Zhu, Y., Duan, W., Feng, C., & He, X. (2015). Allicin induces apoptosis of the MGC-803 human gastric carcinoma cell line through the p38 mitogen-activated protein kinase/caspase-3 signaling pathway. *Molecular Medicine Reports, 11*(4), 2755–2760.
95. Zhu, X., Jiang, X., Li, A., Sun, Y., Liu, Y., Sun, X., Feng, X., Li, S., & Zhao, Z. (2017). S-allylmercaptocysteine suppresses the growth of human gastric cancer xenografts through induction of apoptosis and regulation of MAPK and PI3K/Akt signaling pathways. *Biochemical and Biophysical Research Communications, 491*(3), 821–826.
96. Zhang, W., Ha, M., Gong, Y., Xu, Y., Dong, N., & Yuan, Y. (2010). Allicin induces apoptosis in gastric cancer cells through activation of both extrinsic and intrinsic pathways. *Oncology Reports, 24*(6), 1585–1592.
97. Liang, W. J., Yan, X., Zhang, W. D., & Luo, R. C. (2007). Garlic oil inhibits cyclin E expression in gastric adenocarcinoma cells. *Nan fang yi ke da xue xue bao = Journal of Southern Medical University, 27*(8), 1241–1243.
98. Zheng, G. H., & Li, H. Q. (2008). Effects of garlic oil combined with resveratrol on inducting of apoptosis and expression of Fas, Bcl-2 and Bax in human gastric cancer cell line. *Zhonghua yu fang yi xue za zhi [Chinese Journal of Preventive Medicine], 42*(1), 39–42.
99. Lee, Y. (2008). Induction of apoptosis by S-allylmercapto-L-cysteine, a biotransformed garlic derivative, on a human gastric cancer cell line. *International Journal of Molecular Medicine, 21*(6), 765–770.
100. Yu, C. S., Huang, A. C., Lai, K. C., Huang, Y. P., Lin, M. W., Yang, J. S., & Chung, J. G. (2012). Diallyl trisulfide induces apoptosis in human primary colorectal cancer cells. *Oncology Reports, 28*(3), 949–954.
101. Lai, K. C., Hsu, S. C., Kuo, C. L., Yang, J. S., Ma, C. Y., Lu, H. F., Tang, N. Y., Hsia, T. C., Ho, H. C., & Chung, J. G. (2013). Diallyl sulfide, diallyl disulfide, and diallyl trisulfide inhibit migration and invasion in human colon cancer Colo 205 cells through the inhibition of matrix metalloproteinase-2, -7, and -9 expressions. *Environmental Toxicology, 28*(9), 479–488.
102. Altonsy, M. O., & Andrews, S. C. (2011). Diallyl disulphide, a beneficial component of garlic oil, causes a redistribution of cell-cycle growth phases, induces apoptosis, and enhances butyrate-induced apoptosis in colorectal adenocarcinoma cells (HT-29). *Nutrition and Cancer, 63*(7), 1104–1113.
103. Jo, H. J., Song, J. D., Kim, K. M., Cho, Y. H., Kim, K. H., & Park, Y. C. (2008). Diallyl disulfide induces reversible G2/M phase arrest on a p53-independent mechanism in human colon cancer HCT-116 cells. *Oncology Reports, 19*(1), 275–280.
104. Nian, H., Delage, B., Pinto, J. T., & Dashwood, R. H. (2008). Allyl mercaptan, a garlic-derived organosulfur compound, inhibits histone deacetylase and enhances Sp3 binding on the P21WAF1 promoter. *Carcinogenesis, 29*(9), 1816–1824.
105. Gerhauser, C. (2013). Cancer chemoprevention and nutriepigenetics: State of the art and future challenges. *Topics in Current Chemistry, 329*, 73–132.
106. Trio, P. Z., You, S., He, X., He, J., Sakao, K., & Hou, D. X. (2014). Chemopreventive functions and molecular mechanisms of garlic organosulfur compounds. *Food & Function, 5* (5), 833–844.
107. Lai, K. C., Kuo, C. L., Ho, H. C., Yang, J. S., Ma, C. Y., Lu, H. F., Huang, H. Y., Chueh, F. S., Yu, C. C., & Chung, J. G. (2012). Diallyl sulfide, diallyl disulfide and diallyl trisulfide affect drug resistant gene expression in Colo 205 human colon cancer cells in vitro and in vivo. *Phytomedicine : International Journal of Phytotherapy and Phytopharmacology, 19*(7), 625–630.

108. Ng, K. T., Guo, D. Y., Cheng, Q., Geng, W., Ling, C. C., Li, C. X., Liu, X. B., Ma, Y. Y., Lo, C. M., Poon, R. T., Fan, S. T., & Man, K. (2012). A garlic derivative, S-allylcysteine (SAC), suppresses proliferation and metastasis of hepatocellular carcinoma. *PLoS One, 7*(2), e31655.
109. Iciek, M., Kwiecien, I., Chwatko, G., Sokolowska-Jezewicz, M., Kowalczyk-Pachel, D., & Rokita, H. (2012). The effects of garlic-derived sulfur compounds on cell proliferation, caspase 3 activity, thiol levels and anaerobic sulfur metabolism in human hepatoblastoma HepG2 cells. *Cell Biochemistry and Function, 30*(3), 198–204.
110. Wu, C. C., Chung, J. G., Tsai, S. J., Yang, J. H., & Sheen, L. Y. (2004). Differential effects of allyl sulfides from garlic essential oil on cell cycle regulation in human liver tumor cells. *Food and Chemical Toxicology : An International Journal Published for the British Industrial Biological Research Association, 42*(12), 1937–1947.
111. De Martino, A., Filomeni, G., Aquilano, K., Ciriolo, M. R., & Rotilio, G. (2006). Effects of water garlic extracts on cell cycle and viability of HepG2 hepatoma cells. *The Journal of Nutritional Biochemistry, 17*(11), 742–749.
112. Tsai, C. W., Chen, H. W., Yang, J. J., Sheen, L. Y., & Lii, C. K. (2007). Diallyl disulfide and diallyl trisulfide up-regulate the expression of the pi class of glutathione S-transferase via an AP-1-dependent pathway. *Journal of Agricultural and Food Chemistry, 55*(3), 1019–1026.
113. Belloir, C., Singh, V., Daurat, C., Siess, M. H., & Le Bon, A. M. (2006). Protective effects of garlic sulfur compounds against DNA damage induced by direct- and indirect-acting genotoxic agents in HepG2 cells. *Food and Chemical Toxicology : An International Journal Published for the British Industrial Biological Research Association, 44*(6), 827–834.
114. Zhang, C. L., Zeng, T., Zhao, X. L., Yu, L. H., Zhu, Z. P., & Xie, K. Q. (2012). Protective effects of garlic oil on hepatocarcinoma induced by N-nitrosodiethylamine in rats. *International Journal of Biological Sciences, 8*(3), 363–374.
115. Khataibeh, M., Abu-Alruz, K., Al-Widyan, O., Abu-Samak, M., & Al-Qudah, J. (2007). Combined supplementation of soy and garlic modulate biochemical parameters of 7,12-dimethylbenz[alpha]anthracene induced mammary cancer in female albino rats. *Pakistan Journal of Biological Sciences : PJBS, 10*(14), 2308–2313.
116. Arora, R., Bhushan, S., Kumar, R., Mannan, R., Kaur, P., Singh, A. P., Singh, B., Vig, A. P., Sharma, D., & Arora, S. (2014). Hepatic dysfunction induced by 7, 12-dimethylbenz(alpha) anthracene and its obviation with erucin using enzymatic and histological changes as indicators. *PLoS One, 9*(11), e112614.
117. Ma, H. B., Huang, S., Yin, X. R., Zhang, Y., & Di, Z. L. (2014). Apoptotic pathway induced by diallyl trisulfide in pancreatic cancer cells. *World Journal of Gastroenterology, 20*(1), 193–203.
118. Wang, W., Cheng, J., & Zhu, Y. (2015). The JNK signaling pathway is a novel molecular target for S-propargyl- L-cysteine, a naturally-occurring garlic derivatives: Link to its anticancer activity in pancreatic cancer in vitro and in vivo. *Current Cancer Drug Targets, 15*(7), 613–623.
119. Xie, K., Nian, J., Zhu, X., Geng, X., & Liu, F. (2015). Modulatory role of garlicin in migration and invasion of intrahepatic cholangiocarcinoma via PI3K/AKT pathway. *International Journal of Clinical and Experimental Pathology, 8*(11), 14028–14033.
120. Chhabria, S. V., Akbarsha, M. A., Li, A. P., Kharkar, P. S., & Desai, K. B. (2015). In situ allicin generation using targeted alliinase delivery for inhibition of MIA PaCa-2 cells via epigenetic changes, oxidative stress and cyclin-dependent kinase inhibitor (CDKI) expression. *Apoptosis : An International Journal on Programmed Cell Death, 20*(10), 1388–1409.
121. Lan, X., Sun, H., Liu, J., Lin, Y., Zhu, Z., Han, X., Sun, X., Li, X., Zhang, H., & Tang, Z. (2013). Effects of garlic oil on pancreatic cancer cells. *Asian Pacific Journal of Cancer Prevention : APJCP, 14*(10), 5905–5910.

Chapter 7
Combination of Phytochemicals with Nanotechnology for Targeting GI Cancer Therapy

Harshvardhan Chauhan and Masood Alam

Abstract Gastrointestinal (GI) cancer is one of the lethal among all cancers which includes different types of cancers of the GI system, i.e., esophagus, liver, gallbladder, small intestine, pancreas, stomach, and bowel (large intestine or colon and rectum). Therefore, several efforts are being made to find more suitable anticancer agents based on synthetic and phytochemical approaches. There is the number of phytochemicals reported with prominent anticancer activities, but they include the number of limitations such as poor bioavailability, pitiable water solubility and low penetration into cells, contracted therapeutic index, and higher hepatic disposition. Therefore, this chapter discusses and summarizes the contemporary advances that have been made for the management of GI cancers in the field of nanotechnology with a combination of phytochemicals.

Keywords Phytochemicals · Nanoparticles · Targeted drug delivery · GI cancer

Abbreviations

Akt	Protein kinase-B
AuNPs	Gold nanoparticles
Bcl-2	B-cell lymphoma-2
BiNRs	Bismuth oxide nanorods
COX-2	Cyclooxygenase-2
DAS	Diallyl sulfide
EAC	Esophageal adenocarcinoma
ERK1/2,	Extracellular signal-regulated kinases 1 and 2
ESCC	Esophageal squamous cell carcinoma
FMNP	Fluorescent magnetic nanoparticle
HCT	Human colon carcinoma cells

H. Chauhan · M. Alam (✉)
Department of Applied Sciences and Humanities, Jamia Millia Islamia (A Central University), New Delhi, India
e-mail: malam@jmi.ac.in

G. P. Nagaraju (ed.), *Phytochemicals Targeting Tumor Microenvironment in Gastrointestinal Cancers*, https://doi.org/10.1007/978-3-030-48405-7_7

HePG-2	Hepatocellular carcinoma
HPMC	Hydroxypropyl methylcellulose
HRT	Hormone replacement therapy
MAPK	Mitogen-activated protein kinase
MMP-9	Matrix metallopeptidase-9
MRI	Magnetic resonance imaging
MRS	Magnetic resonance spectroscopy
MSCs	Marked mesenchymal stem cells
NF-κB	Nuclear factor kappa B
NIR	Near-infrared
P13K	Phosphatidylinositol 3-kinase
PEG	Polyethylene glycol
PET	Positron-emission tomography
PtNDs	Platinum nanodendrites
PVA	Polyvinyl alcohol
QDs	Quantum dots
SCC	Squamous cell carcinoma
SPECT	Single-photon emission computed tomography
SPIONs	Superparamagnetic iron oxide nanoparticles
STAT3	Signal transducer and activator of transcription 3
TNF-α	Tumor necrosis factor-alpha

1 Introduction

Cancer is a broad term that includes more than 200 types. It is known as one of the most deadly diseases to living organisms affecting not only humans but also animals and other living organisms [1]. It could be easily understood in general terms as uncontrolled and abnormal growth or division of cells in the body which may result in the form of tumors, can damage the immune system, and can be fatal [2]. Moreover, cancer cells may also move from affected original sites and travel through the bloodstream and lymph systems, lodge in other organs where they grow, and repeat uncontrolled cell division, known as metastasis. The majority of cancers, i.e., around 90–95%, could be observed due to genetic mutations from environmental and lifestyle factors [1, 3], i.e., pollution, radiation, infections, unhealthy diet, use of tobacco and alcohol, and lack of physical activities. The rest of the cases were observed due to inherited genes [4].

According to the WHO report published in 2018, cancer is the second deadly disease globally which is responsible for 9.6 million mortality worldwide with the highest economic impact. It is estimated that one death among each six was due to cancer and a total of around $1.16 trillion of the economy was spent on cancer in 2010. WHO data show that around 22% of cancer deaths occurred due to the use of tobacco and around 25% of cases were observed due to infections in low- and middle-income countries [5]. Cancer factsheet 2018 of WHO also includes the most common types of cancer which were found more responsible for mortality including lung cancer (2.09 million cases), prostate cancer (1.28 million cases), breast cancer (2.09 million cases), colorectal cancer (1.80 million cases), stomach cancer (1.03 million cases), and skin cancer (non-melanoma) (1.04 million cases).

2 Gastrointestinal Cancer (GI Cancer)

The primary purpose of the gastrointestinal tract is to break down the food from a complex structure to a simple one, so nutrients can be absorbed to provide energy. GI cancer includes a broad group of cancers which include different cancers of the GI system, i.e., esophagus, small intestine, gallbladder, liver, stomach, pancreas, bowel (large intestine or colon and rectum), and anus cancer. It also includes other rare cancers such as neuroendocrine tumors and gastrointestinal stromal tumors which could be found throughout the whole GI system. The frequency of GI cancer is very high in industrialized realms. There are some common risk factors associated with GI cancer, i.e., smoking, drinking alcohol, high-fat diet, gender, age, race, infection, geographical location, and family history [6].

Sentinel lymph node (SLN) plotting evidently has converted to a highly practical and accurate method in performing GI cancer and may be very convenient for personalizing multimodal management for esophageal cancer which might be usually accepted smoothly for GI cancer [7]. Integrated ultrasound, OCT, PA, and/or fluorescence imaging endoscope and biopsy [8] are helpful in diagnosing cancers in the gastrointestinal tract. There are diverse methods used to treat cancer in the human body, *viz.* chemotherapy, radiation therapy, and surgery. The selection of the method for treatment of GI cancer depends on the variety of cancer, the stage of its enlargement, and related health elements. The treatment in which synthetic or phytochemicals are practiced to deal with the cancerous cell is known as chemotherapy. Chemotherapy contains the treatment of cancer cells by delivering anticancer agents. While a large assortment of chemopreventive and chemotherapeutic agents in vitro as well as in vivo have been familiarized since the last few periods to fight GI cancer, most of them are exorbitant and have side effects. Hence some phytochemicals were extracted from the plants which are tested to be safe and economical and exert anticancer activities against GI cancer including 6-gingerol, 6-shogaol, resveratrol, damnacanthal, zerumbone, and diallyl sulfide (DAS) [9].

The National Cancer Institute has recognized about 35 plant-based foodstuffs that have cancer-preventive properties, including garlic, soybean, onion, ginger, tomatoes, turmeric, and cruciferous vegetables [10]. Anticancer agents have the ability to modify numerous signaling biomolecules like NF-κB,P13K, STAT3, ERK1/2, Akt, cyclin D1, TNF-α, COX-2, cdk, MMP-9, caspases, survivin, cIAP-1, MAPK, XIAP, Bcl-2, and other cell growth-regulatory proteins [6].

At presently nanotechnology has grown into a very useful technique in diagnosis as well as in treatment process; it has the potential to unravel big challenges in cancer diagnosis and treatment [11]. Delivery of numerous anticancer drugs including phytochemicals was testified in the latest years used for the treatment of GI cancer using quantum dots, polymeric nanoparticles, metallic nanoparticles, and nanoformulation of therapeutic agents [12].

3 Types of GI Cancer

The different types of GI cancer are shown in Fig. 7.1.

3.1 Esophagus Cancer

The esophagus is the region of food pipe between the throat and stomach. When cells that line the esophagus change or mutate and grows out of control to form a mass or

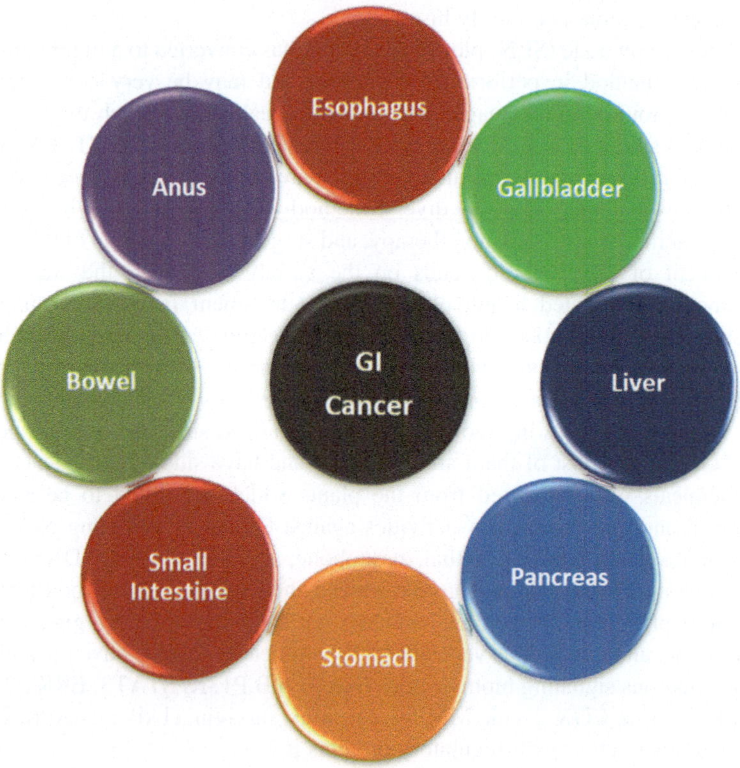

Fig. 7.1 Different types of GI cancer

tumor, it is known as esophagus cancer. The common symptoms of this type of cancer include pain when swallowing, heavy voice, abnormally large lymph nodes, vomiting blood, etc. The esophagus cancer is categorized into subtypes, i.e., esophageal squamous cell carcinoma (ESCC) which begins in the epithelial cells that link the esophagus and esophageal adenocarcinoma (EAC) which come to light from glandular cells in the lower third of the esophagus [13].

3.2 Stomach Cancer

Stomach cancer is as well a known gastric cancer which develops in the lining of the gastric by the growth of cancerous cells. This cancer may spread to other organs of the body, i.e., liver, bones, and abdomen [14]. It is difficult to diagnose it because most of the people do not show symptoms in the earlier stages. Some earlier symptoms may be helpful in its diagnosis such as heartburn, nausea, loss of appetite, and upper abdominal pain. Other symptoms of stomach cancer consist of blood in the stool, vomiting, weight loss, and yellowness of the skin [15]. Established in GLOBOCAN 2018 data, stomach cancer is the fifth common neoplasm and the third most lethal cancer, with a likely 783,000 deaths in 2018 [16].

3.3 Gallbladder Cancer

According to autopsy studies, gallbladder cancer is the sixth-rank cancer of the GI tract which represents 80–95% of GI cancers globally [17]. The highest mortality had been reported in Chile, Poland, India, Japan, and Israel with an average incidence of 27, 14, 10, 7, and 5 out of 100,000 cases, respectively, including some other risk areas such as Pakistan, Korea, and Spain [18, 19]. The causes of this cancer are complex but there is a strong relation with gallstones. The most common symptoms are abdominal pain, vomiting, and jaundice. It has the ability to spread to other organs such as liver [20].

3.4 Liver Cancer

American Institute for Cancer Research marked liver cancer as the fifth most ordinarily taking place cancer in males and the ninth most happening cancer in females with above 840,000 new cases in the year of 2018. Liver cancer starts in the liver and may spread to other organs. The most common causes of liver cancer are excessive use of alcohol, diabetes, obesity, and having the condition of hemochromatosis in which the body takes up and stores more iron than its essentials' limit, taking foodstuffs that have aflatoxin [21].

3.5 *Pancreas Cancer*

Pancreatic cancer (PC) occurs when cells in the pancreas which is a glandular organ behind the stomach begin to proliferate out of control and make a mass or tumor. Most pancreatic cancers begin from minuscular noninvasive epithelial proliferation inside the pancreatic ducts as pancreatic intraepithelial neoplasia [22]. These cancerous cells have the capability to overrun other parts of the body. It is more common in aged persons than in the younger one. It was observed that several factors are responsible for it such as the use of tobacco, use of aspirin, and intake of alcohol and coffee. About 5 to 10% of patients with pancreatic cancer have family antiquity of the disease [23]. PC poorly responds to most chemotherapeutic agents and becomes deadly in the form of pancreatic ductal adenocarcinoma [24].

3.6 *Small Intestine Cancer*

Small intestine cancer comprises the irregular and uncontrolled growth of cells in the inner line of the small intestine (SI) which consists of 75% of the total length and more than 90% of the mucosal surface of the gastrointestinal tract (GIT). It is very uncommon among GI cancer. The foremost clinical signs are weight loss, abdominal pain, lassitude, and discomfort [25]. There are 40 different types of intestine cancer but the 4 most common cancers are carcinoid tumors, adenocarcinomas, sarcoma, and lymphoma. Small intestine cancer has several menace issues which include consumption of red or smoked meat, obesity, smoking, and saturated fat [26].

3.7 *Colon Cancer (CC)*

Colon cancer is the third most occurring cancer globally and the major reason for tumor-related passing away in the USA. Colon cancer (CC) begins in the large intestine (colon) which is the final segment of the digestive tract and typically affects older adults. In the beginning, small noncancerous clumps of cells appear, called polyps inside the colon. This type of cancer is a biologically heterogeneous disease characterized by neoplasms [27, 28].

3.8 *Bowel or Colorectal Cancer (CRC)*

Uncontrolled arising in the internal lining of the bowel or rectum is known as colorectal cancer and such growths are called polyps. Depending on where cancer begins, CRC may be called bowel cancer, colon cancer, or rectal cancer. This is the third most common malignancy in both genders, and the second principal cause of cancer-related death in the Western world [29]. The occurrence of CRC is mostly higher for men, and the hazard of the disease increases with time [30].

3.9 Anus Cancer

Anal cancer is also an unwanted growth in the squamous and glandular epithelia of the anus. It is the distal opening of the gastrointestinal tract. According to anatomical and histological differences, anal cancer is mainly of two types such as squamous cell carcinoma (SCC) and adenocarcinoma. SCC comprises more than 70% of cases compared to the other [31]. It occurs in smoking persons, males who practice anal intercourse, and immunosuppressed patients, including HIV patients and transplant recipients [32].

4 Treatment of GI Cancer

Gastrointestinal stromal tumors (GIST) are unusual lumps of the gastrointestinal (GI) tract that appear in embryonic mesenchymal cells. GISTs arise all over the GI tract. It is positioned in the gastric region and small intestine mainly [33]. GI cancer can be cured with surgery, immunotherapy, targeted therapy, chemotherapy, and radiation therapy.

In the case of GI cancer handling, surgery is one of the methods but the recurrence of GI cancer is a dangerous problem because the resection site and peritoneal surfaces are very common places for reappearance. Disease extends to the polyp bed and to peritoneal surfaces [34]. Surgery may be curative only when the tumor is localized [35]. The other method available is radiation therapy in which the controlled dose of high-energy radiation is given to the tumor site to kill or damage cancer cells. It may be given before or after surgery with the aim of trying to diminish the threat of recurrence of cancer after surgery [36].

In hormonal therapy, oncologist identifies some points as baseline predictors for discontinuation, including the use of hormone replacement therapy (HRT). Several peptide hormones can control the expansion of GI tumors like breast and prostate cancer through all-specific receptors and signal transduction alleyways [37, 38]. Disruption or amendment of these growth-governing mechanisms, such as hormonal centered treatment, may be remedial of advanced GI cancer [35].

Chemotherapy includes the use of chemicals, i.e., anticancer agents or cytotoxic drugs to kill the cancerous cell in the GI tract. They could be given as parenteral and/or oral which depends on the kind and stage of cancer. The main disadvantage of this method is that the anticancer agents also affect healthy tissues of the body [39]. The different methods which are currently in use for the cure of GI cancer are shown in Fig. 7.2.

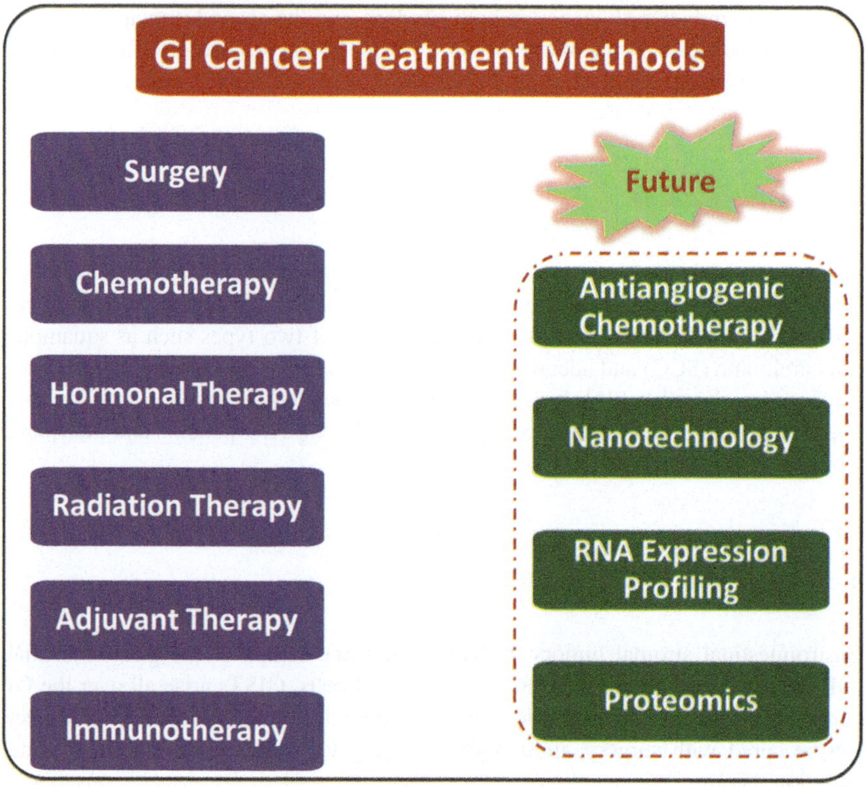

Fig. 7.2 Techniques for the treatment of GI cancer, present and future

4.1 Phytochemicals for GI Cancer Treatment

Phytochemicals are biomolecules that are derived from the plants including nonedible plants. They are secondary metabolites, generally nonnutritive compounds, which have several biological activities in humans including anticancer properties. There is a wide range of phytochemicals and their synthetic derivatives, which are used in cancer prevention and treatment. Some examples of phytochemical-derived biomolecules from eatable and non-eatable plants are rottlerin, sparstolonin B, berbamine, plumbagin, 6-shogaol, and sulforaphane; some of the phytochemicals with their source and anticancer uses are reported in Table 7.1.

Phytochemicals are used as bioactive markers for cytotoxicity counter to tumors and anticancer activity of phytochemicals which mostly depend on their multi-target tool of action, comprising antimutagenic, antiproliferative, and antioxidant deeds. It has been assessed that at present 25–48% of appropriate therapies by the Food and Drug Administration (FDA) are derivative of plants [67, 68].

Table 7.1 Phytochemicals utilized for the treatment of cancer

Phytochemicals	Source	Type of cancer	Reference
Curcumin	Rhizome of turmeric	Multiple myelomas, pancreatic and colon cancers	[40]
Epigallocatechin gallate (EGCG)	Extract of green tea	Brain, prostate, cervical, bladder, and colon cancers	[41]
Crocin	Callus of saffron (*Crocus sativus*)	Human lung cancer, skin carcinoma, pancreatic cancer, colorectal cancer, and breast cancer	[42]
Fisetin	Strawberries, apples, and grapes	Human colon cancer	[43]
Kaempferol	Apples, grapes, tomatoes, broccoli, cucumbers, peaches, blackberries, raspberries, green tea, potatoes, onions, lettuce, green beans, and spinach	Pancreatic cancer and lung cancer	[44]
Lycopene	Tomatoes, red papayas, watermelons, and red carrots	Breast cancer, prostate cancer, endometrial cancer, and colon cancer	[45]
Sulforaphane	Cruciferous vegetables such as broccoli, cabbages, and Brussels sprouts	Human colon cancer	[39]
Tocopherols/ tocotrienols (vitamin E)	Wheat germ oil, safflower oil, and sunflower oil	Liver, stomach, skin, colon, prostate, lung, and pancreatic cancers	[40]
Apigenin	Parsley, celery, chamomile, Egyptian plant, and *Moringa peregrina*	Breast, colon, and pancreatic cancers	[41]
Plumbagin	Drosera and Nepenthes	Ovarian cancer cells, colon cancer, breast cancer, and cervical cancer	[42]
Vitamin D (calcitriol)	Mushroom, soy milk, and cereals	Colon, breast, ovarian, and prostate cancer	[43]
Phenethyl isothiocyanate (PEITC)	Cruciferous vegetables, such as broccoli, cabbage, watercress	Breast, osteogenic sarcoma U-2 OS, lung, cervical, and prostate cancer	[44]
Cyanidin-3-glucoside	Grapes, raspberry, apples, plums, red cabbage, blackberry, cranberry, and red onion	Breast apocrine carcinomas, colon cancer	[45]
Diindolylmethane (DIM), (I3C) (indole-3-carbinol)	Broccoli, cauliflower, collard greens	Breast, colon, prostate, and endometrial cancer	[46]
Genistein	Fava beans, kudzu, coffee, psoralea, *Flemingia vestita*, and soybeans	Gastric cancer, breast cancer, and colorectal cancer	[47]

(continued)

Table 7.1 (continued)

Phytochemicals	Source	Type of cancer	Reference
Gingerol	Ginger	Breast cancer, retinoblastoma cancer, renal, melanoma, colon cancer, and colorectal cancer	[48]
Resveratrol	The skin of red grapes and peanuts	Colon cancer, human breast cancer, and liver cancer	[49]
Rosmarinic acid	Lemon balm, peppermint, sage, thyme, oregano, and rosemary	Human colon carcinoma cell and gastric cancer	[50]
Tocotrienols/vitamin E	Plant oils as barley, coconut, sesame, and wheat germ	Pancreatic cancer, prostate cancer, breast cancer, lung and brain cancer	[50]
Delphinidin	Cranberry and pomegranate	Lung cancer	[51]
3,3′-Diindolylmethane (DIM)	Brussels sprout and fermented cabbage	Breast cancer, colon cancer, and prostate cancer	[52]
Naringenin	Grapefruit and orange skin	Colon cancer and breast cancer	[53]
Proanthocyanidin	Berries	Colon cancer and ovarian cancer	[54]
Pterostilbene	Blueberries	Breast cancer and prostate cancer	[55]
Quercetin	Onions	Ovarian cancer, gastric cancer, breast cancer, and colon cancer	[56]
Retinoic acid	Carrots	Acute promyelocytic leukemia (APL), oral, lung, prostate, skin, breast, bladder, and ovarian cancers	[57]
Silibinin	Milk thistle (*Silybum marianum*)	Skin, prostate, breast, lung, kidney carcinomas, bladder cancer, and colon cancer	[58]
Zerumbone	Gingers	Colon cancer	[59]
Diallyl sulfide (DAS)	Garlic	Colon cancer	[60]
Lappaconitine sulfate	Roots of *Aconitum sinomontanum*	Colon cancer	[61]
Berbamine	Chinese herb *Berberis amurensis*	Human lung cancer and ovarian cancer	[62]
Rottlerin	Kamala tree (*Mallotus philippinensis*)	Colon, breast, prostate, and pancreatic cancers	[63]
Podophyllotoxin	*Podophyllum emodi* Wall (syn. p. hexandrum Royle) or *P. peltatum L.*	Lung cancer and testicular cancer	[64]
Glyceollins	Cruciferous vegetables, beans, soybean, rice, garlic, tomato, and potatoes	Prostate cancer and breast cancer	[65]
Damnacanthal (noni)	Roots of *Morinda citrifolia L.* (noni)	Human colorectal cancer and breast cancer	[66]

5 Nanotechnology and Cancer Treatment

The term nanotechnology has defined the control of the size of matter on the nanosize scale within the range of 1–100 nm. It is a multidisciplinary and emerging area of research, employed in diverse fields, i.e., engineering, biology, chemistry, physics, space, and medicine [69–75]. Nanotechnology becomes very useful in the arena of cancer diagnosis and cures with the hope that it will solve big challenges in the diagnosis and treatment of cancer [11].

The usage of nanotechnology in the field of medicine is very useful because, at the nanoscale level, it paves great advantages in terms of target-specific drug delivery which also reduces the concentration of drugs and reduces toxicity. The use of nanoparticles as a drug carrier could boost up the process of drug delivery with one of the deadly diseases like GI cancer [76]. Nanotechnology involves the synthesis of different types of nanoparticles, their characterizations, and the applications to deal with different cancerous cells and cancers. Selective production of nanoparticles with pointing biological methods has proved extremely leading because it leads to higher efficacy associated with fewer side effects [77].

Nanoparticles were used in numerous techniques for the treatment of GI cancer such as in chemotherapy, targeted drug delivery, imaging, theranostic, and diagnosis. The details are discussed in this chapter.

5.1 Nanoparticles in Cancer Imaging

In the field of cancer diagnosis, the nanoparticles are developing as a new way of molecular imaging (MI) in different problems [78]. During the previous decade, the application of nanotechnology in MI provided several significant benefits and openings for the imaging of living objects. They have potential in precise cancer diagnosis through active targeting and/or passive accumulation methodologies [79]. Nanoparticles can deliver the imaging agents inadequate concentration at targeted tumor sites because they are typically smaller in size when compared to proteins and cells [80]. There are different methods available for MI which include targeted ultrasound, bioluminescence, fluorescence, magnetic resonance spectroscopy (MRS), positron-emission tomography (PET), single-photon emission computed tomography (SPECT), and molecular magnetic resonance imaging (MRI) [81].

Quantum dots (QDs) are unique types of nanoparticles which are extensively studied for preclinical optical imaging techniques [82, 83] due to their tremendous properties for biological imaging, durable endurance to chemical degradation, photobleaching, good UV, high quantum yield, NIR (near-infrared) absorption, and large Stokes shifts [84]. They also proved poor retention in the tumor cell and were able to wash back easily into the bloodstream due to their smaller size which is also one of the major advantages [84].

Geng *et al.* [85] used quantum dot-based molecular targeted imaging methods to inspect the discrete tendency, cell morphology, clone formation rate, and Ki67 expression as well as distribution in clones. They were helpful in the investigation of the morphology of clones of MCF 7 human breast cancer cell line, SGC7901 human gastric cancer cell line, and SW480 human colon cancer cell line. They observed that SW480, MCF-7, and SGC7901 cells have more nuclear:cytoplasmic ratios, heterogeneous morphology, and noticeable pathological mitotic types. They concluded that quantum dot molecular imaging-mediated cell clone formation assay presented a unique method to understand the proliferative features of cancer cells. Liu *et al.* [86] synthesized PEGylated near-infrared QDs, $Zn_x Hg_{1-x} Se_y S_{1-y}$ QDs (ZHS-QDs) consisting of zinc (Zn^{2+}), S^{2-}, Se^{2-}, and mercury (Hg^{2+}), for tumor-specific imaging and delivered intravenously into orthotopic pancreas tumors and breast in mice taking the tumor-penetrating iRGD peptide. The results of transmission electron microscopy (TEM) study showed that the core thickness of the synthesized QDs was 6.6 ± 2.3 nm (mean $\pm$ standard deviation). The study comprises in vitro and in vivo positive ion-exchange actions in ZHS-QDs, slaking of many QDs prompted by Ag-TS. They also analyzed in vivo imaging of pancreatic cancer through ZHS-QDs. The study showed no toxicity and concluded that in vivo positive ion exchange might be a hopeful scheme to boost the specificity of tumor imaging. Another study of Brunetti *et al.* [87] consisted of the synthesis of NIR QDs functionalized with the NT4 cancer-selective tetrabranched peptides (NT4-QDs) and reported that NT4-QDs had a very favorable performance for selectively addressing tumor cells in vitro as well as in vivo, and confirming growing features of NT4-QDs such as theranostics.

The nanoparticles with incorporation or encapsulation of dyes were also reported promising in MI with respect to cancer theranostics [88]. The US Food and Drug Administration (FDA) approved nanoparticles encapsulated/incorporated with NIR region fluorescent cyanine 7 (Cy7), indocyanine green (ICG) [89], and dialkylcarbocyanine fluorophores [81]. A number of nanoparticles were studied for the imaging of tumors by the supply of NIR dye toward the tumor site. Li *et al.* [90] developed phospholipid micelles to assist the usage of IR780 dye for fluorescent imaging of malignant brain tumor. This study included the in vivo brain tumor targeting and NIRF imaging ability to use U87MG glioma ectopic and orthotopic xenograft models and an impatient glioma mouse model obsessed by RAS/RTK initiation. The observations have shown that IR780-phospholipid micelles exhibited intracranial tumor accretion and effective NIRF signal intensity in glioma orthotopic models in a real-time, noninvasive manner. Chansaenpak *et al.* [91] encapsulated NIR-light-activating aza-BODIPY (AZB-NO_2) in polymeric nanoparticles for cancer cell imaging. It was perceived through SEM results that the AZB-NO_2 formed a sphere shape with a hydrodynamic ordinary size of 201 nm. The study indicated that the nanoparticles were equipped by spending 0.8 mg dye and displayed the highest fluorescence quantum yield. It was also testified that AZB-NO_2@PCL nanoparticles demonstrated bright fluorescence from U-251 cells inside 3D Ca-alginate scaffolds after 24-h incubation. It was concluded that the reported nanoparticles might be efficiently used in cancer cell imaging applications.

The nanoparticles are of great significance in the magnetic resonance imaging (MRI) with respect to gastric cancer cell imaging and treating [92]. Iron oxide nanoparticles were extensively studied in this domain [93]. Recently, iron oxide-loaded PLGA-based nanoparticles were reported for magnetic resonance imaging and cancer therapy [94]. Ruan *et al.* synthesized amino-modified fluorescent magnetic nanoparticle (FMNP)-marked mesenchymal stem cells (MSCs) to recognize targeted imaging and hyperthermia therapy of in vivo gastric cancer [95]. They reported that the MNP-tagged MSCs considerably inhibited the development of in vivo gastric cancer due to hyperthermia effects and suggested that CCL19/CCR7 and CXCL12/CXCR4 axis loops may play crucial roles in the targeting of MSCs to in vivo gastric cancer. Deserno *et al.* [96] stated the usage of ferumoxtran-10 (a superparamagnetic iron oxide) [97] for MR imaging. It was concluded that ferumoxtran-10-enhanced MR imaging significantly upgraded nodal performance in patients with bladder cancer by portraying metastases even in normal-sized lymph nodes. Another study of Jalalian *et al.* [98] reported the preparation of epirubicin-loaded superparamagnetic iron oxide nanoparticle-aptamer bioconjugate and their applications for united in vivo colon cancer therapy and imaging through murine colon carcinoma cells (C26 cells, target). They reported that the complex could competently identify tumors when inspected by MRI and constrain tumor growth in vivo. The use of cetuximab-conjugated magneto-fluorescent silica nanoparticles for directing and imaging of in vivo colon cancer was also evidenced [99].

During the uses of nanoparticles in imaging as well as photodynamic therapy of cancer, poor biocompatibility, foreseeable requisite of external irradiation, and depth of tissue penetration of the nanoparticles were some of the major problems, but they could be rectified by using biodegradable and biocompatible nanoparticles. In continuation of this, Xu *et al.* [100] synthesized biodegradable luminescent nanoparticles with an amphiphilic polymeric conjugate and a luminescent giver (luminol) and a fluorescent receiver [chlorin e6 (Ce6)] for in vivo luminescence imaging and photodynamic remedy in deep tissues. They observed that the nanoparticles have shown vivid in vivo imaging capability with apposite tissue penetration.

5.2 *Treating Cancer Cells with Nanoparticles*

Nanoparticles were also used to treat the cancer cell called nanoparticle-mediated chemotherapy. Chemotherapy is utilized for years to cure cancer, but it can also be the root of severe damages to the noncancerous cells of the human body. The use of nanoparticles can be more beneficial in terms of destroying the cancerous cells with a marginal loss to well tissue, with preventing of harmful effects of traditional chemotherapy. Evidence showed that albumin-bound paclitaxel nanoparticles were used as second-line chemotherapy for unresectable or repeated gastric cancer [101]. It exposed auspicious activity against formerly treated unresectable or periodic gastric cancers, with well-tolerated noxiousness. Another evidence showed that paclitaxel/tetrandrine-co-loaded nanoparticles efficiently supported the apoptosis of gastric cancer cells which was centered on "oxidation therapy" [102]. Sun *et al.* [103] reported a poly (ethylene glycol) (PEG)-coated Fe_3O_4 nanoparticles as miRNA supply method to reduce drug resistance of gastric cancer cells through imposing miR16 expression in SGC7901/ADR cells. They perceived that miR16/MNPs were capable to significantly overwhelm SGC7901/ADR tumor growth and suggested that it might be through enhancing SGC7901/ADR cell sensitivity to ADR. In another study, Zheng *et al.* [104] synthesized nanoparticles of poly (lactide)–vitamin E TPGS (PLA–TPGS) copolymers using the dialysis technique to formulate paclitaxel for oral chemotherapy with Caco-2 cells of the gastrointestinal (GI) drug barricade. Wu *et al.* [105] reported the usage of smart gelatinase-stimuli nanoparticles to supply 5-aza-2′-deoxycytidine and 5-fluorouridine to gastric cancer cells and observed that the assimilation of 5-aza-2′-deoxycytidine into NPs expressively enriched the sensitivity of gastric cancer cells to 5-fluorouridine. Li *et al.* [106] testified the use of metal-phenolic nanoparticles of samarium (Sm^{3+}) ions as well as (−)-epicatechin (EC) for therapy against colon cancer. They compared Sm^{III}-EC nanoparticles with a clinic anticancer drug 5-fluorouracil and observed that Sm^{III}-EC nanoparticles not only diminished the tumor volume but also did not affect the bodyweight of mice and ordinary organs presenting significant benefits over clinic equivalent.

In continuation of this, Rashid *et al.* [107] investigated the radiosensitization effects caused by gold nanoparticles (AuNPs), platinum nanodendrites (PtNDs), bismuth oxide nanorods (BiNRs), and superparamagnetic iron oxide nanoparticles (SPIONs) on human colon carcinoma cells (HCT 116) illumined with 150 MeV proton beams. This study indicated that BiNRs demonstrated the maximum sensitization enrichment ratio (SER) of 4.93 and ROS generation corresponding to the level of radiosensitization with the maximum ROS achieved for BiNRs. It was suggested that as-prepared nanoparticles influenced the potential of being clinically applied in proton beam therapy. Karuppaiya *et al.* [108] manufactured silver nanoparticles by rhizome abstract of *Dysosma pleiantha* and studied their antiproliferative effect against breast and human gastric cancer cells. They observed that the synthesized AgNPs demonstrated to be dose-dependent cytotoxic against human gastric cancer cell lines with IC_{50} at 7.14 μM and concluded that biosynthesized AgNPs can be used in the advanced development of anticancer drugs. Al-Radadi [109] synthesized nanoparticles of platinum expending Saudi's dates extract; studied their influence on the hepatocellular carcinoma (HePG-2) cancer cells, breast cells (MCF-7), and colon carcinoma cells (HCT-116); and obtained promising results. Jain *et al.* [110] also reported the derivation and characterization of Eudragit S100-coated mini-capsules packed with chitosan nanoparticles unconjugated and folic acid (FA) conjugated put in a nutshell caspase-3 activator (7-hydroxystaurosporine) used for targeting, treatment of colon cancer, and apoptosis induction. They observed that the equipped nanoparticles were approximately sphere shaped with positive zeta potential. This study indicated through In vitro, ex vivo, as well as in vivo studies that the layered mini-capsules specifically supply the drug in the colon showing great therapeutic importance with low side effects. The metallic nanoparticles were also used in targeting autophagy which is an auspicious approach for cancer treatment [111]. Flavonoid nanoparticles were also evidenced in usage for the cure of cancer [112].

5.3 Nanoparticles for Targeted Drug Delivery

There are different methods used to cure cancer in the human body in which the field where the synthetic or phytochemicals are employed to treat the cancerous cell is called chemotherapy. Chemotherapy comprises the treatment of cancer cells by delivering anticancer agents systemically to patients for reducing the uninhibited growth of cancerous cells. Unluckily, these anticancer agents not only damage the cancer cell, but also create harmful effects on healthy tissues of the body which is due to the toxic nature of anticancer agents and poor drug delivery of these agents to the targeted tumor site. Thus there arise grim side effects containing organ damage, causing impaired treatment with minor dosage and finally low persistence rates [113].

The drug development process is a very complex and interdisciplinary process that includes chemistry, biology, computational design, and clinical study. The easiest way to prevent healthy tissue from anticancer agents is therefore to segregate the cancerous cells and the typical body cells. Then the drug is delivered to specifically targeted tumor sites so the remedy can diminish the growth and proliferation of only cancer cells. To overwhelm these limits of drug delivery, there has been increased interest in nanotechnology in the last decade [114]. Nanoparticles have been widely studied for drug and gene delivery uses by varying their composition and biological properties [115, 116]. NPs also play a significant part in controlled drug delivery or sustained drug release [117].

The consumption of nanoparticles as a drug carrier has a number of advantages such as (i) improvement in water solubility of poorly soluble drugs and their protection in the bloodstream which also improves pharmacological and pharmacokinetic properties of drugs; (ii) delivery of drugs to specific tumor target in controlled manner by limiting the drug accumulation in other organs which also enhances the efficacy and reduces the toxicity; and (iii) being helpful in real-time monitoring of anticancer agents by delivering the combination of imaging agents with drugs [118]. Delivery of several anticancer drugs including phytochemicals was conveyed in recent years for the handling of GI cancer using quantum dots, polymeric nanoparticles, metallic nanoparticles, and nanoformulation of therapeutic agents [119]. Recently the nanoparticles of chitosan, PEG-conjugated chitosan, and chitosan complexed using gelatin were testified intended for the site-specific release and supply of green tea polyphenol extract epigallocatechin-3-gallate through gastric cancer cells via oral administration. The nanoparticles effectively reduced drug release within gastric acids stopping reduced vascular endothelial growth factor protein, gastric cancer cell growth, and induced cell apoptosis [12]. The phase II reading of NK105, which is a paclitaxel-incorporating micellar nanoparticle, used for gastric cancer treatment was also reported [120].

6 Nanoparticle-Mediated Phytochemical Delivery for GI Cancer Therapy

There is a plethora of phytochemicals that play an important role as therapeutic agents also showing promising results in GI cancer treatment. The targeted delivery of these phytochemicals is also possible by using nanoparticles as a nanocarrier [121]. There is a number of reported researches [122] related to the delivery of phytochemicals for GI cancer treatment and few of them are detailed below:

Thipe *et al.* [123] informed the synthesis of resveratrol-conjugated gold nanoparticles and investigated their antitumor usefulness contrary to breast, prostate, and pancreatic cancers. The study shows that resveratrol reduced Au^{3+} to Au^0 to synthesize Res-AuNPs and the encapsulation of gum arabic increased their stability. The in vitro anticancer studies counter to the human breast (MDAMB-231), prostate (PC-3), and pancreatic (PANC-1) cancers showed that the corona of resveratrol was systematically increased on Res-AuNPs. It showed synergetic anticancer effects on selected cancers. The researchers concluded that the improved corona of resveratrol on AuNPs enhances the bioavailability of resveratrol so that therapeutically active species can be optimally accessible in vivo for solicitations in cancer therapy.

The study of Brian [124] included the synthesis of silver nanoparticles through *Ceiba pentandra* bark extract (ethanolic) and their anticancer activities on colorectal cancer cells (HCT-116) with an emphasis on cell cytotoxicity, quantification of ROS, and determination of mitochondria membrane potential. The result of the study indicated that as-prepared nanoparticles exhibited IC_{50} value at 60 μg/mL that significantly inhibited cell viability and changed the morphology of HCT-116 colon cancer cells. Elbialy *et al.* [125] synthesized curcumin-mediated AuNPs and studied the effect of AuNPs on increasing the efficacy of curcumin as an anticancer agent counter to the colon (HCT-116) as well as breast (MCF-7) human cancer cell lines. Their results indicated that the equipped AuNPs-Cur (0.72 $\mu g\ mL^{-1}$) have greater antiproliferative and apoptotic properties against MCF-7 as well as HCT-116 cells, related to free curcumin. Mariadoss *et al.* [126] synthesized phloretin-loaded chitosan nanoparticles (PhCsNPs) and investigated their anticancer properties. They observed that the prepared PhCsNPs have shown major antioxidant and detoxification effects in investigational carcinogenesis as well as it significantly decreased the tumor volume and neoplastic alterations through oral administration in various doses.

The polymeric nanoparticles have also gained interest in the delivery of therapeutic phytochemicals for targeted drug delivery. Zhou *et al.* [127] synthesized mucus-penetrating curcumin-loaded PLGA nanoparticles with different amounts of Pluronic F127 for oral supply to swollen colon tissues. They observed that nanoparticles functionalized with F127 showed improved mucus-penetrating ability with negative cytotoxicity. It was reported that the prepared nanoparticle showed a particularly stronger ability to reduce the secretion of TNF-α from macrophages. The nanoparticles also demonstrated the best therapeutic efficacy against ulcerative colitis. Hajizadeh *et al.* [128] loaded diosgenin (a phytochemical) into noisome by thin-film hydration method to increase its solubility and hence efficiency and investigated the cytotoxicity assay on HepG2 cell line. The results indicated that the prepared nanodrug-delivery system was normal in size and spherical in morphology. They calculated the loading proficiency of diosgenin and obtained 89% with a maintainable and governable release rate. Anter *et al.* [129] prepared chitosan oligosaccharide-based nanoparticles (COS-NPs) by ionic gelation method for gastric mucosal administration of the biomolecules "apocynin" (APO). They analyzed in vivo antiulcerogenic activity counter to ketoprofen (KP)-induced gastrointestinal ulceration in rats and observed that APO-loaded COS-NPs triggered splendid antiulcerogenic activity contrary to KP-induced digestive ulceration in rats compared with free APO-treated group. They concluded that the prepared nanoparticles could be measured as an auspicious oral phytopharmaceutical nanoparticulate scheme for the organization of gastrointestinal ulceration. Maity *et al.* [130] testified the production of nanoconjugates of Au nanoparticles (AuNPs) conjugated through theaflavin (AuNP@TfQ) by a subsequent one-step green synthesis by reacting $HAuCl_4$ and theaflavin at room temperature. They observed that the occurrence of the quinone motif in AuNP@TfQ induced an improved level of ROS generation and resulted in the caspase-mediated apoptotic cell demise which might grip the potential for a "magic bullet"-mediated ovarian cancer treatment.

PEGylated lipid bilayer mesoporous silica nanoparticles were also reported for the supply of two phytochemicals, i.e., paclitaxel and curcumin, simultaneously at the tumor site [131]. This delivery system effectively carries medications into cancer cells with the persistent release, and better controlled the tumor weight.

Sweety *et al.* [132] nanoformulated thymoquinone with three various hydrophilic polymers hydroxypropyl methylcellulose (HPMC), chitosan, as well as polyvinyl alcohol (PVA) and then coated with Eudragit L100 for site-specific supply for colon cancer management. The pitiable physicochemical properties of thymoquinone were overcome by three different nanoformulations and observed that chitosan-based nanoformulation showed great cytotoxicity in colon cancer because of the formation of an oxime bond and sialic acid binding. They reported that the nominal dosage mandatory for killing the colon cancer cells was 10 μg/mL.

Saraf *et al.* [133] developed curcumin-loaded Eudragit S100 nanoparticles using the Box-Behnken experimental design for site-specific supply in colon cancer. They observed the average particle size of nanoparticles in the range of 122.38 ± 0.75 nm and the minimum drug release at pH 1.2, and higher at pH 6.8, and continued drug discharge was found at pH 7.4, corresponding to pH of colon. Udompornmongkol *et al.* [134] equipped curcumin-loaded polymeric nanoparticles of chitosan and gum arabic via an emulsification solvent diffusion technique and studied their anti-colorectal cancer applications. They observed that curcumin was entangled in polymeric nanoparticles with +48 mV and 136 nm size, with high encapsulation proficiency (95%). This study shows that curcumin nanoparticles were able to endure hydrolysis due to digestive juice or small intestinal enzymes, and therefore it should blow out in the colon mainly intact. Moreover, the prepared encapsulated nanoparticles were reported with greater anti-colorectal cancer properties than free curcumin due to bigger cellular uptake. Anitha *et al.* [135] reported the In vitro combinatorial anticancer effects of 5-fluorouracil and curcumin-loaded N, O-carboxymethyl chitosan nanoparticles on colon cancer with in vivo pharmacokinetic results. They observed the sustained-release profile of therapeutic drugs at pH 4.5 and 7.4 outlined above for a period of 4 days and joined disclosure of colon cancer cells (HT29). As per in vivo results, they reported the upgraded plasma concentrations of 5-FU and CUR which sustained up to 72 h dissimilar to the basic drugs. Another study showed the delivery of gambogic acid by telodendrimers and vitamin E (VE) composed of linear polyethylene glycol (PEG)-blocking dendritic oligomer of cholic acid (CA) for colon cancer handling [136]. This study reported that the reported nanoformulation was found to parade analogous In vitro cytotoxic activity contrary to colon cancer cells as the permitted drug. Lotfi-Attari *et al.* [137] studied co-delivery of curcumin as well as chrysin by PEGylated PLGA NPs and inspected their synergistic inhibitory effect counter to human colorectal (Caco-2) cancer cells. Their results indicated that nanoformulations showed dose-dependent cytotoxicity against Caco-2 cells and had an additional synergistic antiproliferative effect which suggestively detained the progress of cancer cells.

Vimala *et al.* [138] testified the anticancer action of doxorubicin-loaded ZnO nanoparticles against Bax and Bcl-2 expression in breast and colon carcinoma. The study reported that the size and shape of nanoparticles depended on the concentrations of the extract and nanoparticles showed a significant decline of Bcl-2 manifestation on MCF-7 cells. They had good biocompatibility without any toxicity in the bloodstream. Dandekar *et al.* [139] inspected the pH-sensitive curcumin-loaded polymeric nanoparticles for the treatment of colon cancer with the HT-29 cell line. They detected that curcumin-encumbered polymeric nanoparticles were homogenous, spherical in size, and negatively surface charged with >99% of drug content. The study reported that nanoparticles were verified virtually to have double obsession of the cancerous cells, as matched to curcumin alone. The authors concluded that the improved action may be accredited to size influencing value-added cellular uptake and may result in the reduction of complete dose necessity. Moreover, the gold nanoparticles produced from *Trichosanthes kirilowii* with ~50 nm in size were also reported as potential anticancer nanomaterials against colon cancer cells through the induction of the apoptotic alley [140]. MTT assay of the reported gold nanoparticles shows that they exhibited the selective, operative anticarcinogenic effect of AuNPs on HCT-116 cells in a dose-dependent style. Moreover, the AuNPs considerably enhanced ROS generation caused by mitochondrial membrane impairment and induced morphological alterations using AO/EtBr yellowing assay. Furthermore, AuNP treatment prompted G0/G1-phase cell cycle detention in HCT-116 cells. Also, AuNP treatment stimulated caspase expression and downregulated the anti-apoptotic expression in HCT-116 cells.

7 Conclusion

It may be concluded that the combination of nanotechnology with phytochemicals into cancer diagnostics and therapeutics is a promptly progressing area. There is a need to address the cost-effectiveness and the understanding of the concepts. Nanotechnology was found to accomplish an essential and effective character in improving efficacy as well as overcoming the limitations of plant-mediated chemotherapy of GI cancers. Nanoparticles were utilized in diverse ways for the treatment of GI cancer such as in chemotherapy, targeted drug delivery, imaging, theranostic, and diagnosis. There are a number of studies reported which indicated that different nanoparticles such as iron oxide nanoparticles, silver nanoparticles, and gold nanoparticles acted as anticancer agents while they also showed promising use in molecular imaging for cancer. The nanoparticles of synthetic and bio-based polymers such as PLGA, PVA, and chitosan were found as efficient nanocarriers that enhanced the therapeutic efficacy, bioavailability, and bioactivity of several phytochemicals with targeted drug delivery and sustained drug release profile. The nanoparticles were also found to reduce the toxicity effect of anticancer agents by delivering them to the tumor-infected site which prevents healthy tissues from exposure to anticancer agents. Moreover, it is expected that the combination of phytochemicals with nanoparticles will constitute the next frontier in clinical improvement. Further advances in the field of nanotechnology research and progress will be associated with the unique and high-impact tactics to cancer diagnosis and treatment.

References

1. Anand, P., Kunnumakara, A. B., Sundaram, C., Harikumar, K. B., Tharakan, S. T., Lai, O. S., Sung, B., & Aggarwal, B. B. (2008). Cancer is a preventable disease that requires major lifestyle changes. *Pharmaceutical Research, 25*(9), 2097–2116.
2. Abbas, Z., & Rehman, S. (2018). An overview of cancer treatment modalities. *Neoplasma, 139.*
3. Khan, N., Afaq, F., & Mukhtar, H. (2010). Lifestyle as risk factor for cancer: Evidence from human studies. *Cancer Letters, 293*(2), 133–143.
4. Parsa, N. (2012). Environmental factors inducing human cancers. *Iranian Journal of Public Health, 41*(11), 1.
5. Choudhury NAB, Selimuzzaman M, Bari MA, Wohab A, Hoque MB: Prevalence and identificationof socio-demographic factors and patterns of childhood cancer: A study in a Dhaka Shishu (Children) Hospital, Dhaka, Bangladesh.
6. Prasad, S., & Tyagi, A. K. (2015). Ginger and its constituents: Role in prevention and treatment of gastrointestinal cancer. *Gastroenterology Research and Practice, 2015.*
7. Aikou, T., Kitagawa, Y., Kitajima, M., Uenosono, Y., Bilchik, A. J., Martinez, S. R., & Saha, S. (2006). Sentinel lymph node mapping with GI cancer. *Cancer and Metastasis Reviews, 25* (2), 269–277.

8. Kaye, P., Lindsay, D., Madhusudan, S., Vohra, R., Catton, J., Platt, C., & Ragunath, K. (2019). Upper GI biopsies for adenocarcinoma – How many biopsies should endoscopists take? *Histopathology, 74*(6), 959–963.
9. Lin, S. Y., Liu, J. D., Chang, H. C., Yeh, S. D., Lin, C. H., & Lee, W. S. (2002). Magnolol suppresses proliferation of cultured human colon and liver cancer cells by inhibiting DNA synthesis and activating apoptosis. *Journal of Cellular Biochemistry, 84*(3), 532–544.
10. Fujiki, H., Sueoka, E., Watanabe, T., & Suganuma, M. (2015). Primary cancer prevention by green tea, and tertiary cancer prevention by the combination of green tea catechins and anticancer compounds. *Journal of Cancer Prevention, 20*(1), 1.
11. Bharali, D. J., Siddiqui, I. A., Adhami, V. M., Chamcheu, J. C., Aldahmash, A. M., Mukhtar, H., & Mousa, S. A. (2011). Nanoparticle delivery of natural products in the prevention and treatment of cancers: Current status and future prospects. *Cancers, 3*(4), 4024–4045.
12. Lin, Y.-H., Chen, Z.-R., Lai, C.-H., Hsieh, C.-H., & Feng, C.-L. (2015). Active targeted nanoparticles for oral administration of gastric cancer therapy. *Biomacromolecules, 16*(9), 3021–3032.
13. Chai, J. (2018). Introductory chapter: Esophagus and esophageal cancer. In *Esophageal Cancer and beyond*. London: IntechOpen.
14. Crew, K. D., & Neugut, A. I. (2006). Epidemiology of gastric cancer. *World journal of gastroenterology: WJG, 12*(3), 354.
15. Brenner, H., Rothenbacher, D., & Arndt, V. (2009). Epidemiology of stomach cancer. In *Cancer epidemiology* (pp. 467–477). Berlin: Springer.
16. Rawla, P., & Barsouk, A. (2019). Epidemiology of gastric cancer: Global trends, risk factors and prevention. *Przeglad Gastroenterologiczny, 14*(1), 26.
17. Hundal, R., & Shaffer, E. A. (2014). Gallbladder cancer: Epidemiology and outcome. *Clinical Epidemiology, 6*, 99.
18. Miller, G., & Jarnagin, W. (2008). Gallbladder carcinoma. *European Journal of Surgical Oncology (EJSO), 34*(3), 306–312.
19. Lazcano-Ponce, E. C., Miquel, J., Muñoz, N., Herrero, R., Ferrecio, C., Wistuba, I. I., De Ruiz, P. A., Urista, G. A., & Nervi, F. (2001). Epidemiology and molecular pathology of gallbladder cancer. *CA: a Cancer Journal for Clinicians, 51*(6), 349–364.
20. Misra, S., Chaturvedi, A., Misra, N. C., & Sharma, I. D. (2003). Carcinoma of the gallbladder. *The Lancet Oncology, 4*(3), 167–176.
21. Kamath, A., Roudenko, A., Hecht, E., Sirlin, C., Chernyak, V., Fowler, K., & Mitchell, D. G. (2019). CT/MR LI-RADS 2018: Clinical implications and management recommendations. *Abdominal Radiology, 44*(4), 1306–1322.
22. Kamisawa, T., Wood, L. D., Itoi, T., & Takaori, K. (2016). Pancreatic cancer. *The Lancet, 388* (10039), 73–85.
23. Xiao, M., Wang, Y., & Gao, Y. (2013). Association between Helicobacter pylori infection and pancreatic cancer development: A meta-analysis. *PLoS One, 8*(9), e75559.
24. Vincent, A., Herman, J., Schulick, R., Hruban, R. H., & Goggins, M. (2011). Pancreatic cancer. *The Lancet, 378*(9791), 607–620.
25. Korman, M. U. (2002). Radiologic evaluation and staging of small intestine neoplasms. *European Journal of Radiology, 42*(3), 193–205.
26. Pan, S. Y., & Morrison, H. (2011). Epidemiology of cancer of the small intestine. *World Journal of Gastrointestinal Oncology, 3*(3), 33.
27. Liu, R., Zhang, W., Liu, Z.-Q., & Zhou, H.-H. (2017). Associating transcriptional modules with colon cancer survival through weighted gene co-expression network analysis. *BMC Genomics, 18*(1), 361.
28. Kumar, K. S., Sastry, N., Polaki, H., & Mishra, V. (2015). Colon cancer prevention through probiotics: An overview. *Journal of Cancer Science and Therapy, 7*(2), 081–092.
29. Song, Y.-X., Gao, P., Wang, Z.-N., Liang, J.-W., Sun, Z., Wang, M.-X., Dong, Y.-L., Wang, X.-F., & Xu, H.-M. (2012). Can the tumor deposits be counted as metastatic lymph nodes in the UICC TNM staging system for colorectal cancer? *PLoS One, 7*(3), e34087.

30. Zavoral, M., Suchanek, S., Zavada, F., Dusek, L., Muzik, J., Seifert, B., & Fric, P. (2009). Colorectal cancer screening in Europe. *World Journal of Gastroenterology: WJG, 15*(47), 5907.
31. Grulich, A. E., Poynten, I. M., Machalek, D. A., Jin, F., Templeton, D. J., & Hillman, R. J. (2012). The epidemiology of anal cancer. *Sexual Health, 9*(6), 504–508.
32. Patel, H. S., Silver, A. R., & Northover, J. M. (2007). Anal cancer in renal transplant patients. *International Journal of Colorectal Disease, 22*(1), 1–5.
33. Pidhorecky, I., Cheney, R. T., Kraybill, W. G., & Gibbs, J. F. (2000). Gastrointestinal stromal tumors: Current diagnosis, biologic behavior, and management. *Annals of Surgical Oncology, 7*(9), 705–712.
34. Sugarbaker, P., Cunliffe, W., Belliveau, J., De Bruijn, E., Graves, T., Mullins, R., Schlag, P., et al. (1991). Rationale for integrating early postoperative intraperitoneal chemotherapy into the surgical treatment of gastrointestinal cancer. In *Proceedings of the 3rd international congress on neo-adjuvant chemotherapy* (pp. 272–275). Berlin: Springer.
35. Bold, R. J., Ishizuka, J., & Townsend, C. M., Jr. (1996). Progress toward hormonal therapy of gastrointestinal cancer. *Annals of Surgery, 223*(1), 4.
36. Hazard, L., O'Connor, J., & Scaife, C. (2006). Role of radiation therapy in gastric adenocarcinoma. *World journal of gastroenterology: WJG, 12*(10), 1511.
37. Barbieri, F., Bajetto, A., Pattarozzi, A., Gatti, M., Würth, R., Thellung, S., Corsaro, A., Villa, V., Nizzari, M., & Florio, T. (2013). Peptide receptor targeting in cancer: The somatostatin paradigm. *International Journal of Peptides, 2013.*
38. Gründker, C., & Emons, G. (2017). The role of gonadotropin-releasing hormone in cancer cell proliferation and metastasis. *Frontiers in Endocrinology, 8*, 187.
39. Ognjenovic, L., Trajkovski, G., Gjoshev, S., Shumkovski, A., Dzambaz, D., Hadzi-Manchev, D., Volcevski, G., Fildishevski, I., Nikolova, D., & Petrushevska, G. (2018). HER2 positive gastric carcinomas and their clinico-pathological characteristics. *Open Access Macedonian Journal of Medical Sciences, 6*(7), 1187.
40. D'Incalci, M., Steward, W. P., & Gescher, A. J. (2005). Use of cancer chemopreventive phytochemicals as antineoplastic agents. *The Lancet Oncology, 6*(11), 899–904.
41. Larsen, C. A., & Dashwood, R. H. (2010). (−)-Epigallocatechin-3-gallate inhibits met signaling, proliferation, and invasiveness in human colon cancer cells. *Archives of Biochemistry and Biophysics, 501*(1), 52–57.
42. Hire, R. R., Srivastava, S., Davis, M. B., Konreddy, A. K., & Panda, D. (2017). Antiproliferative activity of crocin involves targeting of microtubules in breast cancer cells. *Scientific Reports, 7*, 44984.
43. Kashyap, D., Sharma, A., Sak, K., Tuli, H. S., Buttar, H. S., & Bishayee, A. (2018). Fisetin: A bioactive phytochemical with potential for cancer prevention and pharmacotherapy. *Life Sciences, 194*, 75–87.
44. Zhang, Y., Chen, A. Y., Li, M., Chen, C., & Yao, Q. (2008). Ginkgo biloba extract kaempferol inhibits cell proliferation and induces apoptosis in pancreatic cancer cells. *Journal of Surgical Research, 148*(1), 17–23.
45. Miller, E. C., Giovannucci, E., Erdman, J. J., Bahnson, R., Schwartz, S. J., & Clinton, S. K. (2002). Tomato products, lycopene, and prostate cancer risk. *The Urologic Clinics of North America, 29*(1), 83–93.
46. Zhang, C., Su, Z.-Y., Khor TO, Shu, L., & Kong, A.-N. T. (2013). Sulforaphane enhances Nrf2 expression in prostate cancer TRAMP C1 cells through epigenetic regulation. *Biochemical Pharmacology, 85*(9), 1398–1404.
47. Spagnuolo, C., Russo, G. L., Orhan, I. E., Habtemariam, S., Daglia, M., Sureda, A., Nabavi, S. F., Devi, K. P., Loizzo, M. R., & Tundis, R. (2015). Genistein and cancer: Current status, challenges, and future directions. *Advances in Nutrition, 6*(4), 408–419.
48. Lee, S. H., Cekanova, M., & Baek, S. J. (2008). Multiple mechanisms are involved in 6-gingerol-induced cell growth arrest and apoptosis in human colorectal cancer cells.

Molecular Carcinogenesis: Published in cooperation with the University of Texas MD Anderson Cancer Center, 47(3), 197–208.

49. Sinha, D., Sarkar, N., Biswas, J., & Bishayee, A. (2016). Resveratrol for breast cancer prevention and therapy: Preclinical evidence and molecular mechanisms. In *Seminars in cancer biology* (pp. 209–232). Amsterdam: Elsevier.
50. Lim, S.-W., Loh, H.-S., Ting, K. N., Bradshaw, T. D., & Zeenathul, N. A. (2014). Antiproliferation and induction of caspase-8-dependent mitochondria-mediated apoptosis by β-tocotrienol in human lung and brain cancer cell lines. *Biomedicine & Pharmacotherapy, 68* (8), 1105–1115.
51. Pal, H. C., Sharma, S., Strickland, L. R., Agarwal, J., Athar, M., Elmets, C. A., & Afaq, F. (2013). Delphinidin reduces cell proliferation and induces apoptosis of non-small-cell lung cancer cells by targeting EGFR/VEGFR2 signaling pathways. *PLoS One, 8*(10), e77270.
52. Ciska, E., Verkerk, R., & Honke, J. (2009). Effect of boiling on the content of ascorbigen, indole-3-carbinol, indole-3-acetonitrile, and 3, 3′-diindolylmethane in fermented cabbage. *Journal of Agricultural and Food Chemistry, 57*(6), 2334–2338.
53. Hatkevich, T., Ramos, J., Santos-Sanchez, I., & Patel, Y. M. (2014). A naringenin–tamoxifen combination impairs cell proliferation and survival of MCF-7 breast cancer cells. *Experimental Cell Research, 327*(2), 331–339.
54. Kim, K. K., Singh, A. P., Singh, R. K., DeMartino, A., Brard, L., Vorsa, N., Lange, T. S., & Moore, R. G. (2012). Anti-angiogenic activity of cranberry proanthocyanidins and cytotoxic properties in ovarian cancer cells. *International Journal of Oncology, 40*(1), 227–235.
55. Li, K., Dias, S. J., Rimando, A. M., Dhar, S., Mizuno, C. S., Penman, A. D., Lewin, J. R., & Levenson, A. S. (2013). Pterostilbene acts through metastasis-associated protein 1 to inhibit tumor growth, progression and metastasis in prostate cancer. *PLoS One, 8*(3), e57542.
56. Dechsupa, S., Kothan, S., Vergote, J., Leger, G., Martineau, A., Beranger, S., Kosanlavit, R., Moretti, J.-L., & Mankhetkorn, S. (2007). Quercetin, Siamois 1 and Siamois 2 induce apoptosis in human breast cancer MDA-mB-435 cells xenograft in vivo. *Cancer Biology & Therapy, 6*(1), 56–61.
57. Chen, M.-C., Hsu, S.-L., Lin, H., & Yang, T.-Y. (2014). Retinoic acid and cancer treatment. *Biomedicine (Taipei), 4*(4), 22–22.
58. Wing Ying Cheung, C., Gibbons, N., Wayne Johnson, D., & Lawrence Nicol, D. (2010). Silibinin-a promising new treatment for cancer. *Anti-Cancer Agents in Medicinal Chemistry (Formerly Current Medicinal Chemistry-Anti-Cancer Agents), 10*(3), 186–195.
59. Girisa, S., Shabnam, B., Monisha, J., Fan, L., Halim, C. E., Arfuso, F., Ahn, K. S., Sethi, G., & Kunnumakkara, A. B. (2019). Potential of zerumbone as an anti-cancer agent. *Molecules, 24* (4), 734.
60. Puccinelli, M. T., & Stan, S. D. (2017). Dietary bioactive diallyl trisulfide in cancer prevention and treatment. *International Journal of Molecular Sciences, 18*(8), 1645.
61. Qu, D., Zhang, X., Sang, C., Zhou, Y., Ma, J., & Hui, L. (2019). Lappaconitine sulfate induces apoptosis in human colon cancer HT-29 cells and down-regulates PI3K/AKT/GSK3β signaling pathway. *Medicinal Chemistry Research, 28*(6), 907–916.
62. Zhang, H., Jiao, Y., Shi, C., Song, X., Chang, Y., Ren, Y., & Shi, X. (2018). Berbamine suppresses cell proliferation and promotes apoptosis in ovarian cancer partially via the inhibition of Wnt/β-catenin signaling. *Acta Biochimica et Biophysica Sinica, 50*(6), 532–539.
63. Maioli, E., Torricelli, C., & Valacchi, G. (2012). Rottlerin and cancer: Novel evidence and mechanisms. *The Scientific World Journal, 2012*.
64. Chen, J.-Y., Tang, Y.-A., Li, W.-S., Chiou, Y.-C., Shieh, J.-M., & Wang, Y.-C. (2013). A synthetic podophyllotoxin derivative exerts anti-cancer effects by inducing mitotic arrest and pro-apoptotic ER stress in lung cancer preclinical models. *PLoS One, 8*(4), e62082.
65. Payton-Stewart, F., Schoene, N. W., Kim, Y. S., Burow, M. E., Cleveland, T. E., Boue, S. M., & Wang, T. T. (2009). Molecular effects of soy phytoalexin glyceollins in human prostate cancer cells LNCaP. *Molecular Carcinogenesis: Published in cooperation with the University of Texas MD Anderson Cancer Center, 48*(9), 862–871.

66. Witayasinthana, W., & Shotipruk, A. (2009). Recovery of anti-cancer damnacanthal from roots of Morinda citrifolia by microwave-assisted extraction. *Separation Science and Technology, 44*(12), 2942–2955.
67. Catalano, E. (2016). Role of phytochemicals in the chemoprevention of tumors. *arXiv preprint arXiv*, 160504519.
68. Tuorkey, M. J. (2015). Cancer therapy with phytochemicals: Present and future perspectives. *Biomedical and Environmental Sciences, 28*(11), 808–819.
69. Singh, D., Madhav, H., & Jaiswar, G. (2016). Effects on zinc oxide on polyacrylic acid: A core–shell nanoparticles. *Science and Engineering Applications, 1*, 36–39.
70. Madhav, H., Singh, N., Singh, P., & Jaiswar, G. (2017). Biological synthesis of nanoparticles and their applications: A review. *Agra University Journal of Research: Science, 1*(2), 25–30.
71. Singh, N., Madhav, H., Yadav, S., & Jaiswar, G. (2018). Critical evaluation of thermal, optical and morphological properties of V, S and Dy doped-ZnO/PVDF/functionalized-PMMA blended Nanocomposites. *Journal of Inorganic and Organometallic Polymers and Materials, 28*(5), 2121–2130.
72. Madhav, H., Singh, N., & Jaiswar, G. (2019). Thermoset, bioactive, metal–polymer composites for medical applications. In *Materials for biomedical engineering* (pp. 105–143). Amsterdam: Elsevier.
73. Madhav, H., Singh, P., Singh, N., & Jaiswar, G. (2017). Evaluations of thermal and antibacterial properties of nanocomposites of functionalized poly (methyl methacrylate) with different amino containing groups. *Macromolecular Research, 25*(7), 689–696.
74. Singh, N., Madhav, H., Yadav, S., & Jaiswar, G. (2019). Impact of vanadium-, sulfur-, and dysprosium-doped zinc oxide nanoparticles on various properties of PVDF/functionalized-PMMA blend nanocomposites: Structural, optical, and morphological studies. *Journal of Applied Polymer Science, 136*(9), 47116.
75. Rathore, S., Madhav, H., & Jaiswar, G. (2019). Efficient nano-filler for the phase transformation in polyvinylidene fluoride nanocomposites by using nanoparticles of stannous sulfate. *Materials Research Innovations, 23*(4), 183–190.
76. Iravani, S., & Varma, R. S. (2019). Plant-derived edible nanoparticles and miRNAs: Emerging frontier for therapeutics and targeted drug-delivery. *ACS Sustainable Chemistry & Engineering, 7*(9), 8055–8069.
77. Rao PV, Nallappan D, Madhavi K, Rahman S, Jun Wei L, Gan SH: Phytochemicals and biogenic metallic nanoparticles as anticancer agents. *Oxidative medicine and cellular longevity* 2016, 2016.
78. Ma, Y.-Y., Jin, K.-T., Wang, S.-B., Wang, H.-J., Tong, X.-M., Huang, D.-S., & Mou, X.-Z. (2017). Molecular imaging of cancer with nanoparticle based theranostic probes. *Contrast Media & Molecular Imaging, 2017.*
79. Bazak, R., Houri, M., El Achy, S., Kamel, S., & Refaat, T. (2015). Cancer active targeting by nanoparticles: A comprehensive review of literature. *Journal of Cancer Research and Clinical Oncology, 141*(5), 769–784.
80. Wiwanitkit, V. (2006). Glomerular pore size corresponding to albumin molecular size, an explanation for underlying structural pathology leading to albuminuria at nanolevel. *Renal Failure, 28*(1), 101–101.
81. Cheng, Z., Yan, X., Sun, X., Shen, B., & Gambhir, S. S. (2016). Tumor molecular imaging with nanoparticles. *Engineering, 2*(1), 132–140.
82. Pericleous, P., Gazouli, M., Lyberopoulou, A., Rizos, S., Nikiteas, N., & Efstathopoulos, E. P. (2012). Quantum dots hold promise for early cancer imaging and detection. *International Journal of Cancer, 131*(3), 519–528.
83. Fang, M., Peng, C.-W., Pang, D.-W., & Li, Y. (2012). Quantum dots for cancer research: Current status, remaining issues, and future perspectives. *Cancer Biology & Medicine, 9*(3), 151.
84. Gao, J., Chen, K., Luong, R., Bouley, D. M., Mao, H., Qiao, T., Gambhir, S. S., & Cheng, Z. (2011). A novel clinically translatable fluorescent nanoparticle for targeted molecular imaging of tumors in living subjects. *Nano Letters, 12*(1), 281–286.

85. Geng, X. F., Fang, M., Liu, S. P., & Li, Y. (2016). Quantum dot-based molecular imaging of cancer cell growth using a clone formation assay. *Molecular Medicine Reports, 14*(4), 3007–3012.
86. Liu, X., Braun, G. B., Qin, M., Ruoslahti, E., & Sugahara, K. N. (2017). In vivo cation exchange in quantum dots for tumor-specific imaging. *Nature Communications, 8*(1), 343.
87. Brunetti, J., Riolo, G., Gentile, M., Bernini, A., Paccagnini, E., Falciani, C., Lozzi, L., Scali, S., Depau, L., & Pini, A. (2018). Near-infrared quantum dots labelled with a tumor selective tetrabranched peptide for in vivo imaging. *Journal of Nanobiotechnology, 16*(1), 21.
88. Silva, C. O., Pinho, J. O., Lopes, J. M., Almeida, A. J., Gaspar, M. M., & Reis, C. (2019). Current trends in cancer nanotheranostics: Metallic, polymeric, and lipid-based systems. *Pharmaceutics, 11*(1), 22.
89. Wang, H., Li, X., Tse, B. W.-C., Yang, H., Thorling, C. A., Liu, Y., Touraud, M., Chouane, J. B., Liu, X., & Roberts, M. S. (2018). Indocyanine green-incorporating nanoparticles for cancer theranostics. *Theranostics, 8*(5), 1227.
90. Li, S., Johnson, J., Peck, A., & Xie, Q. (2017). Near infrared fluorescent imaging of brain tumor with IR780 dye incorporated phospholipid nanoparticles. *Journal of Translational Medicine, 15*(1), 18.
91. Chansaenpak, K., Tanjindaprateep, S., Chaicharoenaudomrung, N., Weeranantanapan, O., Noisa, P., & Kamkaew, A. (2018). Aza-BODIPY based polymeric nanoparticles for cancer cell imaging. *RSC Advances, 8*(69), 39248–39255.
92. Yang, Y., & Cui, D. (2017). Upconversion nanoparticles for gastric cancer targeted imaging and therapy. In *Gastric cancer prewarning and early diagnosis system* (pp. 239–270). Berlin: Springer.
93. Thomas, R., Park, I.-K., & Jeong, Y. Y. (2013). Magnetic iron oxide nanoparticles for multimodal imaging and therapy of cancer. *International Journal of Molecular Sciences, 14* (8), 15910–15930.
94. Schleich, N., Sibret, P., Danhier, P., Ucakar, B., Laurent, S., Muller, R. N., Jérôme, C., Gallez, B., Préat, V., & Danhier, F. (2013). Dual anticancer drug/superparamagnetic iron oxide-loaded PLGA-based nanoparticles for cancer therapy and magnetic resonance imaging. *International Journal of Pharmaceutics, 447*(1), 94–101.
95. Ruan, J., Ji, J., Song, H., Qian, Q., Wang, K., Wang, C., & Cui, D. (2012). Fluorescent magnetic nanoparticle-labeled mesenchymal stem cells for targeted imaging and hyperthermia therapy of in vivo gastric cancer. *Nanoscale Research Letters, 7*, 309.
96. Deserno, W. M. L. L. G., Harisinghani, M. G., Taupitz, M., Jager, G. J., Witjes, J. A., Mulders, P. F., CAHVD, K., Kaufmann, D., & Barentsz, J. O. (2004). Urinary bladder cancer: Preoperative nodal staging with ferumoxtran-10-enhanced MR imaging. *Radiology, 233*(2), 449–456.
97. Hudgins, P. A., Anzai, Y., Morris, M. R., & Lucas, M. A. (2002). Ferumoxtran-10, a superparamagnetic iron oxide as a magnetic resonance enhancement agent for imaging lymph nodes: A phase 2 dose study. *American Journal of Neuroradiology, 23*(4), 649–656.
98. Jalalian, S. H., Taghdisi, S. M., Hamedani, N. S., Kalat, S. A. M., Lavaee, P., ZandKarimi, M., Ghows, N., Jaafari, M. R., Naghibi, S., & Danesh, N. M. (2013). Epirubicin loaded super paramagnetic iron oxide nanoparticle-aptamer bioconjugate for combined colon cancer therapy and imaging in vivo. *European Journal of Pharmaceutical Sciences, 50*(2), 191–197.
99. Cho, Y.-S., Yoon, T.-J., Jang, E.-S., Hong, K. S., Lee, S. Y., Kim, O. R., Park, C., Kim, Y.-J., Yi, G.-C., & Chang, K. (2010). Cetuximab-conjugated magneto-fluorescent silica nanoparticles for in vivo colon cancer targeting and imaging. *Cancer Letters, 299*(1), 63–71.
100. Xu, X., An, H., Zhang, D., Tao, H., Dou, Y., Li, X., Huang, J., & Zhang, J. (2019). A self-illuminating nanoparticle for inflammation imaging and cancer therapy. *Science Advances, 5* (1), eaat2953.
101. Sasaki, Y., Nishina, T., Yasui, H., Goto, M., Muro, K., Tsuji, A., Koizumi, W., Toh, Y., Hara, T., & Miyata, Y. (2014). Phase II trial of nanoparticle albumin-bound paclitaxel as second-line chemotherapy for unresectable or recurrent gastric cancer. *Cancer Science, 105*(7), 812–817.

102. Li, X., Lu, X., Xu, H., Zhu, Z., Yin, H., Qian, X., Li, R., Jiang, X., & Liu, B. (2011). Paclitaxel/tetrandrine coloaded nanoparticles effectively promote the apoptosis of gastric cancer cells based on "oxidation therapy". *Molecular Pharmaceutics, 9*(2), 222–229.
103. Sun, Z., Song, X., Li, X., Su, T., Qi, S., Qiao, R., Wang, F., Huan, Y., Yang, W., & Wang, J. (2014). In vivo multimodality imaging of miRNA-16 iron nanoparticle reversing drug resistance to chemotherapy in a mouse gastric cancer model. *Nanoscale, 6*(23), 14343–14353.
104. Zhang, Z., & Feng, S.-S. (2006). Self-assembled nanoparticles of poly (lactide)–vitamin E TPGS copolymers for oral chemotherapy. *International Journal of Pharmaceutics, 324*(2), 191–198.
105. Wu, F.-l., Li, R.-T., Yang, M., Yue, G.-F., Wang, H.-Y., Liu, Q., Cui, F.-B., Wu, P.-Y., Ding, H., & Yu, L.-X. (2015). Gelatinases-stimuli nanoparticles encapsulating 5-fluorouridine and 5-aza-2′-deoxycytidine enhance the sensitivity of gastric cancer cells to chemical therapeutics. *Cancer Letters, 363*(1), 7–16.
106. Li, K., Dai, Y., Chen, W., Yu, K., Xiao, G., Richardson, J. J., Huang, W., Guo, J., Liao, X., & Shi, B. (2019). Self-assembled metal-phenolic nanoparticles for enhanced synergistic combination therapy against colon cancer. *Advanced Biosystems, 3*(2), 1800241.
107. Rashid, R. A., Abidin, S. Z., Anuar, M. A. K., Tominaga, T., Akasaka, H., Sasaki, R., Kie, K., Razak, K. A., Pham, B. T., & Hawkett, B. S. (2019). Radiosensitization effects and ROS generation by high Z metallic nanoparticles on human colon carcinoma cell (HCT116) irradiated under 150 MeV proton beam. *OpenNano, 4*, 100027.
108. Karuppaiya, P., Satheeshkumar, E., & Tsay, H. S. (2019). Biogenic synthesis of silver nanoparticles using rhizome extract of Dysosma pleiantha and its antiproliferative effect against breast and human gastric cancer cells. *Molecular Biology Reports*, 1–10.
109. Al-Radadi, N. S. (2019). Green synthesis of platinum nanoparticles using Saudi's dates extract and their usage on the cancer cell treatment. *Arabian Journal of Chemistry, 12*(3), 330–349.
110. Jain, A., Jain, R., Jain, S., Khatik, R., & Veer Kohli, D. (2019). Minicapsules encapsulating nanoparticles for targeting, apoptosis induction and treatment of colon cancer. *Artificial Cells, Nanomedicine, and Biotechnology, 47*(1), 1085–1093.
111. Cordani, M., & Somoza, Á. (2019). Targeting autophagy using metallic nanoparticles: A promising strategy for cancer treatment. *Cellular and Molecular Life Sciences, 76*(7), 1215–1242.
112. Khan, H., Ullah, H., Martorell, M., Valdes, S. E., Belwal, T., Tejada, S., Sureda, A., & Kamal, M. A. (2019). Flavonoids nanoparticles in cancer: Treatment, prevention and clinical prospects. *Seminars in Cancer Biology*.
113. Sutradhar, K. B., & Amin, M. L. (2014). Nanotechnology in cancer drug delivery and selective targeting. *ISRN Nanotechnology, 2014*, 12.
114. Dadwal, A., Baldi, A., & Kumar Narang, R. (2018). Nanoparticles as carriers for drug delivery in cancer. *Artificial Cells, Nanomedicine, and Biotechnology, 46*(sup2), 295–305.
115. Liyanage, P. Y., Hettiarachchi, S. D., Zhou, Y., Ouhtit, A., Seven, E. S., Oztan, C. Y., Celik, E., & Leblanc, R. M. (2019). Nanoparticle-mediated targeted drug delivery for breast cancer treatment. *Biochimica et Biophysica Acta (BBA) - Reviews on Cancer, 1871*(2), 419–433.
116. Lombardo, D., Kiselev, M. A., & Caccamo, M. T. (2019). Smart nanoparticles for drug delivery application: Development of versatile nanocarrier platforms in biotechnology and nanomedicine. *Journal of Nanomaterials, 2019*, 26.
117. Senapati, S., Mahanta, A. K., Kumar, S., & Maiti, P. (2018). Controlled drug delivery vehicles for cancer treatment and their performance. *Signal Transduction and Targeted Therapy, 3*, 7–7.
118. Li, Z., Tan, S., Li, S., Shen, Q., & Wang, K. (2017). Cancer drug delivery in the nano era: An overview and perspectives. *Oncology Reports, 38*(2), 611–624.
119. Suri, S. S., Fenniri, H., & Singh, B. (2007). Nanotechnology-based drug delivery systems. *Journal of Occupational Medicine and Toxicology, 2*(1), 16.
120. Kato, K., Chin, K., Yoshikawa, T., Yamaguchi, K., Tsuji, Y., Esaki, T., Sakai, K., Kimura, M., Hamaguchi, T., & Shimada, Y. (2012). Phase II study of NK105, a paclitaxel-incorporating

micellar nanoparticle, for previously treated advanced or recurrent gastric cancer. *Investigational New Drugs, 30*(4), 1621–1627.
121. Xie, J., Yang, Z., Zhou, C., Zhu, J., Lee, R. J., & Teng, L. (2016). Nanotechnology for the delivery of phytochemicals in cancer therapy. *Biotechnology Advances, 34*(4), 343–353.
122. Arora, D., Saneja, A., & Jaglan, S. (2019). Cyclodextrin-based delivery systems for dietary pharmaceuticals. *Environmental Chemistry Letters*, 1–8.
123. Thipe, V. C., Amiri, K. P., Bloebaum, P., Karikachery, A. R., Khoobchandani, M., Katti, K. K., Jurisson, S. S., & Katti, K. V. (2019). Development of resveratrol-conjugated gold nanoparticles: Interrelationship of increased resveratrol corona on anti-tumor efficacy against breast, pancreatic and prostate cancers. *International Journal of Nanomedicine, 14*, 4413.
124. Brian, M. O., & Selvi, S. (2019). Cytotoxic effects of Ceiba pentandra L. mediated silver nanoparticles on HCT-116 colon cancer cell lines through ROS generation and cell membrane damage. *International Journal of Research in Pharmaceutical Sciences, 10*(4), 3236–3243.
125. Elbialy, N. S., Abdelfatah, E. A., & Khalil, W. A. (2019). Antitumor activity of curcumin-green synthesized gold nanoparticles: In vitro study. *BioNanoScience*, 1–8.
126. Mariadoss, A. V. A., Vinayagam, R., Xu, B., Venkatachalam, K., Sankaran, V., Vijayakumar, S., Bakthavatsalam, S. R., Mohamed, S. A., & David, E. (2019). Phloretin loaded chitosan nanoparticles enhance the antioxidants and apoptotic mechanisms in DMBA induced experimental carcinogenesis. *Chemico-Biological Interactions, 308*, 11–19.
127. Zhou, X., Liu, Y., Huang, Y., Ma, Y., Lv, J., & Xiao, B. (2019). Mucus-penetrating polymeric nanoparticles for oral delivery of curcumin to inflamed colon tissue. *Journal of Drug Delivery Science and Technology, 52*, 157–164.
128. Hajizadeh, M. R., Parvaz, N., Barani, M., Khoshdel, A., Fahmidehkar, M. A., Mahmoodi, M., & Torkzadeh-Mahani, M. (2019). Diosgenin-loaded niosome as an effective phytochemical nanocarrier: Physicochemical characterization, loading efficiency, and cytotoxicity assay. *DARU Journal of Pharmaceutical Sciences*, 1–11.
129. Anter, H. M., Hashim, I. I. A., Awadin, W., & Meshali, M. M. (2019). Novel chitosan oligosaccharide-based nanoparticles for gastric mucosal administration of the phytochemical "apocynin". *International Journal of Nanomedicine, 14*, 4911.
130. Maity, R., Chatterjee, M., Banerjee, A., Das, A., Mishra, R., Mazumder, S., & Chanda, N. (2019). Gold nanoparticle-assisted enhancement in the anti-cancer properties of theaflavin against human ovarian cancer cells. *Materials Science and Engineering: C, 109909.*
131. Gao, J., Fan, K., Jin, Y., Zhao, L., Wang, Q., Tang, Y., Xu, H., Liu, Z., Wang, S., & Lin, J. (2019). PEGylated lipid bilayer coated mesoporous silica nanoparticles co-delivery of paclitaxel and curcumin leads to increased tumor site drug accumulation and reduced tumor burden. *European Journal of Pharmaceutical Sciences, 140*, 105070.
132. Sweety, J. P., Sowparani, S., Mahalakshmi, P., Selvasudha, N., Yamini, D., Geetha, K., & Ruckmani, K. (2020). Fabrication of stimuli gated nanoformulation for site-specific delivery of thymoquinone for colon cancer treatment – insight into thymoquinone's improved physicochemical properties. *Journal of Drug Delivery Science and Technology, 55*, 101334.
133. Saraf, A., Dubey, N., Dubey, N., & Sharma, M. (2019). Box Behnken design based development of curcumin loaded Eudragit S100 nanoparticles for site-spcific delivery in colon cancer. *Research Journal of Pharmacy and Technology, 12*(8), 3672–3678.
134. Udompornmongkol, P., & Chiang, B.-H. (2015). Curcumin-loaded polymeric nanoparticles for enhanced anti-colorectal cancer applications. *Journal of Biomaterials Applications, 30*(5), 537–546.
135. Anitha, A., Sreeranganathan, M., Chennazhi, K. P., Lakshmanan, V.-K., & Jayakumar, R. (2014). In vitro combinatorial anticancer effects of 5-fluorouracil and curcumin loaded N, O-carboxymethyl chitosan nanoparticles toward colon cancer and in vivo pharmacokinetic studies. *European Journal of Pharmaceutics and Biopharmaceutics, 88*(1), 238–251.
136. Huang, W., Wang, X., Shi, C., Guo, D., Xu, G., Wang, L., Bodman, A., & Luo, J. (2015). Fine-tuning vitamin E-containing telodendrimers for efficient delivery of gambogic acid in colon cancer treatment. *Molecular Pharmaceutics, 12*(4), 1216–1229.

137. Lotfi-Attari, J., Pilehvar-Soltanahmadi, Y., Dadashpour, M., Alipour, S., Farajzadeh, R., Javidfar, S., & Zarghami, N. (2017). Co-delivery of curcumin and chrysin by polymeric nanoparticles inhibit synergistically growth and hTERT gene expression in human colorectal cancer cells. *Nutrition and Cancer, 69*(8), 1290–1299.
138. Vimala, K., Sundarraj, S., Paulpandi, M., Vengatesan, S., & Kannan, S. (2014). Green synthesized doxorubicin loaded zinc oxide nanoparticles regulates the Bax and Bcl-2 expression in breast and colon carcinoma. *Process Biochemistry, 49*(1), 160–172.
139. Prajakta, D., Ratnesh, J., Chandan, K., Suresh, S., Grace, S., Meera, V., & Vandana, P. (2009). Curcumin loaded pH-sensitive nanoparticles for the treatment of colon cancer. *Journal of Biomedical Nanotechnology, 5*(5), 445–455.
140. Han, X., Jiang, X., Guo, L., Wang, Y., Veeraraghavan, V. P., Krishna Mohan, S., Wang, Z., & Cao, D. (2019). Anticarcinogenic potential of gold nanoparticles synthesized from Trichosanthes kirilowii in colon cancer cells through the induction of apoptotic pathway. *Artificial Cells, Nanomedicine, and Biotechnology, 47*(1), 3577–3584.

Chapter 8
Emerging Roles of Phytochemicals in the Pathobiology and Management of Esophageal Cancer

Asad ur Rahman, Deepika Sarvepalli, Mamoon Ur Rashid, Saeed Ali, Awais Naeem, Asif Imran, Effa Zahid, and Sarfraz Ahmad

Abstract Esophageal cancer demonstrates varying epidemiology across the globe. Over the last 30 years, esophageal adenocarcinoma has overtaken esophageal squamous cell cancer as the most common histologic variety in the Western hemisphere. However, esophageal squamous cell cancer remains the predominant type in Asia. Despite an increase in our understanding of its pathophysiology, varying chemotherapeutic regimens have not made any significant impact on the survival of patients with this disease. These chemotherapeutic agents have potentially severe adverse effects which affect the patient adherence to the given treatment. As an alternative modality of the disease treatment, various phytochemicals have been studied as therapeutic and prophylactic entities for esophageal cancer. Most of these agents exert their effect using antioxidant and anti-inflammatory pathways. In this chapter, we discuss the roles of curcumin, flavonoids, and other agents in terms of the available data. As we move towards preventative care among the high-risk

A. u. Rahman (✉)
Department of Gastroenterology, Cleveland Clinic Florida, Weston, FL, USA
e-mail: rahmanf3@ccf.org

D. Sarvepalli · M. U. Rashid
Department of Internal Medicine, Advent Health, Orlando, FL, USA

S. Ali
Department of Internal Medicine, University of Iowa, Iowa City, IA, USA

A. Naeem
Department of Medicine, Khyber Teaching Hospital, Peshawar, Pakistan

A. Imran
Department of Gastroenterology, Rehman Medical Institute, Peshawar, Pakistan

E. Zahid
Services Institute of Medical Sciences, Lahore, Pakistan

S. Ahmad (✉)
AdventHealth Cancer Institute, FSU and UCF Colleges of Medicine, Orlando, FL, USA
e-mail: sarfraz.ahmad@adventhealth.com

G. P. Nagaraju (ed.), *Phytochemicals Targeting Tumor Microenvironment in Gastrointestinal Cancers*, https://doi.org/10.1007/978-3-030-48405-7_8

patients with conditions such as Barrett's esophagus, supplementation of these phytochemicals may lead to halting and decrease in the progression towards malignancy. More robust studies are needed prior to recommending their widespread application; however, in the era of cost-effective medicine, introducing such options in the care of patients will have a significant impact in the long run. We also briefly discuss the current state of chemotherapeutic and immune therapeutic options for patients with esophageal cancer.

Keywords Phytochemicals · Cancer · Esophagus · Targeted therapies · Pathobiology · Management · Clinical outcomes

Abbreviations

BSC	Best supportive care
CD	Cluster differentiation
COX	Cyclooxygenase
CSC	Cancer stem cells
CTLA-4	Cytotoxic T-lymphocyte-associated protein 4
EAC	Esophageal adenocarcinoma
EGCG	Epigallocatechin gallate
EGFR	Epidermal growth factor receptor
ESC	Esophageal squamous cell cancer
FDA	Food and Drug Administration (USA)
FGFR	Fibroblast growth factor receptor
5-FU	5-Fluorouracil
GEJ	Gastroesophageal junctional carcinoma
GERD	Gastroesophageal reflux disease
HER2	Human epidermal growth factor receptor 2
IL	Interleukin
NF-kB	Nuclear factor-kB
OR	Odds ratio
ORR	Objective response rate
OS	Overall survival
PD-1	Programmed cell death protein 1
PDGFR	Platelet-derived growth factor receptor
PD-L1	Programmed death-ligand 1
PFS	Progression-free survival
PGE-2	Prostaglandin E-2
ROS	Reactive oxygen species
RTK	Receptor tyrosine kinase
TKI	Tyrosine kinase inhibitors
VEGFR	Vascular endothelial growth factor receptor

1 Epidemiology of Esophageal Cancer

Esophageal cancer is one of the most common malignancies in the world and is the ninth most common malignancy overall [1]. However, in the United States, it accounts for nearly 1% of all the cancer diagnoses and is currently the 11th leading cause of cancer-related deaths [2]. In the United States, it is diagnosed most commonly in patients between the age of 65 and 74 years.

The two major subtypes of esophageal cancer are esophageal adenocarcinoma (EAC) and esophageal squamous cell cancer (ESC). Although globally 95% of all esophageal cancers are ESC, there are significant worldwide geographic differences. EAC has overtaken ESC as the predominant type in the developed countries, while ESC is still the most common variety in the African and East Asian countries [3]. Although the incidence of esophageal cancer in the United States has increased from 1975 till 2006, since then it has shown a steady decline. Both major varieties of esophageal cancers more commonly occur in men compared to women. The current age-adjusted annual incidence is 4.3 cases per 100,000 people [2]. This is in stark contrast to the "esophageal cancer belt" of Northern Iran, Northern China, Kazakhstan, and Uzbekistan, where the incidence of esophageal cancer (predominantly ESC) has been reported to be as high as 800 cases per 100,000 population [4].

The predominant risk factors for ESC include cigarette smoking, alcohol consumption, dietary use of N-nitroso compounds, deficiency of zinc, selenium, caustic strictures, Plummer-Vinson syndrome, and tylosis [5]. Comparatively, the predominant risk factors for EAC are gastroesophageal reflux disease (GERD) and metabolic syndrome since they increase the risk of Barrett's esophagus [6]. About 40% of the diagnosed cases have distant metastatic disease, and these patients have a 5-year survival of 19.9%. However, the 5-year survival is much better (46.7%) in patients with localized esophageal cancer. Despite the decline seen in the incidence of esophageal cancer over the last decade, the mortality rate and 5-year survival have not changed significantly. This has led to significant research to explore newer treatment strategies, including the use of phytochemicals, for the management of esophageal cancer.

2 The Role of Phytochemicals in the Treatment of Esophageal Cancer

Although the localized esophageal cancer is being increasingly managed with endoscopic resection strategies, the mainstay of the treatment for advanced esophageal cancer comprises a combination of surgery, chemotherapy, and/or radiation [7]. Despite significant advances in the diagnosis and treatment, the 5-year survival rate for the disease remains relatively low. The modalities in use for the treatment of esophageal cancers are known to have numerous side effects and, at times, limited efficacy given the usual late stage at which the disease is detected owing to the slow onset of symptoms, a factor that significantly contributes to the dismal survival rate [8, 9]. Therefore, the need to identify novel treatment modalities remains high, not only in complementing the currently available treatment options but also in playing possible role(s) towards the prevention and management of the disease.

One such area of promise is the use of phytochemicals. The word phytochemical is originally derived from phyto which in Greek means related to plants. Phytochemicals are nonessential plant-based compounds found abundantly in fruits, vegetables, grains, etc. [10]. Though used for various ailments over centuries, the role of phytochemicals is only now being elucidated scientifically. Over the past few decades, numerous studies have identified a wide array of pharmacological effects for phytochemicals, particularly as antioxidants and anti-inflammatory agents while also possessing significant anticancer properties [11–14].

Phytochemicals are primarily classified into five groups, namely carotenoids, phenolics, alkaloids, nitrogen-containing compounds, and organo-sulfides [10]. Among these, most studies have been done on phenolics and carotenoids. The anticancer roles/properties of various phytochemicals are well documented in peer-reviewed studies pertaining to cancers of the gastrointestinal tract [11]. Here, we therefore discuss the role(s) of some of the most well-studied phytochemicals in the potential treatment and management of esophageal cancer.

3 Curcumin

Turmeric is a major spice in Asian cuisines and has been used for centuries in herbal medicine. By virtue of its antioxidant properties, it acts as an anti-inflammatory agent; studies have documented its role(s) in lowering the incidence of cancer [12]. It is one of the three curcuminoids in the spice, belonging to the subcategory of phenolic acids under the group phenolics [10, 13]. Curcumin possesses a significant anti-oncogenic profile owing to its effects on multiple molecular pathways involved in carcinogenesis such as its regulation of an array of membrane receptors, transcription factors, cytokines, kinases, and other enzymes [14–16]. The anticancer effects of curcumin in gastrointestinal malignancies such as esophageal, gastric, and colon cancers are well documented [11, 17–19]. Interestingly, a comparison of the effect of curcumin and 5-fluorouracil (5-FU) on esophageal squamous cell carcinoma found curcumin to be more effective [20].

In esophageal cancers, multiple molecular pathways are involved in the pathogenesis and progression of the disease (Fig. 8.1). The efficacy of curcumin on esophageal malignancies has been evaluated through various angles. Oxidative stress produced by reactive oxygen species (ROS) plays a significant role(s) in the development of many cancers, including those of the esophagus [21]. One study identified curcumin to exert an antioxidant and an anti-inflammatory effect on esophageal cell lines as a result of induction of the activity of superoxide dismutase-1, a potent antioxidant enzyme, and inhibition of the activity of cyclooxygenase-2, a pro-inflammatory protein, respectively [22]. Another study

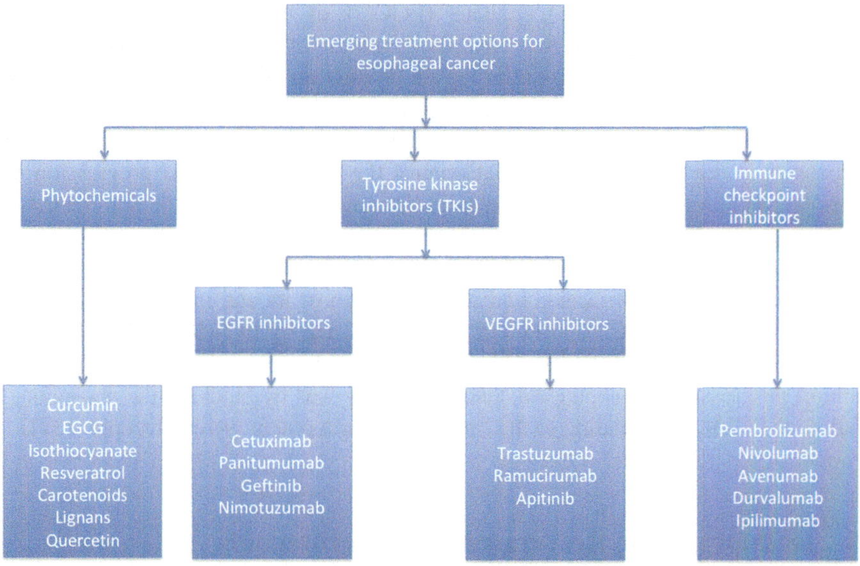

Fig. 8.1 Schematic representation of some of the emerging treatment options for the management of esophageal cancer

further expanded upon curcumin's anti-inflammatory role in esophageal tumorigenesis by highlighting its inhibition of nuclear factor (NF)-kB activity and interleukin (IL)-8 mRNA expression [23].

Curcumin promotes apoptosis and cell cycle arrest in esophageal cancer cells by inhibiting the Notch signaling pathway, a process known to be upregulated in many cases of esophageal cancers [24, 25]. In many tumors, such as esophageal squamous cell carcinoma, cancer stem cells (CSCs) are known to contribute to the poor prognosis of the disease [26, 27]. The CSCs differentiate into non-CSCs making up the bulk of these tumors [28]. Moreover, CSCs have also been found to add to the resistance of tumors towards the traditional chemo- and radiotherapies [29]. Curcumin has shown efficacy in targeting these CSCs in esophageal cancer [18].

4 Epigallocatechin Gallate

Besides phenolic acids from which curcumin traces its origin, another very-well-studied subcategory of phenolics is the flavonoids [10]. Flavonoids are found abundantly in fruits and tea [13]. Historically, green tea has been infamous in possessing numerous health benefits, ranging from its roles as an antibacterial and anti-inflammatory agent to its effects in cardioprotection and cancer prevention [30]. As far as green tea's anticancer role is concerned, researchers have identified the catechin epigallocatechin gallate (EGCG) as the primary active agent [31]. Although abundant in green tea, the levels of EGCG in black tea are much lower as the catechin is oxidized during the production process of black tea leaves, explaining the difference in the anticancer effects of the two types of teas [32]. Studies have also found EGCG to exert its anticancer effects through a myriad of processes at the molecular level that control the development and progression of cancers, including but not restricted to proliferation of cancer cells, angiogenesis, metastasis, and oxidative stress [33–35] (Fig. 8.1).

Studies have identified the mechanism behind EGCG's anticancer role in esophageal cancer to be multifaceted and a combination of its anti-inflammatory effect, such as decreased COX-2 and PGE-2 production, and by inducing cell cycle arrest by inhibition of cyclin D1 [36]. Other mechanisms by which EGCG was found to inhibit progression of esophageal cancer cell lines was by blocking the phosphorylation of EGFR, thus leading to the inactivation of a potent growth receptor [37].

5 Isothiocyanate, Resveratrol, and Carotenoids

Besides curcumin and EGCG, other phytochemicals have also shown promise as anticancer agents against not just esophageal cancers but other cancers as well. Among these are the carotenoids, other flavonoids such as resveratrol and organosulfide isothiocyanate, etc. A meta-analysis conducted to study the association between the consumed amount of carotenoids and risk of developing esophageal cancers concluded that the risk of esophageal cancers is lowered with a higher intake of carotenoids [38]. Although the anticancer role of resveratrol for other gastrointestinal cancers is well established [11], recent studies have also identified its role against esophageal cancer, possibly by upregulating cancer cell apoptosis [39]. Similarly, isothiocyanate has also shown promise in combating esophageal cancer in mice; however, more investigations are needed to elucidate more about the precise molecular mechanisms involved in bringing about the effect [11, 40].

6 Lignans, Quercetin

The Western diet is rich in three phytochemicals that possess estrogenic properties, namely lignans, quercetin, and resveratrol [41–44]. A diet rich in wine, tea, vegetables, lettuce, whole-grain bread, and tomatoes and decreased intake of milk are a great source of all the three phytochemicals. These phytochemicals have a chemical structure similar to female hormones resulting in being able to bind to estrogenic receptors, and thus produce estrogenic effects [45–47]. Interestingly, in vitro studies have found estrogenic receptors in the esophageal tissue [48]. This is intriguing because the presence of estrogen has been postulated to be an important factor for the lower incidence of esophageal adenocarcinoma in females when compared to men (women-to-men ratio of 9:1) [49]. Studies have also shown strong negative correlation between a diet rich in lignans, quercetin, and resveratrol and the incidence of various histological patterns of esophageal cancer [50]. Tea is a good source of lignans and quercetin, and animal studies have demonstrated anticancer properties of black tea [51]. In the European countries, whole-grain bread is found to be a good source of lignans, and the consumption of whole-grain bread has been associated with a relatively lower incidence of esophageal adenocarcinoma [50].

Quercetin is thought to facilitate lipolysis in adipocytes, which can further cause cell apoptosis [52]. Animal studies lead to hypothesis that a diet rich in combined intake of these three phytochemicals might exert antitumor properties based on this synergistic effect on the downregulation of adipogenesis and further facilitation of cell death [53]. A 2013 case-controlled study in Sweden consisted of 181 patients of esophageal adenocarcinoma, 158 cases of esophageal squamous cell carcinoma, 255 cases of gastroesophageal junctional (GEJ) carcinoma, and 806 control cases [50]. The study assessed the intake of lignans, quercetin, and resveratrol in the study population by using simplified dietary pattern in quintiles. A diet rich in lignans, quercetin, and resveratrol has been characterized by the high intake of lettuce, wine, tea, tomatoes, and whole-grain bread and a low intake of milk [50]. The study demonstrated a dose-dependent correlation between the dietary score and all varieties of esophageal cancers. The adjusted odds ratio (OR) for the types of cancer was as follows: OR 0–24 for esophageal adenocarcinoma, OR 0–31 for squamous cell cancer, and OR 0–49 for gastroesophageal junction cancer [50]. The positive results of the study demonstrate that a diet high in lignans, quercetin, and resveratrol may have a protective effect in the incidence of esophageal cancer in the Swedish people [50].

7 Pharmacologic Agents Used in the Treatment of Esophageal Cancer (Table 8.1)

7.1 Tyrosine Kinase Inhibitors (TKIs)

Receptor tyrosine kinases (RTKs) are transmembrane glycoproteins that comprise three parts: an extracellular domain for ligand attachment, a transmembrane domain, and a tyrosine kinase motif [54, 55]. The extracellular domain of the RTK helps in the identification of various subfamilies of the kinases. Binding of the corresponding ligands to the RTKs results in their activation via phosphorylation of tyrosine residues on the receptor and through intracellular signaling proteins [56]. The activated RTKs play an important role in the regulation of many cellular processes, such as cellular proliferation, adhesion, differentiation, migration, and survival [57]. RTKs are classified into at least 21 groups, such as the vascular endothelial growth factor receptor (VEGFR), epidermal growth factor receptor (EGFR), fibroblast growth factor receptor (FGFR), and platelet-derived growth factor receptor

Table 8.1 Summary of a select group of pharmacologic agents used in the treatment of esophageal cancer

Sl. No.	Study authors (year)	Drug tested	Phase of the study	Study population	Clinical outcomes
EGFR inhibitors					
1.	Dutton et al. (2014)	Gefitinib	Phase III	Patients with esophageal cancer progression after chemotherapy	In all the patients, gefitinib as a second-line therapy did not improve the overall survival
2.	Zhai et al. (2010)	Erlotinib	Phase II pilot study	Concurrent erlotinib and radiation therapy in patients intolerant to chemoradiotherapy	Erlotinib + radiotherapy was effective and tolerable in esophageal squamous cell carcinoma patients
3.	Huang et al. (2016)	Icotinib	Phase II	Patients with pretreated advanced esophageal squamous cell cancer and EGFR overexpression	Icotinib showed positive results in terms of overall survival and progression-free survival
VEGFR inhibitors					
4.	Horgan et al. (2016)	Sunitinib	Phase II	Patients who underwent chemoradiotherapy and surgery for locally advanced esophageal cancer	Adjuvant sunitinib resulted in median survival of 26 months and a 2-year survival rate of 52%
5.	Janjigan et al. (2015)	Sorafenib	Phase II	Patients with chemotherapy-refractory esophageal carcinoma	In all the patients, the median overall survival was 9.7 months and median progression-free survival was 3.6 months

(PDGFR) families [58]. In cancer cells, multiple signaling processes including cellular proliferation, differentiation, and metabolic pathways are activated by dimerization of RTK. Studies have shown that monoclonal antibodies can inhibit the activation and overexpression of kinases in cancer cells. Some of the RTK inhibitors that have been approved by regulatory agencies for the treatment of cancers include trastuzumab for advanced-stage breast cancer [59], gefitinib used in the treatment of non-small cell lung carcinoma [60], and cetuximab for metastatic colon cancer [61]. The benefits of targeted therapy in esophageal cancer are rather limited. The application of molecular targeted drugs is also rather limited in esophageal cancer, and is restricted to the inhibition of EGFR, VEGFR, or HER-2.

8 EGFR Inhibitors

The EGFR is a tyrosine kinase receptor that helps in cell growth, cell differentiation, migration of cells, and metastasis. Studies have shown that EGFR overexpression is noticed in about 30–90% of esophageal cancers [62]. A 2004 study in patients diagnosed with esophageal cancer has shown a correlation between the EGFRs and overall survival (OS) [63]. In that study, the median OS was 16 months in the EGFR-positive cases whereas the median OS was 35 months in the EGFR-negative patients [63]. This signifies the importance of targeting EGFR in esophageal cancer, and to that aim, various drugs have been tested such as cetuximab, panitumumab, and gefitinib. Cetuximab has shown survival benefits in different malignancies such as cancers such as colon cancer and head-and-neck cancers, when combined with chemotherapy [64]. Unfortunately, it failed to produce any positive results in esophageal cancer. Since the year 2010, many clinical trials have been conducted regarding the efficacy of cetuximab and a meta-analysis including ten trials has shown that cetuximab combined with chemotherapy did not have any appreciable survival benefits in either local or advanced esophageal cancer [65]. Panitumumab is another EGFR inhibitor that also failed to show improvement in overall survival in phase III clinical trials [66]. Similarly, gefitinib and nimotuzumab were tested for esophageal cancer, but these agents also failed to demonstrate any positive outcomes in phase III trials [67, 68].

9 VEGFR Inhibitors

The VEGFRs play major role(s) in tumor angiogenesis, which helps in cancer cell invasion and metastasis. Studies have demonstrated that up to 30–60% of advanced esophageal cancer cases have upregulation of VEGFR [69]. Ramucirumab, a VEGFR/HER2 inhibitor, when used as a second-line monotherapy showed promising results in gastric cancer, including gastroesophageal junction carcinoma. The HER2 receptor is upregulated in 20% of esophageal cancers. Ramucirumab is FDA approved as second-line therapy of advanced esophageal cancer, either as a single agent or when used with abraxane [70]. Similarly, trastuzumab, another HER2 inhibitor, has also been approved for the first-line treatment of esophageal cancer in combination with chemotherapy [71]. Apatinib, a VEGFR/HER2 inhibitor, has shown positive results in terms of overall survival as well as progression-free survival in comparison with placebo in the Asian patients with advanced GE junction cancer [72].

10 Immunotherapy

Immunotherapies act by boosting the body's innate immune response by enabling destruction of tumor cells. Cytotoxic cluster differentiation (CD) 8 T cells recognize and destroy cancer cells through apoptosis. When cancer cells undergo mutation, they develop immunosuppressive mechanisms that either inhibit or anergize cytotoxic T cells [73]. Below we summarize some of the key immunotherapeutic studies related to esophageal and related cancers.

10.1 Immune Checkpoint Inhibitors

Programmed cell death protein 1 (PD-1) is an immune checkpoint-signaling molecule, which functions as an inhibitory signaling receptor on T-lymphocytes. Studies have demonstrated that tumor cells have overexpression of programmed cell death-ligand 1 (PD-L1) that helps in the suppression of lymphocyte activation and further cell destruction by T cells [74]. Targeting PD-L1 or PD-1 has demonstrated benefits in the treatment of various cancers such as lymphomas, lung, melanoma, head and neck, and some gynecologic malignancies [73]. Studies have shown that the majority of esophageal cancers present with *p53* gene mutations presumably due to the impact of chronic gastroesophageal reflux and inflammation resulting in continuing cell turnover, eventually resulting in tumorigenesis [75]. Furthermore, PD-L1 is detected in around 40% of the GEJ adenocarcinomas and esophageal adenocarcinomas, thus making them vulnerable to the checkpoint inhibitor therapies [76].

10.2 Pembrolizumab

Pembrolizumab is a monoclonal antibody that aims to inhibit PD-1. A phase Ib trial consisting of 39 patients (KEYNOTE-012) [77] was conducted to assess the effects of pembrolizumab as a first-line medication in metastatic or recurrent gastric and GEJ PD-L1-positive adenocarcinomas. In that study, pembrolizumab showed positive results in terms of objective response rate (ORR) (22%) and OS (11.4 months), and 12-month survival rate (42%) [77].

10.3 Nivolumab

Nivolumab is a monoclonal antibody that inhibits PD-1. It was evaluated for metastatic GEJ and gastric cancers in a randomized, phase III trial (ATTRACTION-2) [78] that recruited patients from Asian countries including

Japan, South Korea, and Taiwan. In that study, nivolumab's overall response rate (ORR) was 11.2% with an OS of 5.3 months in comparison to 4.1 months for patients receiving placebo. In the ATTRACTION-04 phase II trial [79], the combination of nivolumab with S-1 and oxaliplatin demonstrated an ORR of 57.1%, with progression-free survival of 9.7 months, while the combination of nivolumab, capecitabine, and oxaliplatin had an ORR of 76.5% and a PFS of 10.6 months. Both combinations were tolerated well and had fewer adverse events and these combinations have been tested in a phase III trial. Nivolumab has been approved for patients with PD-L1-positive GE junction and gastric cancer in Japan. This is expected to receive approval for esophageal cancer therapy. Another study (CheckMate 032) [80] assessed nivolumab in 160 patients with metastatic esophagogastric or advanced cancer refractory to chemotherapy. The study showed a 12% ORR and a 1-year survival rate of 39%, with a median OS of around 7 months for nivolumab alone [80]. Interestingly, the study also concluded that the PD-L1 status did not have a significant association with the antitumor response.

10.4 Avelumab

Avelumab is an anti-PD-L1 monoclonal antibody. A phase III trial (JAVELIN 300) [81] evaluated the potential of avelumab in advanced gastric and GEJ cancers that was refractory to chemotherapy. Unfortunately, results from this trial were discouraging as the ORR for avelumab was worse than that from the treatment with paclitaxel (4% vs. 8%) when considered as a third-line treatment option [81].

10.5 Durvalumab

Durvalumab is a high-affinity, selective human IgG1κ monoclonal antibody that functions by blocking PD-L1 binding to CD80 and PD-1. Studies utilizing a dose of 10 mg/kg of durvalumab administered intravenously biweekly for 12 months can have a positive impact on gastroesophageal cancers [82]. A phase II open-label study consisting of 23 patients is investigating treatment with 1500 mg of maintenance durvalumab offered intravenously every 4 weeks to patients with persistent residual esophageal cancer after definitive surgery following concurrent chemoradiation (NCT02639065). Another ongoing study consists of a phase Ib/II study on GEJ or gastric adenocarcinoma patients in the second- and third-line metastatic settings for treatment with durvalumab alone, single-agent tremelimumab, or combination therapy with durvalumab and tremelimumab [anti-CTLA-4 (cytotoxic T-lymphocyte-associated protein 4)] [83].

11 Combination Drugs

The CTLA-4 is a receptor located on the surface of T cells. Attachment of CTLA-4 to CD80 or CD86 results in downregulation of immune system. Ipilimumab, the powerful anti-CTLA-4 drug, failed to show any benefits when used alone in advanced gastric or GEJ adenocarcinomas when compared to best supportive care (BSC) [84]. This poor response was also demonstrated by another phase II trial, this time using a different anti-CTLA-4 monoclonal antibody (i.e., tremenumab) that was tried as a second-line treatment for metastatic gastric and esophageal adenocarcinoma [85]. Combination therapy consisting of anti-PD-1 (nivolumab) and anti-CTLA-4 (ipilimumab) checkpoint inhibitors has shown efficacy in phase I and phase II studies and this combination is currently being evaluated in a phase III trial [86].

A non-randomized study, KEYNOTE-059 [87], assessed the efficacy of pembrolizumab as a third-line therapy in patients with advanced and chemotherapy-refractory gastric and GEJ adenocarcinomas. In that study, the ORR was 11.6% for all patients. Interestingly, the drug efficacy was dependent on the PD-L1 status; the ORR for the PD-L1-positive cases was 15.5% whereas it was only 6.4% for the PD-L1-negative cases. Furthermore, the combination of pembrolizumab with chemotherapeutic agents (i.e., cisplatin plus 5-FU or capecitabine) resulted in an overall response rate of 60% for all patients, with PD-L1-positive cases again displaying higher ORR compared to the PD-L1-negative cases (69% vs. 38%). Additionally, when the single-agent pembrolizumab was used as a first-line treatment in patients with PD-L1-positive status, the ORR was 26%, which was considered promising [88]; however, the medication had significant adverse effects. Based on the results of the KEYNOTE-059 trial, pembrolizumab was approved by the FDA as a third-line option for PD-L1-positive, metastatic, or locally advanced gastric and GEJ adenocarcinomas [89]. Contrary to the above results, a phase III randomized trial (KEYNOTE-061) [90] compared the efficacy of pembrolizumab with paclitaxel in patients with advanced gastric and GEJ cancer and a positive PD-L1 status. In that study, pembrolizumab did not show any positive results. This finding suggested that the PD-L1 status may not serve as a reliable prognostic biomarker for making ideal treatment choices.

Other recent trials on the efficacy of pembrolizumab in PD-L1-positive esophageal squamous cell cancers include the KEYNOTE-180 phase II and KEYNOTE-181 phase III trials. Pembrolizumab showed positive response in metastatic ESC patients who underwent >2 lines of standard therapy, in terms of the ORR (14.3%). For esophageal adenocarcinoma, the results were more evident in those with positive PD-L1 status (13.8% vs. 6.3%) [91]. Later, the KEYNOTE-181 trial demonstrated that pembrolizumab when used in metastatic ESC as a second-line treatment resulted in a slightly improved OS when compared to chemotherapy, but this effect was not found to be statistically significant [92]. In July 2019, pembrolizumab received FDA approval as a second-line agent for the PD-L1-positive ESC. In addition, these results have paved the way for further trials that worked on analyzing the combination of pembrolizumab and chemotherapy as a first-line treatment of advanced esophageal cancer. Recently, a phase II trial analyzed the effects of pembrolizumab in combination with trastuzumab, capecitabine, and oxaliplatin as the first-line therapy for EAC. The study demonstrated positive results in terms of ORR (83%) and progression-free survival (11.4 months) in subjects with metastatic esophageal adenocarcinoma and positive HER-2 status [93].

12 Conclusions and Future Perspectives

Despite the ever-growing list of phytochemicals as potential novel anticancer agents, further conclusive studies are needed to strengthen their beneficial role(s) in the management of esophageal cancer. The lack of control groups and relatively small sample sizes are some of the issues that need to be addressed in future studies. Although the molecular mechanisms behind the functions of many phytochemicals have successfully been identified, much more needs to be done in identifying the pharmacokinetics, interactions, and side effect profiles of these substances. It can be deduced from the current evidence that phytochemicals still have a long way to go before ever being formally inducted as treatment options for cancers. Even their role (s) in the prevention of cancers, at the moment, remains somewhat questionable given the low concentration and possibly inactive forms of most of these compounds in natural dietary sources. However, based on the studies conducted so far, the initial results are indeed promising and warrant further translational studies that may become more effectively implemented in clinical practice.

Acknowledgements *Author Contributions*: Dr. Asad ur Rahman conceived the idea and subsequently all the authors have diligently contributed to the development and preparation of this research work (book chapter), including the literature search, concept organization, data interpretation, and writings. All the authors have read and approved the final draft for publication.

Conflict of Interest: The authors declare that they have no conflicts of interest associated with this book chapter.

Financial Disclosures: None to disclose.

References

1. Accessed March 3, 2020 from https://www.wcrf.org/dietandcancer/cancer-trends/oesophageal-cancer-statistics.
2. van Hagen, P., Hulshof, M. C., van Lanschot, J. J., Steyerberg, E. W., van Berge, et al. (2012). Preoperative chemoradiotherapy for esophageal or junctional cancer. *The New England Journal of Medicine, 366*(22), 2074–2084.
3. Kato, H., & Nakajima, M. (2013). Treatments for esophageal cancer: A review. *General Thoracic and Cardiovascular Surgery, 61*(6), 330–335.
4. Zhang, Y. (2013). Epidemiology of esophageal cancer. *World Journal of Gastroenterology, 19* (34), 5598–5606.

5. Cesas, A., & Bagajevas, A. (2004). Combined treatment of esophageal cancer: A review. *Medicina (Kaunas, Lithuania), 40.*
6. Lee, M. T., Lin, W. C., Yu, B., & Lee, T. T. (2017). Antioxidant capacity of phytochemicals and their potential effects on oxidative status in animals: A review. *Asian-Australasian Journal of Animal Sciences, 30*(3), 299–308.
7. Zhu, F., Du, B., & Xu, B. (2018). Anti-inflammatory effects of phytochemicals from fruits, vegetables, and food legumes: A review. *Critical Reviews in Food Science and Nutrition, 58*(8), 1260–1270.
8. Wang, H., Khor, T. O., Shu, L., Su, Z., Fuentes, F., Lee, J. J.-H., & Kong, A.-N. T. (2012). Plants against cancer: A review on natural phytochemicals in preventing and treating cancers and their druggability. *Anti-Cancer Agents in Medicinal Chemistry, 12*(10), 1281–1305.
9. Dutt, R., Garg, V., Khatri, N., & Madan, A. K. (2019). Phytochemicals in anticancer drug development. *Anti-Cancer Agents in Medicinal Chemistry, 19*(2), 172–183.
10. Liu, R. H. (2004). Potential synergy of phytochemicals in cancer prevention: Mechanism of action. *The Journal of Nutrition, 134*(12 Suppl), 3479S–3485S.
11. Chung, M.-Y., Lim, T. G., & Lee, K. W. (2013). Molecular mechanisms of chemopreventive phytochemicals against gastroenterological cancer development. *World Journal of Gastroenterology, 19*(7), 984–993.
12. Wargovich, M. J. (1997). Experimental evidence for cancer preventive elements in foods. *Cancer Letters, 114*(1-2), 11–17.
13. Phytochemicals directory. Accessed March 3, 2020 from https://www.phytochemicals.info/phytochemicals/curcumin.php.
14. Shehzad, A., Wahid, F., & Lee, Y. S. (2010). Curcumin in cancer chemoprevention: Molecular targets, pharmacokinetics, bioavailability, and clinical trials. *Archiv der Pharmazie (Weinheim), 343*(9), 489–499.
15. Anand, P., Sundaram, C., Jhurani, S., Kunnumakkara, A. B., & Aggarwal, B. B. (2008). Curcumin and cancer: An 'old-age' disease with an 'age-old' solution. *Cancer Letters, 267* (1), 133–164.
16. Lee, K. W., Bode, A. M., & Dong, Z. (2011). Molecular targets of phytochemicals for cancer prevention. *Nature Reviews. Cancer, 11*(3), 211–218.
17. Guo, Y., Shu, L., Zhang, C., Su, Z. Y., & Kong, A. N. (2015). Curcumin inhibits anchorage-independent growth of HT29 human colon cancer cells by targeting epigenetic restoration of the tumor suppressor gene DLEC1. *Biochemical Pharmacology, 94*(2), 69–78.
18. Almanaa, T. N., Geusz, M. E., & Jamasbi, R. J. (2012). Effects of curcumin on stem-like cells in human esophageal squamous carcinoma cell lines. *BMC Complementary and Alternative Medicine, 12*, 195.
19. Sullivan-Coyne, G., Sullivan, G. C., Donovan, T. R., Piwocka, K., & McKenna, S. L. (2009). Curcumin induces apoptosis-independent death in oesophageal cancer cells. *British Journal of Cancer, 101*(9), 1585–1595.
20. Pendleton, E. G., Jamasbi, R. J., & Geusz, M. E. (2019). Tetrahydrocurcumin, curcumin, and 5-fluorouracil effects on human esophageal carcinoma cells. *Anti-Cancer Agents in Medicinal Chemistry, 19*(8), 1012–1020.
21. Valko, M., Rhodes, C. J., Moncol, J., Izakovic, M., & Mazur, M. (2006). Free radicals, metals and antioxidants in oxidative stress-induced cancer. *Chemico-Biological Interactions, 160*(1), 1–40.
22. Bower, M. R., Aiyer, H. S., Li, Y., & Martin, R. C. G. (2010). Chemoprotective effects of curcumin in esophageal epithelial cells exposed to bile acids. *World Journal of Gastroenterology, 16*(33), 4152–4158.
23. Rawat, N., Alhamdani, A., McAdam, E., Cronin, J., Eltahir, Z., Lewis, P., Griffiths, P., Baxter, J. N., & Jenkins, G. J. (2012). Curcumin abrogates bile-induced NF-κB activity and DNA damage in vitro and suppresses NF-κB activity whilst promoting apoptosis in vivo, suggesting chemopreventative potential in Barrett's oesophagus. *Clinical & Translational Oncology, 14* (4), 302–311.

24. Liao, S., Xia, J., Chen, Z., Zhang, S., Ahmad, A., Miele, L., Sarkar, F. H., & Wang, Z. (2011). Inhibitory effect of curcumin on oral carcinoma CAL-27 cells via suppression of Notch-1 and NF-κB signaling pathways. *Journal of Cellular Biochemistry, 112*(4), 1055–1065.
25. Masuda, S. (2012). Dysfunctional transforming growth factor-β signaling with constitutively active notch signaling in Barrett's esophageal adenocarcinoma. *Cancer, 118*(7), 1956–1957.
26. Haraguchi, N., Utsunomiya, T., Inoue, H., Tanaka, F., Mimori, K., Barnard, G. F., & Mori, M. (2006). Characterization of a side population of cancer cells from human gastrointestinal system. *Stem Cells, 24*(3), 506–513.
27. Ricci-Vitiani, L., Lombardi, D. G., Pilozzi, E., Biffoni, M., Todaro, M., Peschle, C., & De Maria, R. (2007). Identification and expansion of human colon-cancer-initiating cells. *Nature, 445*(7123), 111–115.
28. D'Angelo, R. C., & Wicha, M. S. (2010). Stem cells in normal development and cancer. *Progress in Molecular Biology and Translational Science, 95*, 113–158.
29. Dean, M., Fojo, T., & Bates, S. (2005). Tumour stem cells and drug resistance. *Nature Reviews. Cancer, 5*(4), 275–284.
30. Chacko, S. M., Thambi, P. T., Kuttan, R., & Nishigaki, I. (2010). Beneficial effects of green tea: A literature review. *Chinese Medicine, 5*, 13.
31. Fujiki, H., Watanabe, T., Sueoka, E., Rawangkan, A., & Suganuma, M. (2018). Cancer prevention with green tea and its principal constituent, EGCG: From early investigations to current focus on human cancer stem cells. *Molecules and Cells, 41*(2), 73–82.
32. Wang, L. X., Shi, Y. L., Zhang, L. J., Wang, K. R., Xiang, L. P., Cai, Z. Y., et al. (2019). Inhibitory effects of (−)-Epigallocatechin-3-gallate on esophageal cancer. *Molecules, 8*, 24(5).
33. Khan, N., Afaq, F., Saleem, M., Ahmad, N., & Mukhtar, H. (2006). Targeting multiple signaling pathways by green tea polyphenol (−)-epigallocatechin-3-gallate. *Cancer Research, 66*(5), 2500–2505.
34. Singh, B. N., Shankar, S., & Srivastava, R. K. (2011). Green tea catechin, epigallocatechin-3-gallate (EGCG): Mechanisms, perspectives and clinical applications. *Biochemical Pharmacology, 82*(12), 1807–1821.
35. Ye, F., Zhang, G.-H., Guan, B.-X., & Xu, X.-C. (2012). Suppression of esophageal cancer cell growth using curcumin, (−)-epigallocatechin-3-gallate and lovastatin. *World Journal of Gastroenterology, 18*(2), 126–135.
36. Li, Z. G., Shimada, Y., Sato, F., Maeda, M., Itami, A., Kaganoi, J., et al. (2002). Inhibitory effects of epigallocatechin-3-gallate on N-nitrosomethylbenzylamine-induced esophageal tumorigenesis in F344 rats. *International Journal of Oncology, 21*(6), 1275–1283.
37. Hou, Z., Sang, S., You, H., Lee, M. J., Hong, J., Chin, K. V., & Yang, C. S. (2005). Mechanism of action of (−)-epigallocatechin-3-gallate: Auto-oxidation-dependent inactivation of epidermal growth factor receptor and direct effects on growth inhibition in human esophageal cancer KYSE 150 cells. *Cancer Research, 65*(17), 8049–8056.
38. Ge, X. X., Xing, M. Y., Yu, L. F., & Shen, P. (2013). Carotenoid intake and esophageal cancer risk: A meta-analysis. *Asian Pacific Journal of Cancer Prevention, 14*(3), 1911–1918.
39. Zhou, H.-B., Yan, Y., Sun, Y.-N., & Zhu, J.-R. (2003). Resveratrol induces apoptosis in human esophageal carcinoma cells. *World Journal of Gastroenterology, 9*(3), 408–411.
40. Stoner, G. D., Kresty, L. A., Carlton, P. S., Siglin, J. C., & Morse, M. A. (1999). Isothiocyanates and freeze-dried strawberries as inhibitors of esophageal cancer. *Toxicological Sciences, 52* (2 Suppl), 95–100.
41. Adlercreutz, H. (2007). Lignans and human health. *Critical Reviews in Clinical Laboratory Sciences, 44*(5-6), 483–525.
42. Hertog, M. G., Hollman, P. C., & Katan, M. B. (1992). Content of potentially anticarcinogenic flavonoids of 28 vegetables and 9 fruits commonly consumed in the Netherlands. *Journal of Agricultural and Food Chemistry, 40*(12), 2379–2383.
43. Peters, P. H., Slimani, N., van der Schouw, Y. T., Grace, P. B., Navarro, C., Tjonneland, A., Olsen, A., Clavel-Chapelon, F., Touillaud, M., Boutron-Ruault, M. C., & Jenab, M. (2007).

Variations in plasma phytoestrogen concentrations in European adults. *The Journal of Nutrition, 137*(5), 1294–1300.
44. Lamuela-Raventos, R. M., Romero-Perez, A. I., Waterhouse, A. L., & de la Torre-Boronat, M. C. (1995). Direct HPLC analysis of cis-and trans-resveratrol and piceid isomers in Spanish red Vitis vinifera wines. *Journal of Agricultural and Food Chemistry, 43*(2), 281–283.
45. Penttinen, P., Jaehrling, J., Damdimopoulos, A. E., Inzunza, J., Lemmen, J. G., van der Saag, P., Pettersson, K., Gauglitz, G., Mäkelä, S., & Pongratz, I. (2007). Diet-derived polyphenol metabolite enterolactone is a tissue-specific estrogen receptor activator. *Endocrinology, 148* (10), 4875–4886.
46. van der Woude, H., ter Veld, M. G., Jacobs, N., van der Saag, P. T., Murk, A. J., & Rietjens, I. M. (2005). The stimulation of cell proliferation by quercetin is mediated by the estrogen receptor. *Molecular Nutrition & Food Research, 49*(8), 763–771.
47. Gehm, B. D., McAndrews, J. M., Chien, P. Y., & Jameson, J. L. (1997). Resveratrol, a polyphenolic compound found in grapes and wine, is an agonist for the estrogen receptor. *Proceedings of the National Academy of Sciences of the United States of America, 94*(25), 14138–14143.
48. Tiffin, N., Suvarna, S. K., Trudgill, N. J., & Riley, S. A. (2003). Sex hormone receptor immunohistochemistry staining in Barrett's oesophagus and adenocarcinoma. *Histopathology, 42*(1), 95–96.
49. Lagergren, J., & Lagergren, P. (2013). Recent developments in esophageal adenocarcinoma. *CA: A Cancer J Clin, 63*(4), 232–248.
50. Lin, Y., Yngve, A., Lagergren, J., & Lu, Y. (2014). A dietary pattern rich in lignans, quercetin and resveratrol decreases the risk of oesophageal cancer. *The British Journal of Nutrition, 112* (12), 2002–2009.
51. Tavani, A., Bertuzzi, M., Talamini, R., Gallus, S., Parpinel, M., Franceschi, S., Levi, F., & La Vecchia, C. (2003). Coffee and tea intake and risk of oral, pharyngeal and esophageal cancer. *Oral Oncology, 39*(7), 695–700.
52. Kuppusamy, U. R., & Das, N. P. (1994). Potentiation of β-adrenoceptor agonist-mediated lipolysis by quercetin and fisetin in isolated rat adipocytes. *Biochemical Pharmacology, 47* (3), 521–529.
53. Park, H. J., Yang, J. Y., Ambati, S., Della-Fera, M. A., Hausman, D. B., Rayalam, S., & Baile, C. A. (2008). Combined effects of genistein, quercetin, and resveratrol in human and 3T3-L1 adipocytes. *Journal of Medicinal Food, 11*(4), 773–783.
54. Robinson, D. R., Wu, Y. M., & Lin, S. F. (2000). The protein tyrosine kinase family of the human genome. *Oncogene, 19*(49), 5548–5557.
55. Schlessinger, J. (2000). Cell signaling by receptor tyrosine kinases. *Cell, 103*(2), 211–225.
56. Morishita, A., Gong, J., & Masaki, T. (2014). Targeting receptor tyrosine kinases in gastric cancer. *World Journal of Gastroenterology, 20*(16), 4536.
57. Hubbard, S. R., & Till, J. H. (2000). Protein tyrosine kinase structure and function. *Annual Review of Biochemistry, 69*(1), 373–398.
58. Becker, J. C., Müller-Tidow, C., Serve, H., Domschke, W., & Pohle, T. (2006). Role of receptor tyrosine kinases in gastric cancer: New targets for a selective therapy. *World Journal of Gastroenterology, 12*(21), 3297–3305.
59. Shawver, L. K., Slamon, D., & Ullrich, A. (2002). Smart drugs: Tyrosine kinase inhibitors in cancer therapy. *Cancer Cell, 1*(2), 117–123.
60. Cohen, M. H., Williams, G. A., Sridhara, R., Chen, G., & Pazdur, R. (2003). FDA drug approval summary: Gefitinib (ZD1839) (Iressa) tablets. *The Oncologist, 8*(4), 303–306.
61. (2004). New treatments for colorectal cancer. *FDA Consumer, 38*(3), 17.
62. Al-Kasspooles, M., Moore, J. H., Orringer, M. B., & Beer, D. G. (1993). Amplification and over-expression of the EGFR and erbB-2 genes in human esophageal adenocarcinomas. *International Journal of Cancer, 54*(2), 213–219.
63. Wilkinson, N. W., Black, J. D., Roukhadze, E., Driscoll, D., Smiley, S., Hoshi, H., Geradts, J., Javle, M., & Brattain, M. (2004). Epidermal growth factor receptor expression correlates with

histologic grade in resected esophageal adenocarcinoma. *Journal of Gastrointestinal Surgery, 8* (4), 448–453.
64. Tew, W. P., Kelsen, D. P., & Ilson, D. H. (2005). Targeted therapies for esophageal cancer. *The Oncologist, 10*(8), 590–601.
65. Huang, Z. H., Ma, X. W., Zhang, J., Li, X., Lai, N. L., & Zhang, S. X. (2018). Cetuximab for esophageal cancer: An updated meta-analysis of randomized controlled trials. *BMC Cancer, 18* (1), 1170.
66. Waddell, T., Chau, I., Cunningham, D., Gonzalez, D., Okines, A. F., Wotherspoon, A., Saffery, C., Middleton, G., Wadsley, J., Ferry, D., & Mansoor, W. (2013). Epirubicin, oxaliplatin, and capecitabine with or without panitumumab for patients with previously untreated advanced oesophagogastric cancer (REAL3): A randomized, open-label phase 3 trial. *The Lancet Oncology, 14*(6), 481–489.
67. Dutton, S. J., Ferry, D. R., Blazeby, J. M., Abbas, H., Dahle-Smith, A., Mansoor, W., Thompson, J., Harrison, M., Chatterjee, A., Falk, S., & Garcia-Alonso, A. (2014). Gefitinib for oesophageal cancer progressing after chemotherapy (COG): A phase 3, multicentre, double-blind, placebo-controlled randomized trial. *The Lancet Oncology, 15*(8), 894–904.
68. Zhang, X., Jia, J., Lu, M., Wang, X., Gong, J., Li, J., Li, J., Li, Y., Zhang, X., Lu, Z., et al. (2017). Nimotuzumab plus paclitaxel and cisplatin as 1st line treatment for unresectable esophageal squamous cell carcinoma: Long term follow-up of survival in a phase II study. *Journal of Clinical Oncology, 35*, e15573.
69. Kleespies, A., Guba, M., Jauch, K. W., & Bruns, C. J. (2004). Vascular endothelial growth factor in esophageal cancer. *Journal of Surgical Oncology, 87*(2), 95–104.
70. Fuchs, C. S., Shitara, K., Di Bartolomeo, M., Lonardi, S., Al-Batran, S. E., Van Cutsem, E., Ilson, D. H., Alsina, M., Chau, I., Lacy, J., & Ducreux, M. (2019). Ramucirumab with cisplatin and fluoropyrimidine as first-line therapy in patients with metastatic gastric or junctional adenocarcinoma (RAINFALL): A double-blind, randomised, placebo-controlled, phase 3 trial. *The Lancet Oncology, 20*(3), 420–435.
71. Creemers, A., Ebbing, E. A., Hooijer, G. K., Stap, L., Jibodh-Mulder, R. A., Gisbertz, S. S., van Berge Henegouwen, M. I., van Montfoort, M. L., Hulshof, M. C., Krishnadath, K. K., & van Oijen, M. G. (2018). The dynamics of HER2 status in esophageal adenocarcinoma. *Oncotarget, 9*(42), 26787.
72. Li, J., Qin, S., Xu, J., Xiong, J., Wu, C., Bai, Y., Liu, W., Tong, J., Liu, Y., Xu, R., & Wang, Z. (2016). Randomized, double-blind, placebo-controlled phase III trial of apatinib in patients with chemotherapy-refractory advanced or metastatic adenocarcinoma of the stomach or gastroesophageal junction. *Journal of Clinical Oncology, 34*(13), 1448–1454.
73. Barsouk, A., Rawla, P., Hadjinicolaou, A. V., Aluru, J. S., & Barsouk, A. (2019). Targeted therapies and immunotherapies in the treatment of esophageal cancers. *Medical Science, 7*(10), 100.
74. Sharpe, A. H., & Pauken, K. E. (2018). The diverse functions of the PD-1 inhibitory pathway. *Nature Reviews. Immunology, 18*(3), 153.
75. Kailasam, A., Mittal, S. K., & Agrawal, D. K. (2015). Epigenetics in the pathogenesis of esophageal adenocarcinoma. *Clinical and Translational Science, 8*(4), 394–402.
76. Raufi, A. G., & Klempner, S. J. (2015). Immunotherapy for advanced gastric and esophageal cancer: Pre-clinical rationale and ongoing clinical investigations. *Journal of Gastrointestinal Oncology Journal of Gastrointestinal Oncology, 6*(5), 561–569.
77. Muro, K., Chung, H. C., Shankaran, V., Geva, R., Catenacci, D., Gupta, S., Eder, J. P., Golan, T., Le, D. T., Burtness, B., & McRee, A. J. (2016). Pembrolizumab for patients with PD-L1-positive advanced gastric cancer (KEYNOTE-012): A multicentre, open-label, phase 1b trial. *The Lancet Oncology, 17*(6), 717–726.
78. Kang, Y. K., Boku, N., Satoh, T., Ryu, M. H., Chao, Y., Kato, K., Chung, H. C., Chen, J. S., Muro, K., Kang, W. K., & Yeh, K. H. (2017). Nivolumab in patients with advanced gastric or gastro-oesophageal junction cancer refractory to, or intolerant of, at least two previous

chemotherapy regimens (ONO-4538-12, ATTRACTION-2): A randomised, double-blind, placebo-controlled, phase 3 trial. *The Lancet, 390*(10111), 2461–2471.

79. Boku, N., Ryu, M. H., Kato, K., Chung, H. C., Minashi, K., Lee, K. W., Cho, H., Kang, W. K., Komatsu, Y., Tsuda, M., & Yamaguchi, K. (2019). Safety and efficacy of nivolumab in combination with S-1/capecitabine plus oxaliplatin in patients with previously untreated, unresectable, advanced, or recurrent gastric/gastroesophageal junction cancer: Interim results of a randomized, phase II trial (ATTRACTION-4). *Annals of Oncology, 30*(2), 250–258.
80. Le, D. T., Bendell, J. C., Calvo, E., Kim, J. W., Ascierto, P. A., Sharma, P., Ott, P. A., Bono, P., Jaeger, D., Evans, T. J., & De Braud, F. G. (2016). Safety and activity of nivolumab monotherapy in advanced and metastatic (A/M) gastric or gastroesophageal junction cancer (GC/GEC): Results from the CheckMate-032 study. *Journal of Clinical Oncology, 21*, 34(6).
81. Bang, Y. J., Ruiz, E. Y., Van Cutsem, E., Lee, K. W., Wyrwicz, L., Schenker, M., Alsina, M., Ryu, M. H., Chung, H. C., Evesque, L., & Al-Batran, S. E. (2018). Phase III, randomised trial of avelumab versus physician's choice of chemotherapy as third-line treatment of patients with advanced gastric or gastro-oesophageal junction cancer: Primary analysis of JAVELIN gastric 300. *Annals of Oncology, 29*(10), 2052–2060.
82. Segal, N. H., Antonia, S. J., Brahmer, J. R., Maio, M., Blake-Haskins, A., Li, X., Vasselli, J., Ibrahim, R. A., Lutzky, J., & Khleif, S. (2014). Preliminary data from a multi-arm expansion study of MEDI4736, an anti-PD-L1 antibody. *Journal of Clinical Oncology, 32*(suppl; Abstr 3002), 5s.
83. Kelly, R. J., Chung, K., Gu, Y., Steele, K. E., Rebelatto, M. C., Robbins, P. B., Tavakkoli, F., Karakunnel, J. J., Lai, D. W., & Almhanna, K. (2015). Phase Ib/II study to evaluate the safety and antitumor activity of durvalumab (MEDI4736) and tremelimumab as monotherapy or in combination, in patients with recurrent or metastatic gastric/gastroesophageal junction adenocarcinoma. *Journal for Immunotherapy of Cancer, 3*(Suppl 2), 157.
84. Bang, Y. J., Cho, J. Y., Kim, Y. H., Kim, J. W., Di Bartolomeo, M., Ajani, J. A., Yamaguchi, K., Balogh, A., Sanchez, T., & Moehler, M. (2017). Efficacy of sequential ipilimumab monotherapy versus best supportive care for unresectable locally advanced/metastatic gastric or gastroesophageal junction cancer. *Clinical Cancer Research, 23*(19), 5671–5678.
85. Ralph, C., Elkord, E., Burt, D. J., O'Dwyer, J. F., Austin, E. B., Stern, P. L., Hawkins, R. E., & Thistlethwaite, F. C. (2010). Modulation of lymphocyte regulation for cancer therapy: A phase II trial of tremelimumab in advanced gastric and esophageal adenocarcinoma. *Clinical Cancer Research, 16*(5), 1662–1672.
86. Janjigian, Y. Y., Bendell, J., Calvo, E., Kim, J. W., Ascierto, P. A., Sharma, P., Ott, P. A., Peltola, K., Jaeger, D., Evans, J., & De Braud, F. (2018). CheckMate-032 study: Efficacy and safety of nivolumab and nivolumab plus ipilimumab in patients with metastatic esophagogastric cancer. *Journal of Clinical Oncology, 36*(28), 2836–2844.
87. Fuchs, C. S., Doi, T., Jang, R. W., Muro, K., Satoh, T., Machado, M., Sun, W., Jalal, S. I., Shah, M. A., Metges, J. P., & Garrido, M. (2018). Safety and efficacy of pembrolizumab monotherapy in patients with previously treated advanced gastric and gastroesophageal junction cancer: Phase 2 clinical KEYNOTE-059 trial. *JAMA Oncology, 4*(5), e180013.
88. Bang, Y. J., Kang, Y. K., Catenacci, D. V., Muro, K., Fuchs, C. S., Geva, R., Hara, H., Golan, T., Garrido, M., Jalal, S. I., & Borg, C. (2019). Pembrolizumab alone or in combination with chemotherapy as first-line therapy for patients with advanced gastric or gastroesophageal junction adenocarcinoma: Results from the phase II nonrandomized KEYNOTE-059 study. *Gastric Cancer, 22*(4), 828–837.
89. Fashoyin-Aje, L., Donoghue, M., Chen, H., He, K., Veeraraghavan, J., Goldberg, K. B., Keegan, P., McKee, A. E., & Pazdur, R. (2019). FDA approval summary: Pembrolizumab for recurrent locally advanced or metastatic gastric or gastroesophageal junction adenocarcinoma expressing PD-L1. *The Oncologist, 24*(1), 103–109.
90. Ohtsu, A., Tabernero, J., Bang, Y. J., Fuchs, C. S., Sun, L., Wang, Z., Csiki, I., Koshiji, M., & Van Cutsem, E. (2016). Pembrolizumab (MK-3475) versus paclitaxel as second-line therapy for

advanced gastric or gastroesophageal junction (GEJ) adenocarcinoma: Phase 3 KEYNOTE-061 study. *Journal of Clinical Oncology, 34*, TPS183.

91. Shah, M. A., Kojima, T., Hochhauser, D., Enzinger, P., Raimbourg, J., Hollebecque, A., Lordick, F., Kim, S. B., Tajika, M., Kim, H. T., & Lockhart, A. C. (2019). Efficacy and safety of pembrolizumab for heavily pretreated patients with advanced, metastatic adenocarcinoma or squamous cell carcinoma of the esophagus: The phase 2 KEYNOTE-180 study. *JAMA Oncology, 5*(4), 546–550.
92. Shah, M. A., Adenis, A., Enzinger, P. C., Kojima, T., Muro, K., Bennouna, J., Francois, E., Hsu, C. H., Moriwaki, T., Kim, S. B., & Lee, S. H. (2019). Pembrolizumab versus chemotherapy as second-line therapy for advanced esophageal cancer: Phase 3 KEYNOTE-181 study. *Journal of Clinical Oncology, 37*, 4010.
93. Kojima, T., Muro, K., Francois, E., Hsu, C.-H., Moriwaki, T., Kim, S.-B., Lee, S.-H., Bennouna, J., Kato, K., Lin, S., et al. (2019). Pembrolizumab versus chemotherapy as second-line therapy for advanced esophageal cancer: Phase III KEYNOTE-181 study. *Journal of Clinical Oncology, 37*(4 Suppl), 2. https://doi.org/10.1200/JCO.2019.37.4_suppl.2.

Chapter 9
Gastric Cancer: Role of Phytochemicals and Tyrosine Kinase Inhibitors

Muzammil Muhammad Khan, Deepika Sarvepalli, Mamoon Ur Rashid, Hammad Zafar, Muhammad Shayan Khan, Effa Zahid, Akash Khetpal, Bayarmaa Mandzhieva, Rima Shobar, Anum Jalil, and Sarfraz Ahmad

Abstract Cancer is one of the prominent causes of mortality in the world while carcinoma of stomach happens to be the seventh most prevalent reason for carcinoma-related mortality worldwide. The development of chemotherapeutic drugs has certainly improved cancer patients' outcomes; however, metastasized cancer remains largely untreatable. Hence, the innovation and research for the effective and safer chemoprevention and treatment of cancers are needed. Cancer chemoprevention and treatments with natural phytochemical compounds is an emerging strategy to potentially cure cancer. For a long time, the study of phytochemicals has shown very encouraging results in clinical trials against cancer cells. Hence, it is recommended that consuming fruits and vegetables by modifying/improving lifestyle can result in the prevention of different gastrointestinal cancers, including gastric carcinoma. In this chapter, we discuss some of the key natural phytochemicals that exercise their antioxidant properties and also act as inhibitors of inflammation and cancer-causing agents by aiming certain pathways and molecules

M. M. Khan
Khyber Teaching Hospital, Peshawar, Khyber Pakhtunkhwa, Pakistan

D. Sarvepalli · M. U. Rashid (✉) · H. Zafar · B. Mandzhieva · R. Shobar · A. Jalil
Department of Internal Medicine, AdventHealth, Orlando, FL, USA
e-mail: mamoon.rashid.MD@adventhealth.com; hammad.zafar.MD@adventhealth.com; bayarmaa.mandzhieva.MD@adventhealth.com; rima.shobar.MD@adventhealth.com; anum.jalil.MD@adventhealth.com

M. S. Khan
Department of Internal Medicine, Mercy Saint Vincent Medical Center, Toledo, OH, USA

E. Zahid
Services Institute of Medical Sciences, Lahore, Punjab, Pakistan

A. Khetpal
Dow University of Health Sciences, Karachi, Pakistan

S. Ahmad (✉)
AdventHealth Cancer Institute, FSU and UCF Colleges of Medicine, Orlando, FL, USA
e-mail: sarfraz.ahmad@adventhealth.com

G. P. Nagaraju (ed.), *Phytochemicals Targeting Tumor Microenvironment in Gastrointestinal Cancers*, https://doi.org/10.1007/978-3-030-48405-7_9

in gastric carcinoma along with newer targeted therapies of gastric cancer. We also highlight the role of inhibitors of receptor tyrosine kinases in the carcinoma of stomach.

Keywords Gastric carcinoma · Phytochemicals · Tyrosine kinase inhibitors · Anticancer mechanisms · Clinical trials

Abbreviations

DNA	Deoxyribonucleic acid
EGFR	Epidermal growth factor receptor
FGFR	Fibroblast growth factor receptor
GEJ	Gastroesophageal junction
GST	Glutathione S transferase
H Pylori	*Helicobacter pylori*
IHC	Immunohistochemistry
IL	Interleukin
ITC	Isothiocyanates
NADPH	Nicotinamide adenine dinucleotide phosphate
OS	Overall survival
PDGFR	Platelet-derived growth factor receptor
PFS	Progression-free survival
ROS	Reactive oxygen species
RTK	Receptor tyrosine kinases
SFN	Sulforaphane
TKI	Tyrosine kinase inhibitor
TNF	Tumor necrosis factor
UDP	Uridine 5′-diphosphate
UGT	UDP-glucuronosyltransferase
VEGFR	Vascular endothelial growth factor receptor

1 Introduction

Cancer remains one of the leading sources of morbidity and death worldwide, and an upsurge in cancer incidence is witnessed in the recent years as well. It is second behind cardiovascular diseases as the leading source of mortality in developed nations [1]. The development of malignancy is marked by uncontrolled and sustained proliferation, notwithstanding apoptosis, which can invade tissues and angiogenesis. Genetic alterations in the cell can produce unstable genetic makeover resulting in normal cells transforming into a malignant cell. These changes consist of alterations in tumor-suppressor genes, oncogenes, and DNA repair genes, which are involved in cell growth and differentiation. Some extrinsic elements (smoking, infectious agents, and radiation) as well as intrinsic causes (immune conditions, and hormones) are responsible for these mutations.

Carcinoma of the stomach stands as the top ten leading sources of carcinoma-related deaths. Studies have shown that factors such as exposure to cancer causing chemical agents and bacteria such as *Helicobacter pylori* are the two main causative factors resulting in the initiation of several events causing gastric carcinoma [2]. Infection by *H. pylori* can result in gastric mucosal infiltration with macrophages and neutrophil cells which further results in the production of harmful free radicals called reactive oxygen species (ROS) including superoxide and nitric oxide, which go on to cause gastric mucosal injury, ulcer, and eventually carcinoma [3]. Phytochemicals with antioxidant properties may help in protecting against carcinoma.

Consumption of fruits and herbal medicine is the most suitable and productive method of taking phytochemicals on a daily basis and in a cost-effective manner. In this chapter, we review the natural phytochemicals that possess antioxidant, anti-oncogenic, or anti-inflammatory properties that function via altering the course of action of different molecules involved in gastric carcinogenesis. We also discuss the newer targeted therapies extensively being studied for gastric cancer with special reference to tyrosine inhibitors that play critical roles in gastric cancer outcomes.

2 Curcumin

Turmeric plants (*Curcuma longa*) contain a bright yellow pigment called curcumin. Curcumin also happens to be the major curcuminoid present in turmeric. There is vast evidence about the numerous advantages of curcumin such as anti-inflammatory, antioxidant, and antitumor properties [4, 5]. The mode of action of curcumin is mainly mediated by targeting multiple intracellular pathways [6]. Over the years, inability to clear *H. pylori* infection has been implicated as the main cause of gastritis, ulcers, and eventually gastric carcinoma. Recently, it has been shown that curcumin is effective in arresting the growth of *H. pylori* [7]. The prospective therapeutic capabilities of curcumin have been assessed through several in vitro studies. The main reason for tumors being resistant to chemotherapy is the overexpression of nuclear transcription factor NF-κB. Curcumin can suppress the NF-κB effects, thereby augmenting chemotherapeutic drug effects. Yu et al. [8] in their studies showed enhanced activity of chemotherapeutic drugs (doxorubicin and etoposide) in combination with curcumin as compared to either of the drugs alone. Studies on the gastric cancer cell cultures (SGC 7901) in humans have shown that curcumin causes downregulation of NF-κB, which further results in the downregulation cell death inhibitor genes such as Bcl-2 and Bcl-xl via inhibition of NF-κB activity [8].

It has been shown previously that curcumin inhibits the receptor tyrosine kinase, EGFR, as well as downstream regulation of EGFR tyrosine kinase, p21-activated tyrosine kinase 1 (PAK1), without affecting its expression. In addition, curcumin causes mRNA suppression, which results in decreased production of cyclin-D1 protein and eventually results in the arrest of cell cycle progression in G1 phase. Consequently, curcumin can inhibit not only the cell proliferation but also the invasion of gastric carcinoma cells [9].

3 Isothiocyanates

Isothiocyanates (ITCs) are plant phytochemicals that are abundantly present in vegetables belonging to the family Cruciferae such as broccoli, Brussels sprouts, wasabi, radish, and turnips [3]. These occur in their inactive form, glucosinolates, and become reactive after coming in contact with an enzyme called myrosinase present in the oral cavity and small intestine. Some of the ITCs consist of aliphatic ITC (AITC) and sulforaphane (SFN) which are aliphatic compounds, and phenethyl ITC (pEITC) and benzyl ITC (BITC) which are aromatic.

Isothiocyanates have been shown to decrease the activity of enzymes that are responsible for the biotransformation of xenobiotics. The oxidative enzyme that facilitates phase one reactions is nicotinamide adenine dinucleotide phosphate (NADPH) cytochrome P450 reductase while glutathione S transferase (GST) and uridine 5′-diphospho (UDP)-glucuronosyltransferase (UGT) enzymes are responsible for second-phase reactions. It is believed that ITCs such as sulforaphane exert its antioxidant effects by stimulating Nrf-2-dependent enzymes, such as GST, thus guarding against the free radicals [10–12]. Sulforaphane can maintain the effect of enzymes such as NADPH, quinone oxidoreductase NQOI, and GST in Nrf-2-deficient mice when injected with foods containing large quantities of salt and *H. pylori* [3]. These results demonstrate the antioxidant potential of sulforaphane on the gastric mucosa.

SFN can also increase the Nrf-2-dependent antioxidant effect. A study by Fahey et al. [10] has shown that sulforaphane can inhibit the development of gastric cancer in the Institute of Cancer Research (ICR) mice which were treated with benzo[a] pyrene. These effects are thought to be facilitated by stimulation of phase two reactions of GST and NQOI, and also by an increase in the production of antioxidant enzymes, which are abolished by the deletion of Nrf-2 gene in the mice [10]. In patients with gastritis due to *H. pylori*, eradication of the bacteria augmented or reinstated the GST enzyme levels, which further reinforces the significance of antioxidants in preventing *H. pylori*-associated gastric tumors [13].

Sulforaphane also possesses chemopreventive activities against *H. pylori* infection [3]. During a study on people infected with *H. pylori*, 48 subjects were followed who ingested 70 g/d of broccoli (precursor of 420 μmol/L sulforaphane) for 8 weeks and were compared with placebo. The study reported a decline in *H. pylori* markers such as stool antigen and urease enzyme when compared to placebo. A decline in gastric inflammation markers such as pepsinogen 1 and 2 was noticed in broccoli group as well compared to placebo [14]. A study in C57BL/6 female mice that were infected with *H. pylori* and were kept on excessive salt regime also established the potential of sulforaphane in bacterial inhibition [14]. Consumption of sulforaphane-enriched broccoli in mice resulted in low levels of interleukin (IL)-1β and tumor necrosis factor (TNF)-α adding to the improvement of inflammation, decrease of bacterial colonization, and thus prevention of gastric corpus atrophy via high-salt diet. Interestingly, there were no effects of sulforaphane on Nrf-2 gene-depleted mice, suggesting that its mechanism of action is Nrf-2 dependent [14].

4 Resveratrol

Resveratrol belongs to the family of a polyphenol commonly found in red wine and red grapes. There has been a widely reported benefit of red wine with the inverse relation of cardiovascular diseases [15]. Studies have also shown beneficial effects of resveratrol on the neuronal cell death [16]. It is also believed that resveratrol is responsible for the benefits of red wine on cardiovascular diseases [17]. This prompted for extensive research on resveratrol in malignancies during the last 20 years focusing on its anti-inflammatory, antioxidant, and anticancer potential [18]. Exposure of gastric cells to *H. pylori* results in elevated IL-8 production and free radical production. Furthermore, *H. pylori* infection resulted in stimulation of gastric motility and phenotype alterations observed in cell lines through humming-bird effect [19]. It was also established that resveratrol possesses antibacterial activity against *H. pylori* infection, resulting in hampering of the *H. pylori* proliferation [20–22]. Treatment with resveratrol significantly reduced IL-8 expression, decreased free radical production, and suppressed the phenotype alterations in *H. pylori*-infected cells. These positive results explain the potential of resveratrol in gastric cancer treatment.

In vitro studies have shown that resveratrol can cause cell cycle arrest in the G0/G1 phase via inhibition of the kinase C-mediated processes and further stimulation of cell apoptosis. This cell cycle inhibition hampers the formation of RF-1 and KATO-III cells [23, 24]. Another critical mechanism by which resveratrol regulates the growth and expansion of gastric adenocarcinoma cells happens to be the MEK1/2-ERK1/2-c-Jun cascade. Studies have postulated that resveratrol causes MEK1/2-ERK1/2 phosphorylation downregulation, thereby further inhibiting c-Jun translocation into the nucleus, ultimately resulting in cell growth inhibition [25]. Furthermore, resveratrol (50–200 μmol/L) can also stimulate cell death by producing ROS in human gastric cancer SGC7901 cells. These effects of resveratrol could be overturned when tumor cells are treated with substances such as superoxide dismutase and catalase, which dilute the apoptotic process [26]. Resveratrol can cause cell death of transplanted tumor cells, most likely mediated by suppression of Bcl2 anti-apoptotic genes and cell death activation via Bax gene in an implanted gastric tumor cells in nude mice [27] (Fig. 9.1).

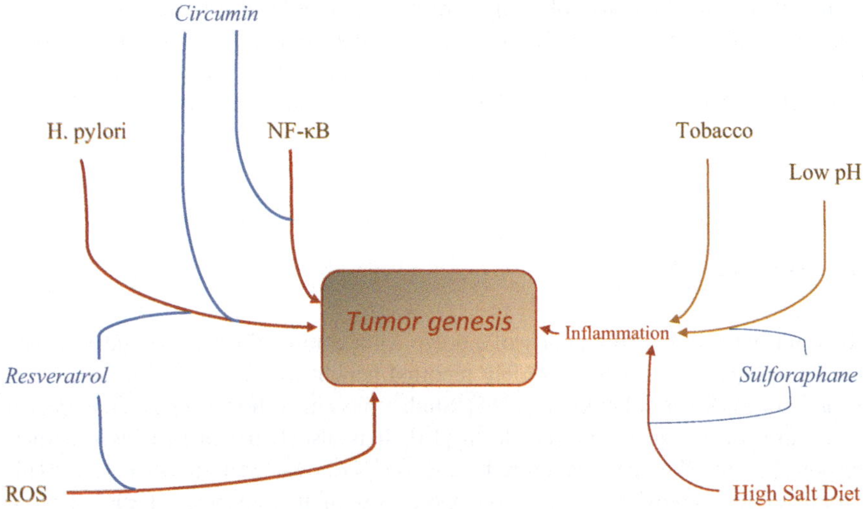

Fig. 9.1 Schematic representation of the mechanisms of action of phytochemicals and pro-cancer/tumor formation agents

5 Receptor Tyrosine Kinases (RTKs) and Tyrosine Kinase Inhibitors (TKIs)

Studies have shown that in gastric cancer, several receptor tyrosine kinases get stimulated and amplified. So, drugs aimed at controlling the RTKs can be beneficial in advanced gastric carcinoma people. RTKs occur as transmembrane glycoproteins that comprise a domain for ligand attachment extracellular, a motif for the tyrosine kinase, and another domain across the membrane [28–30]. The extracellular domain of the RTK helps in the identification of various subfamilies of the kinases. Binding of the corresponding ligands to the RTKs results in their activation via tyrosine molecule phosphorylation and further activation of cellular proteins [31]. Activated RTKs play a major regulatory role in a variety of cellular processes including proliferation, differentiation, migration, and survival [32]. When some of the bivalent ligands bind to two receptor molecules, it forms a dimer, which results in the activation of the kinases [33]. The activation of kinases is dependent on two key steps; the first step is augmentation of catalysis intrinsically while the second step consists of formation of protein attachment sites intracellularly, both of which are dependent on tyrosine autophosphorylation. While phosphorylation of tyrosine molecules near the enzyme's activation loop upregulates kinase actions, phosphorylation of the enzyme adjacent to the membrane helps in the formation of anchors for the attachment of modules, which identify the phosphotyrosine molecules in precise patterns [34] (Fig. 9.2).

Tyrosine kinase receptors are classified into 21 groups, such as the epidermal growth factor receptor (EGFR), vascular endothelial growth factor receptor

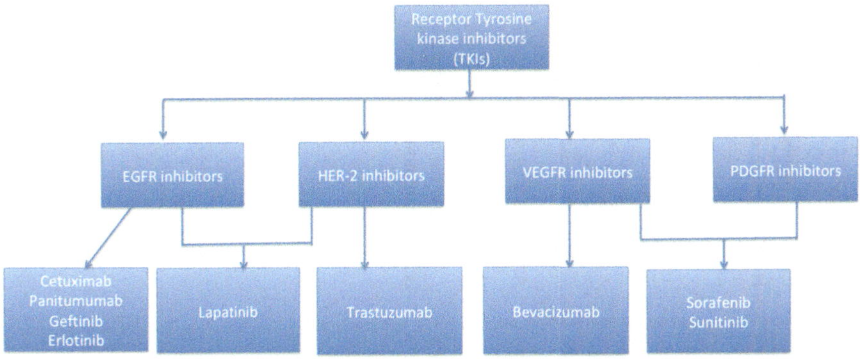

Fig. 9.2 Selected tyrosine kinase inhibitors and their relationship with gastric cancer

(VEGFR), fibroblast growth factor receptor (FGFR), and platelet-derived growth factor receptor (PDGFR) families [35]. In cancer cells, RTKs play a major role in various cellular processes such as growth, differentiation, and metabolism. Studies have also shown that monoclonal antibodies can inhibit the activation and overexpression of kinases in cancer cells. Some of the RTK inhibitors that became standard treatment options in various malignancies include trastuzumab in carcinoma of breast [36], gefitinib in lung cancer [37], and cetuximab in advanced colorectal carcinoma [38].

Studies have shown that RTKs exhibit various mutations and changes in gastric cancer patients. Mutations and overexpression of RTKs were observed in 37% of people diagnosed with gastric carcinoma [39]. The study has also reported the family of kinases that were amplified including KRAS in 8.8% of people with gastric cancer, FGFR2 in 9.3%, EGFR in 7.7%, and ErbB2 in 7.2% of the diagnosed patients. Moreover, upregulation of RTKs was found to be associated with patient prognosis; higher RTK levels correlated with inferior patient outcomes. Later, in a study by Morishita et al. [31], the levels of various RTKs (EGFR, FGFR1/2, ErbB2) were amplified in tumor cells in contrast with healthy gastric cells. The findings of these studies propose that drugs targeting kinase receptors can be beneficial in patients with gastric malignancies.

There are many monoclonal antibodies under various phases of clinical trials such as trastuzumab, cetuximab, and lapatinib, which are classified based on their ability of inhibition of various families of RTKs (Table 9.1). Below we summarize the biological and clinical applications of these monoclonal antibodies in gastric cancer.

Table 9.1 An updated summary of the current clinical trials studying tyrosine kinase inhibitors in gastric cancer

Sl. No.	Name of the study	Drug evaluated	Country, trial is conducted	Status of the trial	Condition treated
1.	Study Evaluating Pyrotinib/Pyrotinib in Combination with Docetaxel in Patients with HER2+ Advanced Gastric Cancer	Pyrotinib/pyrotinib with docetaxel	• Beijing Cancer Hospital, Peking University, Beijing, China • Cancer Hospital, Chinese Academy of Medical Sciences, Beijing, China • Chinese PLA General Hospital, Beijing, China • Cancer Center, Sun Yet-Sen University, Guangzhou, Guangdong, China	Unknown	HER2-positive gastric cancer
2.	FLO +/– Pazopanib as First-line Treatment in Advanced Gastric Cancer	• Pazopanib • 5-FU, oxaliplatin, leucovorin (FLO)	Charite University Medicine, Berlin, Germany	Completed	Advanced gastric cancer
3.	Exploratory Clinical Study of Apatinib and SHR-1210 in Treating Advanced Hepatocellular Carcinoma or Gastric Cancer	• Apatinib • SHR-1210	The Affiliated Hospital of the Chinese Academy of Military Medical Sciences, Beijing, China	Unknown	• Gastric cancer • Hepatocellular carcinoma
4.	A Study to Evaluate the Clinical Efficacy of JNJ-42756493 (Erdafitinib), A Pan-Fibroblast Growth Factor Receptor (FGFR) Tyrosine Kinase Inhibitor, in Asian Participants with Advanced Non-small-Cell Lung Cancer, Urothelial Cancer, Esophageal Cancer or Cholangiocarcinoma	Erdafitinib	• Cancer Hospital, Chinese Academy of Medical Sciences, Beijing, China • Beijing Cancer Hospital of Peking University, Beijing, China • Beijing Cancer Hospital of Peking University, Beijing, China • (and 33 more . . .)	Recruiting	Neoplasm
5.					

	Study of GSK1363089 in Metastatic Gastric Cancer	GSK1363089 (formerly XL880)	• GSK Investigational Site, Birmingham, Alabama, USA • GSK Investigational Site, Scottsdale, Arizona, USA • GSK Investigational Site, Los Angeles, California, USA • (and 14 more . . .)	Completed. Has results	Neoplasms, gastrointestinal tract
6.	Apatinib Combined with Capecitabine Second-line Treatment of Advanced Gastric Cancer: A Single-Arm Exploratory Clinical Pilot Trial	Apatinib/capecitabine	First Affiliated Hospital of Xiamen University, Xiamen, Fujian, China	Not yet recruiting	Progression-free survival; disease control rate; safety
7.	Conversion Therapy of Sintilimab in Combination with Apatinib and Chemotherapy in Unresectable Gastric Cancer	• Sintilimab • Apatinib • S1 • Nab paclitaxel	Department of Gastrointestinal Medical Oncology, Tianjin Medical University Cancer Hospital, Tianjin, China	Recruiting	Gastric cancer stage
8.	Cabozantinib in Combination with Durvalumab in Patients with Gastroesophageal Cancer and Other Gastrointestinal Malignancies (CAMILLA)	• Cabozantinib • Durvalumab	The University of Kansas Cancer Center, Fairway, Kansas, USA	Recruiting	• Gastric cancer • Esophageal adenocarcinoma • Hepatocellular carcinoma • Colorectal cancer
9.	Prognostic Value and Clinical Pathology of c-MET Expression and Amplification in Gastric Carcinoma	Prognostic markers/values	Sun Yat-sen University Cancer Center, Guangzhou, Guangdong, China	Unknown	Gastric cancer
10.	Cabozantinib S-malate in Treating Patients with Neuroendocrine Tumors Previously Treated with Everolimus That Are Locally Advanced,	• Cabozantinib S-malate • Laboratory biomarker analysis • Placebo administration • Quality-of-life assessment	• Katmai Oncology Group, Anchorage, Alaska, USA • Kingman Regional Medical Center, Kingman, Arizona, USA • University of Arkansas for Medical Sciences, Little	Recruiting	• Atypical carcinoid tumor • Carcinoid tumor • Digestive system neuroendocrine neoplasm • (and 13 more...)

(continued)

Table 9.1 (continued)

Sl. No.	Name of the study	Drug evaluated	Country, trial is conducted	Status of the trial	Condition treated
	Metastatic, or Cannot Be Removed by Surgery		Rock, Arkansas, USA • (and 347 more . . .)		
11.	Capecitabine and Cisplatin (XP) + Sorafenib in Advanced Gastric Cancer (AGC): Sorafenib + XP	Capecitabine, cisplatin, sorafenib	Asan Medical Center, Seoul, Korea	Completed. Has results	Advanced gastric cancer
12.	Patterns of Care and Outcomes of Patients with METAstatic Gastrointestinal Stromal Tumors (METAGIST)	Oral tyrosine-kinase inhibitors (TKI) of KIT and PDGFR as per recommendations	Institut Bergonié, Comprehensive Cancer Center, Bordeaux, France	Recruiting	Gastrointestinal stromal tumor
13.	Efficacy and Safety of Pembrolizumab (MK-3475) Plus Lenvatinib (E7080/MK-7902) in Previously Treated Participants with Select Solid Tumors (MK-7902-005/E7080-G000–224/LEAP-005)	• Pembrolizumab • Lenvatinib	• City of Hope (Site 0002), Duarte, California, USA • Cedars Sinai Medical Center (Site 0003), Los Angeles, California, USA • University of California, Davis Comprehensive Cancer Center (Site 0005), Sacramento, California, USA • (and 45 more . . .)	Active, not recruiting	• Advanced solid tumors • Triple-negative breast cancer • Ovarian cancer • (and 4 more . . .)
14.	Targeted Therapy Directed by Genetic Testing in Treating Patients with Advanced Refractory Solid Tumors, Lymphomas, or Multiple Myeloma (the MATCH Screening Trial)	• Adavosertib • Afatinib • Afatinib Dimaleate • (and 30 more . . .)	• University of Alabama at Birmingham Cancer CenterBirmingham, Alabama, USA • Mobile Infirmary Medical Center, Mobile, Alabama, USA • University of South Alabama Mitchell Cancer Institute, Mobile, Alabama, USA • (and 1312 more . . .)	Recruiting	• Advanced malignant solid neoplasm • Bladder carcinoma • Breast carcinoma • (and 47 more . . .)

15.	GIST: Assessment of Tumor Mutations and TKI Plasma Exposure	• Vena puncture for blood collection • Tumor biopsy	• Antoni van Leeuwenhoek Hospital, Amsterdam, The Netherlands • University Medical Center Groningen, The Netherlands • Leiden University Medical Center, Leiden, The Netherlands • (and 2 more . . .)	Recruiting	Gastrointestinal stromal tumor
16.	Multi-center Placebo-Controlled Double-blinded Phase II Study of Lenvatinib Efficacy in Patients with Locally Advanced or Metastatic GIST (Gastrointestinal Stromal Tumor) After Imatinib/Sunitinib Failure	Lenvatinib	• Centre Léon BérardLyon, France • Institut Gustave Roussy, Villejuif, France	Not yet recruiting	Gastrointestinal stromal tumor
17	A Phase 1 Study of KBP-5209 in Patients with Advanced Solid Tumors	KBP-5209	• Indiana University, Melvin and Bren Simon Cancer Center, Indianapolis, Indiana, USA • University of Texas, MD Anderson Cancer CenterHouston, Texas, USA • University of Utah Huntsman Cancer Institute, Salt Lake City, Utah, USA	Unknown	Advanced solid tumors

5.1 HER-2 Inhibitors

5.1.1 Trastuzumab

Trastuzumab is a monoclonal antibody which targets HER-2 and causes inhibition of its downward signaling. ErbB2/HER cluster comprises four different receptors and HER-2 (ErbB2) is one among them. Studies have demonstrated that 10–38% of people with gastric malignancies present with amplification of HER-2; inhibition of HER-2 has demonstrated successful results in metastatic gastric carcinoma cases [40–42]. Nevertheless, the study was unable to show clear results regarding the relationship between HER-2 amplification and clinical outcome in advanced gastric cancer [43, 44].

Bang et al. [45] in the ToGA trial reported that patients who were HER-2 positive had a greater benefit [based on the immunohistochemistry (IHC) scoring system] when managed with trastuzumab. In 2006, the results of clinical trials on the effects of trastuzumab in late stages of gastric cancer got published. In the first phase II clinical trials, the combination of trastuzumab with cisplatin and docetaxel showed improved response on radiological findings in four out of five patients with advanced gastric carcinoma and cancer of gastroesophageal junction (GEJ) who are HER-2 positive [46]. Another phase II study was conducted in people who presented with metastatic gastric cancer or GEJ cancer and are HER-2 positive. During the study, the patients were put on a combination therapy consisting of trastuzumab (8 mg/kg loading dose followed by 6 mg/kg) and cisplatin (75 mg/m^2) every 3 weeks until relapse. The study reported positive results in terms of patient response (35% out of 17 people) at the end of an average of two treatment cycles [47].

An open-label, global, phase III, clinical trial (the ToGA study) was conducted including many countries where the people with gastric cancer were randomly given either combination therapy with trastuzumab + chemotherapy or chemotherapy monotherapy. The study demonstrated positive results in terms of median overall survival (OS) in the combination therapy arm which was 13.8 months, whereas in the second group the median OS was only 11.1 months. The combination arm also showed an improved OS and progression-free survival (PFS); an increase in median survival by almost 2.7 months was witnessed in the trastuzumab group [45]. However, it was worth noting that trastuzumab was associated with an elevated probability of type 2 chemotherapy-related cardiac issues, which were managed by the removal of the antibody [48]. Nevertheless, the patients in the trastuzumab group did not report any positive results in terms of quality of life [49].

5.2 EGFR Inhibitors

EGFR amplification and activation happened in significant number of patients (27–64%) with gastric carcinoma, more predominantly for proximally located cancers. The EGFR amplification was correlated with poor prognosis as well [50, 51]. Other factors that were associated with EGFR overexpression were elderly people, infiltrative pathologies, and advanced cancers. Drugs that are aimed against EGFR include the following:

5.2.1 Cetuximab

Cetuximab is a monoclonal antibody (mAb) that inhibits EGFR. It also remains the most frequently studied EGFR inhibitor in people with gastric carcinoma. In gastric cancer patients, several studies were conducted to understand the impact of cetuximab. A total of six clinical studies reported that the combination therapy of cetuximab and chemotherapy resulted in positive results in terms of response rate (41–63%) and median OS (9–16.6 months) [52–55]. Contrary to this, the initial results from a phase II study in 2011 [56] showed that the combination therapy consisting of cetuximab and docetaxel + oxaliplatin failed to produce positive results. Later, a phase III clinical study (NCT00678535) [57] that examined the effects of cetuximab in combination with cisplatin + capecitabine also reported similar results in 2013. The combination therapy reported no benefit in terms of PFS (4.4 months in combination therapy vs. 5.6 months in chemotherapy alone). Furthermore, majority of the patients in the study (83% in combination therapy group and 77% in chemotherapy alone) suffered from adverse events including diarrhea, dermatitis, low potassium and magnesium levels, and hand-foot syndrome.

5.2.2 Gefitinib and Erlotinib

EGFR inhibitors, gefitinib and erlotinib, are frontline drugs used in the management of GEJ cancer. However, in patients with advanced gastric cancer, both the drugs failed to produce positive results when used as monotherapy during the phase II clinical trials [58].

5.2.3 Panitumumab

There are very few study results regarding the effect of panitumumab in advanced gastric carcinoma therapy. REAL3, a phase III clinical study [59], classified and studied esophagogastric carcinoma patients based on the treatment received; the first group received combination therapy consisting of chemotherapeutic agents epirubicin, oxaliplatin, and capecitabine (EOC) and panitumumab whereas the second set of patients received chemotherapy alone. The median overall survival in the chemotherapy-alone (EOC) group was 11.3 months whereas the median OS was 8.8 months in the combination (mEOC plus P) group. The patients in the combination therapy arm also suffered from drug side effects such as diarrhea, rash, mucositis, and neutropenia.

Matuzumab and nimotuzumab are other EGFR inhibitors that were tested in combination with chemotherapy during phase II clinical studies. Unfortunately, both the drugs produced unsatisfactory clinical outcomes in terms of PFS [60, 61].

5.3 Combined EGFR and HER-2 Inhibitor

Lapatinib is a dual inhibitor of RTKs acting on HER-2 and EGFR. The efficacy of lapatinib in gastric carcinoma patients was tested in a phase II trial where the drug demonstrated positive clinical outcomes in terms of overall reduction rate (ORR), which was 7%, and disease stabilization rate of 20%. Adverse effects included grade 4 fatigue (two patients) and vomiting [62]. In patients with metastatic gastric cancer, the efficacy of lapatinib is being tested in two current phase III clinical studies. In the first study (LoG-IC trial) [63], lapatinib is being tested as a frontline drug in combination with chemotherapeutic agents oxaliplatin and capecitabine. The second clinical trial (TYTAN) [64] is being conducted on Asian population who are diagnosed with HER-2-positive gastric cancer. In this trial, paclitaxel is tested as a second-line drug with/without lapatinib combination. The results of both these studies are expected to help establish lapatinib as an option for metastatic gastric carcinoma treatment.

5.4 VEGFR Inhibitor

Bevacizumab (Avastin) is a monoclonal antibody, which suppresses angiogenesis via inhibition of vascular endothelial growth factor-A (VEGF-A). In advanced gastric cancer patients, bevacizumab has shown an ORR of 42–67% and an OS of 8.9–16.2 months, during the phase II clinical trials. Adverse events consisted of grade 3–4 thromboembolic disease (25%) and gastric perforation (8%) [65–67]. The phase III clinical trial (AVAGAST) [68] focused on assessing the effectiveness of bevacizumab as second-line therapy in metastatic gastric cancer patients. Patients were classified into two groups; the first set of patients were put on bevacizumab in addition to frontline therapy with capecitabine-cisplatin whereas the second group received chemotherapy alone. The overall survival drastically enhanced after bevacizumab incorporation (46% vs. 37%) and the median PFS got notably prolonged as well (6.7 vs. 5.3 months). Moreover, the results varied based on the geographical location.

An increase in the OS was also seen in all the patients of American origin whereas no significant survival benefits were observed in the Asian and European patients. However, the authors reported a prognostic benefit with bevacizumab. These results could be due to alterations in patient selection, genetic variations within populations, and intake of second-line drugs in those patients. During the AVAGAST study, Ohtsu et al. stated that the prognosis of patients with metastatic gastric cancer could be associated with the levels of angiogenic factors, such as tumor neuropilin-1 and plasma VEGF-A [68, 69]. Unfortunately, patients in both the study arms experienced side effects such as anemia, neutropenia, and anorexia [68].

5.5 *Dual Inhibitors of VEGFR and PDGFR*

Sorafenib suppresses a variety of RTKs such as VEGF, PDGFR, and BRAF. Sunitinib causes inhibition of VEGFR, PDGFR, c-Kit, and Flt-3. Both the antibodies did not show any significant survival benefits in phase II studies [70–72] (Table 9.1).

6 Conclusion

Phytochemicals are abundantly found in fruits and vegetables and have been valuable in gastric cancer. While the combination of phytochemicals could augment antitumor effects on gastric cancer through multiple prevention mechanisms, additional translational and clinical outcome researches are necessary to greatly understand their potential benefits in cancer prevention and prognosis. In addition, several receptor tyrosine kinases are stimulated in gastric malignancies; therefore identification of kinase inhibitors can be potentially beneficial in providing tailored treatment to the patients. Several clinical trials are in development and are anticipated to provide benefits in clinical practice.

Acknowledgements *Author Contributions*: Drs. Muzammil M. Khan, Deepika Sarvepalli, and Mamoon Ur Rashid conceived the idea, and subsequently all the authors have diligently contributed to the development and preparation of this research manuscript (book chapter), including the literature search, concept organization, data interpretation, and writings. All the authors have read and approved the final draft for publication.

Conflict of Interest: The authors declare that they have no conflicts of interest associated with this research manuscript (book chapter).

Financial Disclosures: None to disclose.

References

1. Siegel, R. L., Miller, K. D., & Jemal, A. (2020). Cancer statistics, 2020. *CA: A Cancer Journal for Clinicians, 70*(1), 7–30.
2. Kuipers, E. J. (1999). Exploring the link between Helicobacter pylori and gastric cancer. *Alimentary Pharmacology & Therapeutics, 13*, 3–11.
3. Yanaka, A. (2011). Sulforaphane enhances protection and repair of gastric mucosa against oxidative stress in vitro, and demonstrates anti-inflammatory effects on helicobacter pylori infected gastric mucosae in mice and human subjects. *Current Pharmaceutical Design, 17*(16), 1532–1540.

4. Esatbeyoglu, T., Huebbe, P., Ernst, I. M., Chin, D., Wagner, A. E., & Rimbach, G. (2012). Curcumin—From molecule to biological function. *Angewandte Chemie International Edition, 51*(22), 5308–5332.
5. Goel, A., & Aggarwal, B. B. (2010). Curcumin, the golden spice from Indian saffron, is a chemosensitizer and radiosensitizer for tumors and chemoprotector and radioprotector for normal organs. *Nutrition and Cancer, 62*(7), 919–930.
6. Lee, K. W., Bode, A. M., & Dong, Z. (2011). Molecular targets of phytochemicals for cancer prevention. *Nature Reviews Cancer, 11*(3), 211.
7. De, R., Kundu, P., Swarnakar, S., Ramamurthy, T., Chowdhury, A., Nair, G. B., & Mukhopadhyay, A. K. (2009). Antimicrobial activity of curcumin against Helicobacter pylori isolates from India and during infections in mice. *Antimicrobial Agents and Chemotherapy, 53* (4), 1592–1597.
8. Yu, L. L., Wu, J. G., Dai, N., Yu, H. G., & Si, J. M. (2011). Curcumin reverses chemoresistance of human gastric cancer cells by downregulating the NF-κB transcription factor. *Oncology Reports, 26*(5), 1197–1203.
9. Cai, X. Z., Wang, J., Xiao-Dong, L., Wang, G. L., Liu, F. N., Cheng, M. S., & Li, F. (2009). Curcumin suppresses proliferation and invasion in human gastric cancer cells by down-regulation of PAK1 activity and cyclin D1 expression. *Cancer Biology & Therapy, 8*(14), 1360–1368.
10. Fahey, J. W., Haristoy, X., Dolan, P. M., Kensler, T. W., Scholtus, I., Stephenson, K. K., Talalay, P., & Lozniewski, A. (2002). Sulforaphane inhibits extracellular, intracellular, and antibiotic-resistant strains of Helicobacter pylori and prevents benzo [a] pyrene-induced stomach tumors. *Proceedings of the National Academy of Sciences USA, 99*(11), 7610–7615.
11. Fahey, J. W., Zhang, Y., & Talalay, P. (1997). Broccoli sprouts: An exceptionally rich source of inducers of enzymes that protect against chemical carcinogens. *Proceedings of the National Academy of Sciences USA, 94*(19), 10367–10372.
12. Ramos-Gomez, M., Kwak, M. K., Dolan, P. M., Itoh, K., Yamamoto, M., Talalay, P., & Kensler, T. W. (2001). Sensitivity to carcinogenesis is increased and chemoprotective efficacy of enzyme inducers is lost in nrf2 transcription factor-deficient mice. *Proceedings of the National Academy of Sciences US, 98*(6), 3410–3415.
13. van Oijen, A. H., Verhulst, M. L., Roelofs, H. M., Peters, W. H., de Boer, W. A., & Jansen, J. B. (2001). Eradication of Helicobacter pylori restores glutathione S-transferase activity and glutathione levels in antral mucosa. *Japanese Journal of Cancer Researc, 92*(12), 1329–1334.
14. Yanaka, A., Fahey, J. W., Fukumoto, A., Nakayama, M., Inoue, S., Zhang, S., Tauchi, M., Suzuki, H., Hyodo, I., & Yamamoto, M. (2009). Dietary sulforaphane-rich broccoli sprouts reduce colonization and attenuate gastritis in Helicobacter pylori-infected mice and humans. *Cancer Prevention Research, 2*(4), 353–360.
15. Kopp, P. (1998). Resveratrol, a phytoestrogen found in red wine. A possible explanation for the conundrum of the 'French paradox'? *European Journal of Endocrinology, 138*(6), 619–620.
16. Sun, A. Y., Simonyi, A., & Sun, G. Y. (2002). The "French paradox" and beyond: Neuroprotective effects of polyphenols. *Free Radical Biology and Medicine, 32*(4), 314–318.
17. Hung, L. M., Chen, J. K., Huang, S. S., Lee, R. S., & Su, M. J. (2000). Cardioprotective effect of resveratrol, a natural antioxidant derived from grapes. *Cardiovascular Research, 47*(3), 549–555.
18. Catalgol, B., Batirel, S., Taga, Y., & Ozer, N. K. (2012). Resveratrol: French paradox revisited. *Frontiers in Pharmacology, 3*, 141.
19. Zaidi, S. F., Ahmed, K., Yamamoto, T., Kondo, T., Usmanghani, K., Kadowaki, M., & Sugiyama, T. (2009). Effect of resveratrol on Helicobacter pylori-induced interleukin-8 secretion, reactive oxygen species generation and morphological changes in human gastric epithelial cells. *Biological and Pharmaceutical Bulletin, 32*(11), 1931–1935.
20. Daroch, F., Hoeneisen, M., González, C. L., Kawaguchi, F., Salgado, F., Solar, H., & García, A. (2001). In vitro antibacterial activity of Chilean red wines against Helicobacter pylori. *Microbios, 104*(408), 79–85.

21. Mahady, G. B., Pendland, S. L., & Chadwick, L. R. (2003). Resveratrol and red wine extracts inhibit the growth of CagA+ strains of Helicobacter pylori in vitro. *The American Journal of Gastroenterology, 98*(6), 1440.
22. Mahady, G. B., & Pendland, S. L. (2000). Resveratrol inhibits the growth of Helicobacter pylori in vitro. *The American Journal of Gastroenterology, 95*(7), 1849.
23. Atten, M. J., Attar, B. M., Milson, T., & Holian, O. (2001). Resveratrol-induced inactivation of human gastric adenocarcinoma cells through a protein kinase C-mediated mechanism. *Biochemical Pharmacology, 62*(10), 1423–1432.
24. Atten, M. J., Godoy-Romero, E., Attar, B. M., Milson, T., Zopel, M., & Holian, O. (2005). Resveratrol regulates cellular PKC α and δ to inhibit growth and induce apoptosis in gastric cancer cells. *Investigational New Drugs, 23*(2), 111–119.
25. Aquilano, K., Baldelli, S., Rotilio, G., & Ciriolo, M. R. (2009). Trans-resveratrol inhibits H_2O_2-induced adenocarcinoma gastric cells proliferation via inactivation of MEK1/2-ERK1/2-c-Jun signalling axis. *Biochemical Pharmacology, 77*(3), 337–347.
26. Wang, Z., Li, W., Meng, X., & Jia, B. (2012). Resveratrol induces gastric cancer cell apoptosis via reactive oxygen species, but independent of sirtuin1. *Clinical and Experimental Pharmacology and Physiology, 39*(3), 227–232.
27. Zhou, H. B., Chen, J. J., Wang, W. X., Cai, J. T., & Du, Q. (2005). Anticancer activity of resveratrol on implanted human primary gastric carcinoma cells in nude mice. *World Journal of Gastroenterology, 11*(2), 280.
28. Robinson, D. R., Wu, Y. M., & Lin, S. F. (2000). The protein tyrosine kinase family of the human genome. *Oncogene, 19*(49), 5548–5557. https://doi.org/10.1038/sj.onc.1203957.
29. Schlessinger, J. (2000). Cell signaling by receptor tyrosine kinases. *Cell, 103*(2), 211–225.
30. Olayioye, M. A., Neve, R. M., Lane, H. A., & Hynes, N. E. (2000). The ErbB signaling network: Receptor heterodimerization in development and cancer. *The EMBO Journal, 19*(13), 3159–3167.
31. Morishita, A., Gong, J., & Masaki, T. (2014). Targeting receptor tyrosine kinases in gastric cancer. *World Journal of Gastroenterology, 20*(16), 4536.
32. Hubbard, S. R., & Till, J. H. (2000). Protein tyrosine kinase structure and function. *Annual Review of Biochemistry, 69*(1), 373–398.
33. Lemmon, M. A., & Schlessinger, J. (2010). Cell signaling by receptor tyrosine kinases. *Cell, 141*(7), 1117–1134.
34. Kuriyan, J., & Cowburn, D. (1997). Modular peptide recognition domains in eukaryotic signaling. *Annual Review of Biophysics and Biomolecular Structure, 26*(1), 259–288.
35. Becker, J. C., Müller-Tidow, C., Serve, H., Domschke, W., & Pohle, T. (2006). Role of receptor tyrosine kinases in gastric cancer: New targets for a selective therapy. *World Journal of Gastroenterology, 12*(21), 3297–3305.
36. Shawver, L. K., Slamon, D., & Ullrich, A. (2002). Smart drugs: Tyrosine kinase inhibitors in cancer therapy. *Cancer Cell, 1*(2), 117–123.
37. Cohen, M. H., Williams, G. A., Sridhara, R., Chen, G., & Pazdur, R. (2003). FDA drug approval summary: Gefitinib (ZD1839) (Iressa) tablets. *The Oncologist, 8*(4), 303–306.
38. (2004). New treatments for colorectal cancer. *FDA Consumer, 38*(3), 17.
39. Deng, N., Goh, L. K., Wang, H., Das, K., Tao, J., Tan, I. B., Zhang, S., Lee, M., Wu, J., Lim, K. H., & Lei, Z. (2012). A comprehensive survey of genomic alterations in gastric cancer reveals systematic patterns of molecular exclusivity and co-occurrence among distinct therapeutic targets. *Gut, 61*(5), 673–684.
40. Yano, T., Ohtsu, A., Boku, N., Hashizume, K., Nakanishi, M., & Ochiai, A. (2006). Comparison of HER2 gene amplification assessed by fluorescence in situ hybridization and HER2 protein expression assessed by immunohistochemistry in gastric cancer. *Oncology Reports, 15*(1), 65–71.
41. Koeppen, H. K., Wright, B. D., Burt, A. D., Quirke, P., McNicol, A. M., Dybdal, N. O., Sliwkowski, M. X., & Hillan, K. J. (2001). Overexpression of HER2/neu in solid tumours: An immunohistochemical survey. *Histopathology, 38*(2), 96–104.

42. Jaehne, J., Urmacher, C., Thaler, H. T., Friedlander-Klar, H., Cordon-Cardo, C., & Meyer, H. J. (1992). Expression of Her2/neu oncogene product p185 in correlation to clinicopathological and prognostic factors of gastric carcinoma. *Journal of Cancer Research and Clinical Oncology, 118*(6), 474–479.
43. Im, S. A., Lee, K. E., Nam, E., Kim, D. Y., Lee, J. H., Han, H. S., Seoh, J. Y., Park, H. Y., Cho, M. S., Han, W. S., & Lee, S. N. (2005). Potential prognostic significance of p185HER2 overexpression with loss of PTEN expression in gastric carcinomas. *Tumori Journal, 91*(6), 513–521.
44. Chua, T. C., & Merrett, N. D. (2012). Clinicopathologic factors associated with HER2-positive gastric cancer and its impact on survival outcomes—A systematic review. *International Journal of Cancer, 130*(12), 2845–2856.
45. Bang, Y. J., Van Cutsem, E., Feyereislova, A., Chung, H. C., Shen, L., Sawaki, A., Lordick, F., Ohtsu, A., Omuro, Y., Satoh, T., & Aprile, G. (2010). Trastuzumab in combination with chemotherapy versus chemotherapy alone for treatment of HER2-positive advanced gastric or gastro-oesophageal junction cancer (ToGA): A phase 3, open-label, randomised controlled trial. *The Lancet, 376*(9742), 687–697.
46. Moelans, C. B., van Diest, P. J., Milne, A. N., & Offerhaus, G. J. (2011). Her-2/neu testing and therapy in gastroesophageal adenocarcinoma. *Pathology Research International, 2011*, 674182.
47. Nicholas, G., Cripps, C., Au, H. J., Jonker, D., Salim, M., Bjarnason, G., Chiritescu, G., & Gallant, V. (2006). Early results of a trial of trastuzumab, cisplatin, and docetaxel (TCD) for the treatment of metastatic gastric cancer overexpressing HER-2. *Annals of Oncology, 17*, 316–316.
48. Ewer, S., & Lippman, S. M. (2005). Type II chemotherapy-related cardiac dysfunction: Time to recognize a new entity by Michael. *Journal of Clinical Oncology, 23*, 2900–2902.
49. Tanaka, Y., Yonetani, Y., Shiozaki, Y., Kitaguchi, T., Sato, N., Takeshita, S., & Horibe, S. (2010). Retear of anterior cruciate ligament grafts in female basketball players: A case series. *BMC Sports Science, Medicine and Rehabilitation, 2*(1), 7.
50. Kim, M. A., Lee, H. S., Lee, H. E., Jeon, Y. K., Yang, H. K., & Kim, W. H. (2008). EGFR in gastric carcinomas: Prognostic significance of protein overexpression and high gene copy number. *Histopathology, 52*(6), 738–746.
51. Ilson, D. H., Kelsen, D., Shah, M., Schwartz, G., Levine, D. A., Boyd, J., Capanu, M., Miron, B., & Klimstra, D. (2011). A phase 2 trial of erlotinib in patients with previously treated squamous cell and adenocarcinoma of the esophagus. *Cancer, 117*(7), 1409–1414.
52. Pinto, C., Di Fabio, F., Barone, C., Siena, S., Falcone, A., Cascinu, S., Llimpe, F. R., Stella, G., Schinzari, G., Artale, S., & Mutri, V. (2009). Phase II study of cetuximab in combination with cisplatin and docetaxel in patients with untreated advanced gastric or gastro-oesophageal junction adenocarcinoma (DOCETUX study). *British Journal of Cancer, 101*(8), 1261–1268.
53. Pinto, C., Di Fabio, F., Siena, S., Cascinu, S., Rojas Llimpe, F. L., Ceccarelli, C., Mutri, V., Giannetta, L., Giaquinta, S., Funaioli, C., & Berardi, R. (2007). Phase II study of cetuximab in combination with FOLFIRI in patients with untreated advanced gastric or gastroesophageal junction adenocarcinoma (FOLCETUX study). *Annals of Oncology, 18*(3), 510–517.
54. Kim, C., Lee, J. L., Ryu, M. H., Chang, H. M., Kim, T. W., Lim, H. Y., Kang, H. J., Park, Y. S., Ryoo, B. Y., & Kang, Y. K. (2011). A prospective phase II study of cetuximab in combination with XELOX (capecitabine and oxaliplatin) in patients with metastatic and/or recurrent advanced gastric cancer. *Investigational New Drugs, 29*(2), 366–373.
55. Han, S. W., Oh, D. Y., Im, S. A., Park, S. R., Lee, K. W., Song, H. S., Lee, N. S., Lee, K. H., Choi, I. S., Lee, M. H., & Kim, M. A. (2009). Phase II study and biomarker analysis of cetuximab combined with modified FOLFOX6 in advanced gastric cancer. *British Journal of Cancer, 100*(2), 298–304.
56. Richards, D., Kocs, D. M., Spira, A. I., McCollum, A. D., Diab, S., Hecker, L. I., Cohn, A., Zhan, F., & Asmar, L. (2013). Results of docetaxel plus oxaliplatin (DOCOX) ± cetuximab in

patients with metastatic gastric and/or gastroesophageal junction adenocarcinoma: Results of a randomised phase 2 study. *European Journal of Cancer, 49*(13), 2823–2831.

57. Lordick, F., Kang, Y. K., Chung, H. C., Salman, P., Oh, S. C., Bodoky, G., Kurteva, G., Volovat, C., Moiseyenko, V. M., Gorbunova, V., & Park, J. O. (2013). Capecitabine and cisplatin with or without cetuximab for patients with previously untreated advanced gastric cancer (EXPAND): A randomised, open-label phase 3 trial. *The Lancet Oncology, 14*(6), 490–499.
58. Dragovich, T., McCoy, S., Fenoglio-Preiser, C. M., Wang, J., Benedetti, J. K., Baker, A. F., Hackett, C. B., Urba, S. G., Zaner, K. S., Blanke, C. D., & Abbruzzese, J. L. (2006). Phase II trial of erlotinib in gastroesophageal junction and gastric adenocarcinomas: SWOG 0127. *Journal of Clinical Oncology, 24*(30), 4922–4927.
59. Waddell, T., Chau, I., Cunningham, D., Gonzalez, D., Okines, A. F., Wotherspoon, A., Saffery, C., Middleton, G., Wadsley, J., Ferry, D., & Mansoor, W. (2013). Epirubicin, oxaliplatin, and capecitabine with or without panitumumab for patients with previously untreated advanced oesophagogastric cancer (REAL3): A randomised, open-label phase 3 trial. *The Lancet Oncology, 14*(6), 481–489.
60. Rao, S., Starling, N., Cunningham, D., Sumpter, K., Gilligan, D., Ruhstaller, T., Valladares-Ayerbes, M., Wilke, H., Archer, C., Kurek, R., & Beadman, C. (2010). Matuzumab plus epirubicin, cisplatin and capecitabine (ECX) compared with epirubicin, cisplatin and capecitabine alone as first-line treatment in patients with advanced oesophago-gastric cancer: A randomised, multicentre open-label phase II study. *Annals of Oncology, 21*(11), 2213–2219.
61. Smolen, G. A., Sordella, R., Muir, B., Mohapatra, G., Barmettler, A., Archibald, H., Kim, W. J., Okimoto, R. A., Bell, D. W., Sgroi, D. C., & Christensen, J. G. (2006). Amplification of MET may identify a subset of cancers with extreme sensitivity to the selective tyrosine kinase inhibitor PHA-665752. *Proceedings of the National Academy of Sciences USA, 103*(7), 2316–2321.
62. Iqbal, S., Goldman, B., Fenoglio-Preiser, C. M., Lenz, H. J., Zhang, W., Danenberg, K. D., Shibata, S. I., & Blanke, C. D. (2011). Southwest Oncology Group study S0413: A phase II trial of lapatinib (GW572016) as first-line therapy in patients with advanced or metastatic gastric cancer. *Annals of Oncology, 22*(12), 2610–2615.
63. LOGiC-Lapatinib Optimization Study in ErbB2 (HER2) Positive Gastric Cancer: A Phase III Global, Blinded Study Designed to Evaluate Clinical Endpoints and Safety of Chemotherapy Plus Lapatinib. ClinicalTrials.gov. accessed January 27, 2020 from https://clinicaltrials.gov/ct2/show/results/NCT00680901.
64. Satoh, T., Bang, Y., Wang, J., Xu, J., Chung, H. C., Yeh, K., Chen, J., Mukaiyama, A., Yoshida, P., & Ohtsu, A. (2010). Interim safety analysis from TYTAN: A phase III Asian study of lapatinib in combination with paclitaxel as second-line therapy in gastric cancer. *Journal of Clinical Oncology, 28*(15_suppl), 4057.
65. Shah, M. A., Ilson, D. H., D'Adamo, D. O., Tse, A. T., Schwartz, L. C., & Schwartz, G. K. (2006). Multicenter phase II study of irinotecan, cisplatin, and bevacizumab in patients with metastatic gastric or gastroesophageal junction adenocarcinoma. *Journal of Clinical Oncology, 24*(33), 5201–5206.
66. Shah, M. A., Jhawer, M., Ilson, D. H., Lefkowitz, R. A., Robinson, E., Capanu, M., & Kelsen, D. P. (2011). Phase II study of modified docetaxel, cisplatin, and fluorouracil with bevacizumab in patients with metastatic gastroesophageal adenocarcinoma. *Journal of Clinical Oncology, 29* (7), 868–874.
67. Cohenuram, M. K., Lacy, J. FOLFOX6 and bevacizumab (FOLFOX6/B) for metastatic esophageal (E), gastroesophageal (GE), and gastric (G) adenocarcinoma: A single institution's initial clinical experience. In: Proceedings of the American Society of Clinical Oncology Gastrointestinal Cancers Symposium. 2008.
68. Ohtsu, A., Shah, M. A., Van Cutsem, E., Rha, S. Y., Sawaki, A., Park, S. R., Lim, H. Y., Yamada, Y., Wu, J., Langer, B., & Starnawski, M. (2011). Bevacizumab in combination with

chemotherapy as first-line therapy in advanced gastric cancer: A randomized, double-blind, placebo-controlled phase III study. *Journal of Clinical Oncology, 29*(30), 3968–3976.
69. Van Cutsem, E., de Haas, S., Kang, Y. K., Ohtsu, A., Tebbutt, N. C., Xu, J. M., Yong, W. P., Langer, B., Delmar, P., Scherer, S. J., & Shah, M. A. (2012). Bevacizumab in combination with chemotherapy as first-line therapy in advanced gastric cancer: A biomarker evaluation from the AVAGAST randomized phase III trial. *Journal of Clinical Oncology, 30*(17), 2119–2127.
70. Martin-Richard, M., Gallego, R., Pericay, C., Foncillas, J. G., Queralt, B., Casado, E., Barriuso, J., Iranzo, V., Juez, I., Visa, L., & Saigi, E. (2013). Multicenter phase II study of oxaliplatin and sorafenib in advanced gastric adenocarcinoma after failure of cisplatin and fluoropyrimidine treatment. *A GEMCAD study. Investigational New Drugs, 31*(6), 1573–1579.
71. Bang, Y. J., Kang, Y. K., Kang, W. K., Boku, N., Chung, H. C., Chen, J. S., Doi, T., Sun, Y., Shen, L., Qin, S., & Ng, W. T. (2011). Phase II study of sunitinib as second-line treatment for advanced gastric cancer. *Investigational New Drugs, 29*(6), 1449–1458.
72. Moehler, M. H., Hartmann, J. T., Lordick, F., Al-Batran, S., Reimer, P., Trarbach, T., Ebert, M. P., Daum, S., Weihrauch, M., Galle, P. R., & Upper GI Group of German AIO. (2010). An open-label, multicenter phase II trial of sunitinib for patients with chemorefractory metastatic gastric cancer. *Journal of Clinical Oncology, 28*(15_suppl), e14503.

Chapter 10
Therapeutic Effects of Curcumin Against Colorectal Cancer

Christoffer Briggs Lambring, Sagar Shelake, Faraz Hasan, and Riyaz Basha

Abstract Colorectal cancer is the third most prevalent cancer in terms of incidences and cancer-related deaths. Surgery, chemotherapy, and radiation are the standard therapeutic options for several cancers including colorectal cancer. Phytochemicals or derivatives such as taxol and vincristine have shown efficacy and are widely used for the treatment of multiple cancers. Since the toxicity associated with the standard chemotherapeutic agents still is a major concern for treating colorectal cancer, alternative strategies using herbal products are extensively tested. Curcumin (cur) is a product of the plant, *Curcuma longa*, which exhibits anti-inflammatory, anti-infectious, and anticancer activities. A wide variety of evidences from numerous studies demonstrated that Cur prevents carcinogenesis, modulates signaling, inhibits angiogenesis and other critical aspects linked to cancer cell survival and proliferation, and induces chemopreventive and anticancer activity against colorectal cancer. Cur also showed improved efficacy of chemotherapeutic agents in combination studies. Bioavailability and distribution, and clearance in tissues, pose some limitations for the therapeutic application of this herbal component. To address such limitations, strategies such as combination with other compounds, synthesis of derivatives, and nanoparticles were tested with some success. Overall, Cur could play a vital role in the prevention and therapy of colorectal cancer.

C. B. Lambring · F. Hasan
Graduate School of Biomedical Sciences, UNT Health Science Center, Fort Worth, TX, USA

S. Shelake
Janssen BioTherapeutics Development, Janssen Research & Development, LLC, Spring House, PA, USA

R. Basha (✉)
Graduate School of Biomedical Sciences, UNT Health Science Center, Fort Worth, TX, USA

Janssen BioTherapeutics Development, Janssen Research & Development, LLC, Spring House, PA, USA

Texas College of Osteopathic Medicine, UNT Health Science Center, Fort Worth, TX, USA
e-mail: Riyaz.Basha@unthsc.edu

G. P. Nagaraju (ed.), *Phytochemicals Targeting Tumor Microenvironment in Gastrointestinal Cancers*, https://doi.org/10.1007/978-3-030-48405-7_10

Keywords Colorectal cancer · Curcumin · Signaling · Anticancer activity · Prevention · Cancer treatment

Abbreviations

5-FU	Fluorouracil
Bcl-2	B-cell lymphoma-2
CCND1	Cyclin D1
COX	Cyclooxygenase
CRC	Colorectal cancer
CSCs	Cancer stem cells
Cur	Curcumin
MRP	Multidrug resistance-associated protein
NF	Nuclear factor
NSCs	Normal stem cells
PARP	Poly (ADP-ribose) polymerase
PD-1	Programmed cell death protein-1
PI3-k	Phosphoinositide 3-kinase
Sp	Specificity protein
TA	Tolfenamic acid

1 Introduction

1.1 Colorectal Cancer (CRC)

CRC is one of the most significant malignancies, with global statistics demonstrating that CRC stands fourth (after lung, breast, and prostate cancers) in incidences but third in deaths [1]. In the United States, it is third in both incidences and cancer-related deaths among men and women [2]. CRC is a slow-growing malignancy originating in the large intestine or rectum and hence screening patients and diagnosis at an early stage are crucial for their prognosis. Typically, surgery is the first option for the removal of tumors, subsequently followed by an adjunctive therapy involving chemo- and radiotherapy. There is slight variation for the chances of developing CRC among men (1:22) and women (1:24). CRC originates from benign polyps in colon or rectum. Alongside colonoscopy, other methods such as stool and blood-based and radiological tests are also used for screening CRC [3–7]. Early detection maximizes patient outcomes and minimizes deaths in CRC patients. The 5-year survival rate for CRC patients with the localized disease in the United States is approximately 90%; the survival of patients diagnosed at later/advanced stages is poor (regional disease: ~70%; one distant metastasis: 4%) [8]. Global data predicts that 2.2 million new cases and 1.1 million deaths may occur by 2030 reaching a CRC burden of 60% [9].

1.2 Curcumin (Cur)

Cur is derived from *Curcuma longa* (turmeric), a spice commonly used in Asian subcontinental foods. It is a unique herbal product with multiple medicinal applications due to its antioxidant properties and upon discovery of its pharmacological safety Cur has undergone testing as an anticancer agent [10–13]. While several mechanisms are suggested to be involved with the anticancer activities exerted by Cur, the overwhelming evidence is pointing towards the activities mediated through the nuclear factor (NF)-κB [14–17]. Cur treatment has been shown to upregulate various factors incluing cleaved poly (ADP-ribose) polymerase (PARP) and resulting in an increase of apoptosis [18–20]. The observed cellular growth reduction and increase of apoptosis may be due to the inhibition of NF-κB, a transcription factor (TF) that among other functions transcribes growth-regulatory genes and promotes cellular proliferation. Therefore, Cur's effect on NF-κB was investigated. The other interesting candidate modulated by Cur is cyclooxygenase (COX)-2, an enzyme that is involved with arachidonic acid metabolism [21–24].

2 Cur: Signaling

2.1 Signaling in Cancer

Cancer is defined as a collection of diseases characterized by cells undergoing uncontrolled growth. Advances in cell and molecular biology over the past decades have helped uncover arrays of signaling pathways that play major roles in cancer initiation, progression, and resistance to standard therapy regimens. Hanahan and Weinberg et al. elucidated six hallmarks of cancer that provide the basic mechanisms of cancer progressiveness [25]. These include sustained proliferative signaling, evasion of growth suppressors, resistance to apoptosis, angiogenesis, cellular replication immortality, and activation of invasion and metastasis. Each of these aforementioned function is highly regulated by a conglomerate of well-controlled signaling pathways.

3 Molecules That Impact Signaling in Cancer

Genetic alternations due to either hereditary or environmental factors such as exposure to radioactive agents result in cancer-inducing events including but not limited to overactivation of additional downstream signaling pathways and inhibition of negative feedback pathways that regulate cell proliferation and tumor-suppressor genes. Important molecules in these pathways are genes labeled as proto-oncogenes. Proto-oncogenes are genes which serve many normal cellular functions, but most importantly in the context of cancer have regulatory roles in the cell cycle and cellular division. Gain-of-function mutations of proto-oncogenes result in oncogenes, which can hyperactivate signaling pathways and drive cell proliferation [26]. Mutations can also occur in tumor-suppressor genes and multiple other molecules and molecular pathways; the culmination of these mutations leads to cancer development. Several of these molecular pathways and their effectors are targets of anticancer agents such as doxorubicin, vincristine, and cisplatin. Below are major signaling molecules that play key roles in cancer.

4 Cell Survival and Cell Cycle Regulators

Several proteins are involved in cell survival such as specificity protein (Sp) family TFs (Sp1 and Sp3), survivin, and apoptosis-regulator proteins such as Bcl2. Initiator and effector caspases are of critical importance for regulating cell health and apoptosis [27, 28]. Other regulators such as cyclin D1 and PCNA proteins are considered to play a pivotal role in cellular growth and cell cycle. However, upregulation of these proteins is found to have strong correlation with cancer progression and chemotherapy resistance [29]. Most importantly, targeting survival regulators, mainly Sp1 and survivin, using small inhibitors like tolfenamic acid (TA) and its copper (II) complex analog Cu-TA is shown to induce anticancer activity in cancer cells [28].

5 TGF-Beta/Smad Signaling Pathway

Dysregulation of transforming growth factor (TGF)-β signaling pathway is involved in many diseases, including cancer. (TGF)-β signaling pathway has tumor-suppressor functions in healthy cells. These functions mainly include apoptosis and cell cycle arrest regulation. However, in cancer cells it acts as a cancer-promoting pathway. The (TGF)-β superfamily consists of several growth factors which include both ligands such as (TGF)-β1, (TGF)-β2, (TGF)-β3, and smad1/3 and their receptors (TGF)-βR1 and (TGF)-βR2. Most importantly, (TGF)-β is seen as an important regulator of epithelial-mesenchymal transition (EMT). In metastatic and chemotherapy-resistant cancers, such as oxaliplatin-resistant colorectal cancer, activation of (TGF)-β EMT is found to be an important mechanism of chemotherapy resistance [30].

6 NF-kappaB Signaling Pathway

6.1 *Cur's Role in Impacting Signaling and How it Affects Anticancer Activity*

The anticancer properties of Cur are mainly believed to be related to its capacity to downregulate cytokines, growth factors, and signaling pathways that activate cancer progression and induce chemotherapy resistance. In chemotherapy-resistant CRC, (TGF)-β/Smad signaling pathway and hyperactivation of NF-kB signaling pathways mediate resistance to oxaliplatin. Interestingly, in two independent studies, Cur combination therapy with oxaliplatin was shown to rescue oxaliplatin-resistant cancer cells by not only downregulating (TGF)-β, an EMT-inducing pathway, and NF-κB signaling pathway, but also increasing apoptotic caspase-3 in CRC cells [30, 31]. In another study reported by Preethi Ravindranathan et al., Cur is shown to promote antitumor activity of oligomeric proanthocyanidins by altering the expression of PCNA and cyclin D1, key cell cycle regulators [29].

7 Cur and Chemotherapy Combination

7.1 *Resistance in CRC*

Colorectal cancer, especially late-stage and metastatic CRC (mCRC), is associated with a high mortality rate due in large part to its ability to respond to and survive chemotherapeutic interactions. Chemo-surviving cells can eventually lead to relapse and a regrowth of chemotherapy-nonrespondent cells. Chemoresistance is suspected to be the cause for treatment failure in over 90% of mCRC cases [32]. Resistance to one drug can also result in multidrug resistance (MDR) leading to CRC gaining the ability to defend against drugs that have different mechanisms of action. Resistance to anticancer drugs is mediated through up- and downregulation of certain pathways, altered levels of gene expression, and other various mechanisms.

7.2 *Mechanisms Associated with Resistance in CRC*

A few of the general mechanisms of chemoresistance in cancer cells involve genetic modifications and DNA repair mechanisms, altered metabolism, trapping the drug in compartments within the cell, and up- and downregulation of signaling pathways that respond to treatment [33, 34] (Fig. 10.1). Cancer cells in general can have innate resistance to targeted drugs. ABC transporters are proteins that participate in the movement of substrates intra- and extracellularly. ABC transporters likely assist in CRC resistance due to their ability to efflux and transport anticancer drugs via ATP

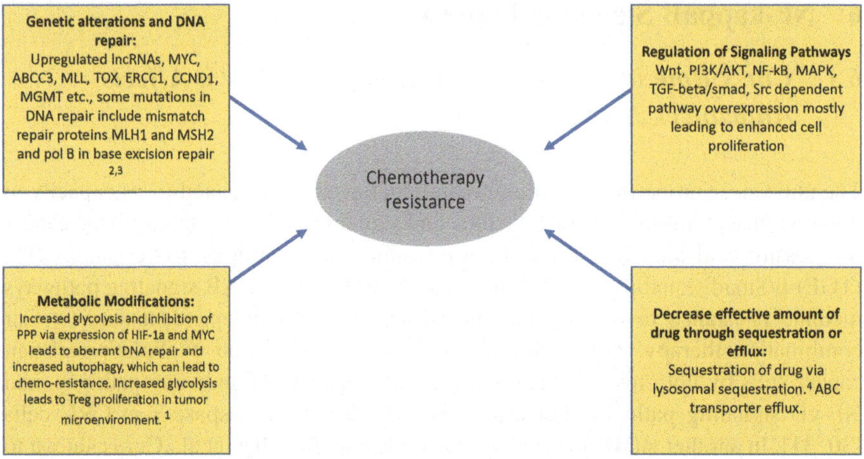

Fig. 10.1 General mechanisms and associated components in chemotherapy resistance in CRC cells. The ability to use one or multiple of these mechanisms can lead to chemo-surviving cells and regrowth

hydrolysis and inhibition of ABC transporters have shown negative effects on tumorigenesis [35]. Multidrug-resistant proteins (MRPs) are a family of proteins under the umbrella of ABC transporters and are thought to be one of the main drivers behind MDR in cancer cells [36]. Knockdown of multidrug-resistant protein-1 (MRP1) showed increased sensitivity in CRC cells to FOLFOX and XELOX, some of the main chemotherapy combinations used in the treatment of CRC [37]. Chemoresistance to treatment by 5-fluorouracil (5-FU) is common among CRC resistance and identification of biomarkers to track the progression of CRC resistance is being elucidated. Long intergenic noncoding RNAs (lincRNAs) have been implicated as important players in CRC cancer. LINC00957 is linked to poor survival rates of CRC patients when it is overexpressed and its inhibition leads to a reversal of resistance to 5-FU, most likely due to its possible regulation of MRP [38]. Another lincRNA, LINC00261, and its overexpression in CRC cells have shown increased sensitivity to cisplatin, possibly through the suppression of nuclear β-catenin, effectively reducing the activation of genes Myc and cyclin D (CCND)1 which are known oncogenic drivers [39]. Multiple pathways have been indicated in resistance to certain chemotherapeutic drugs; as mentioned in the previous chapter, NF-κB-mediated resistance acts through its activation of the NF-κB pathway upon stimulation, by oxaliplatin or other chemotherapeutic interactions, and subsequent phosphorylation of p65, resulting in an upregulation of B-cell lymphoma (Bcl)-2 and survivin [31]. Src-dependent pathways are evident in 5-FU resistance in CRC cells. Src pathways involve multiple downstream effectors that have relevance in CRC and Src dysregulation can result in uncontrolled proliferation and metastasis. Allgayer et al. reported Src activation at nearly a twofold increase in CRC tumors and suggest that Src elevation could be used as a prognostic marker [40].

8 Combination Treatments to Address Resistance to Chemotherapy

Mounting efforts to combat resistance to chemotherapy and radiation in CRC are becoming more focused on options that offer fewer adverse effects. Combinational therapies offer multiple advantages in chemotherapy because they offer multiple modes of action in the targeting of cancers and a decrease in the dosage of medications which could result in curbing the negative effects of conventional chemotherapy. In the case of CRC, the most prominent medications, oxaliplatin and fluorouracil (5-FU) or Xeloda, are used in combinations like XELOX (Xel: Xeloda; OX: oxaliplatin), a combination of capecitabine and oxaliplatin, and FOLFOX which contains 5-FU and leucovorin [41]. But as described above resistance to these first-line drugs is common and avenues to circumvent this are necessary for treatment. Immunotherapy medications are available to be used in combination with classical drugs in the hope of providing a different approach for the treatment of CRC. The aim of immunotherapy combinations in CRC is to increase the immune response of the body and sensitize the tumor to attack by eliminating factors that may create a positive microenvironment for the growth of CRC cells; this provides another mechanism to combat the ability of a tumor cell to proliferate and acquire resistance. An immunotherapy medication that is used synergistically with a conventional drug is atezolizumab, a monoclonal antibody and programmed cell death protein-1 or PD-L1 inhibitor that is used in combination with cobimetinib [42]. Studies into natural products to combat chemoresistance are also underway. *Hedyotis diffusa*, a plant used in traditional Chinese medicine, shows the ability to sensitize CRC to 5-FU treatment possibly through regulation of multidrug resistance-associated protein (MRP)1 [43]. NSAIDs have also been used in combinational therapy with chemotherapy in order to address resistance in CRC. Celecoxib has been shown to have synergistic effects with multiple drugs including cetuximab which is used in the treatment of metastatic CRC. Celecoxib and cetuximab were shown to decrease the levels of nuclear β-catenin [44], which as mentioned before is associated with MDR through regulation by lincRNAs.

Several options are in testing to address drug resistance in cancer treatment [45–47], in emerging combinatorial therapies, Cur has been tested as an option in combination treatments for resistant CRC [30, 31, 48–50]. Cur's ability to reverse oxaliplatin resistance in CRC has already been discussed, but Cur has also been shown to increase sensitization to 5-FU. Cur and 5-FU combination treatment was shown to increase pro-apoptotic proteins Bax, PARP, and caspases-8, -9, and -3 and subsequently the combination decreased anti-apoptotic proteins like BCL-xL [51]. Cur also suppressed 5-FU's induction of NF-κB and phosphoinositide 3-kinase (PI-3 K)/Src enhancement when compared to 5-FU treatment alone [51]. Cur-induced up- and downregulation of relevant cellular constituents are shown in Fig. 10.2. Cur has also been used in combination with other natural molecules including silymarin which is a phytochemical and the bioactive component of milk thistle [52]. Silymarin has an inhibiting effect on β-catenin/TCF4 in

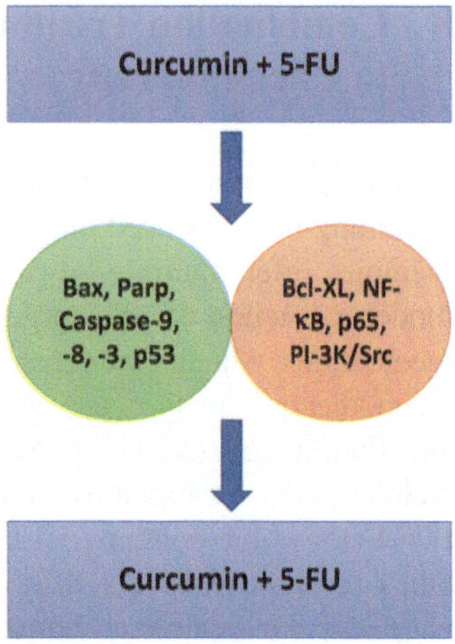

Fig. 10.2 Cur and 5-FU combination treatment for CRC. The pathways associated with cellular growth are affected by Cur and induce sensitivity to 5-FU. The critical markers that are upregulated or downregulated by Cur are given inside green or red circles, respectively

CRC cells [53]. Montgomery et al. showed that Cur effectively sensitized CRC cells to silymarin, leading to a higher rate of apoptosis in three CRC cell lines [52]. Combinational therapy based solely on natural compounds like Cur and silymarin avoids both the negative side effects and possibility of resistance in conventional chemotherapy for CRC.

9 Cancer Stem Cells

Cancer stem cells (CSCs) are distinct from normal stem cells (NSCs) which can be formed due to mutated genes in NSCs or progenitor cells [54–57]. Similar to other cancers, CRC cells are driven by these tumor-initiating CSCs [58, 59]. CSCs exhibit less ability for cell differentiation and a high level of activity for self-renewal [60]. Even though CSCs are only a fraction (~1%) of cancer cell population, they are critical for the formation of tumors due to their higher proliferative ability [61, 62]. These cells can also play a role in a tumor's ability to develop resistance to therapies and also spread to local or distant organs [63, 64].

CSCs can influence the response to therapy and outcomes in cancer treatment [65, 66]. About 50% of CRC patients experience reoccurrence of the disease and CSCs are believed to play a role in cancer reoccurrence. Since the first report on CSCs in CRC [67], there is an increasing interest to test strategies to target CSCs for therapy. Cur has been shown to affect CSCs in human cancers including CRC [62, 68–70]. Interestingly, Cur exhibited a distinct effect on NSCs and CSCs by inhibiting cytokines, Wnt, and Notch pathways [71]. Several mechanisms have been attributed to describe the cellular resistance and attenuation in response to chemotherapy including the modulation of apoptosis and epigenetic reprogramming [72] and Cur has been demonstrated to affect most of such mechanisms (Fig. 10.3) and induce CSC death.

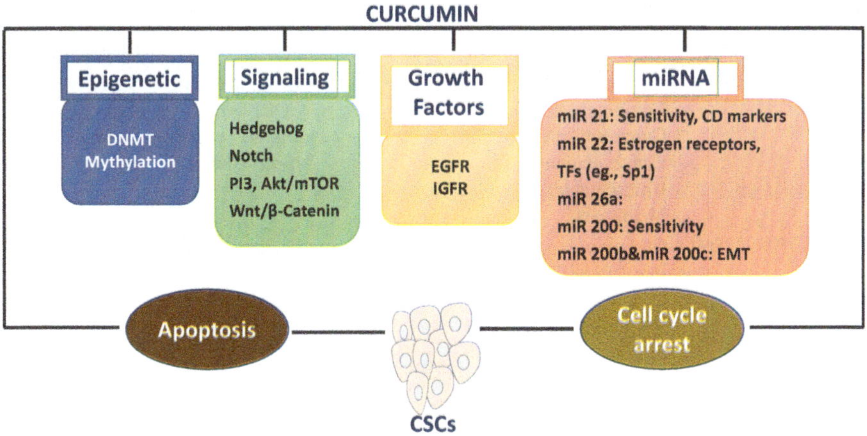

Fig. 10.3 Effect of Cur on CSCs. Research showed distinct effect of Cur against NSCs and CSCs. Cur modulates apoptosis, cell cycle phase distribution, miRNAs, cytokines, and signaling molecules; promotes CSC death; and sensitizes CRC cells against chemotherapy

10 Clinical Trials

Cur has been tested and currently under clinical testing for multiple cancers. A search on "clinicaltrials.gov" revealed eight studies (completed: four; active (not recruiting): one; unknown status: one; and terminated: two) focused on CRC. Two studies (NCT00003365: Sulindac and Plant Compounds in Preventing Colon Cancer, and NCT00118989: Curcumin for the Chemoprevention of Colorectal Cancer) are terminated and results are not available yet at "clinicaltrials.gov." The other six studies with details are listed in Table 10.1.

11 Conclusion

Current options for treating advanced or distant metastatic CRC result in modest benefits. Cytotoxic therapies using chemotherapeutic agents cause morbidity and have not provided much improvement as outcomes and survival rates remain low. Cur, a natural compound shown to induce anticancer activity against several cancer models, is a viable addition for use in current cancer therapy. Due to the morbidity associated with traditional highly toxic cancer therapy, reducing toxicity in CRC is very important. A few natural agents have been evaluated in combination with standard chemotherapeutic agents. Preclinical and clinical studies provide strong evidence that Cur is effective in both CRC prevention and therapy. Most importantly Cur's ability to fight against resistance to chemotherapy is well established. The mechanisms associated with the anticancer activity of Cur include epigenetic modifications, signaling, miRNAs, etc. Typically, similar mechanisms are contributed to

Table 10.1 Clinical trials: curcumin and colorectal cancer (clinicaltrials.gov)

	NCT number	Title	Status	Interventions	Characteristics
1	NCT02439385	Avastin/FOLFIRI in Combination with Curcumin in Colorectal Cancer Patients with Unresectable Metastasis	Completed	• Drug: avastin/ FOLFIRI • Dietary supplement: curcumin	Study type: interventional Phase: phase 2
2	NCT00973869	Curcumin in Preventing Colorectal Cancer in Patients Undergoing Colorectal Endoscopy or Colorectal Surgery	Unknown	• Dietary supplement: curcumin • Other: high-performance liquid chromatography • Other: laboratory biomarker analysis • Other: pharmacological study • Procedure: diagnostic endoscopic procedure • Procedure: therapeutic conventional surgery	Study type: interventional Phase: phase 1
3	NCT01859858	Effect of Curcumin on Dose Limiting Toxicity and Pharmacokinetics of Irinotecan in Patients with Solid Tumors	Active (not recruiting)	• Dietary supplement: curcumin • Drug: irinotecan	Study type: interventional Phase: phase 1
4	NCT01333917	Curcumin Biomarkers	Completed	• Drug: curcumin C3 tablet	Study type: interventional Phase: phase 1
5	NCT01490996	Combining curcumin with FOLFOX Chemotherapy in Patients with Inoperable Colorectal Cancer	Completed	• Drug: oral complex C3 curcumin + chemotherapy • Drug: chemotherapy only	Study type: interventional Phase: • Phase 1 • Phase 2
6	NCT00027495	Curcumin for the Prevention of Colon Cancer	Completed	• Dietary supplement: curcumin	Study type: interventional

(continued)

affect CRC cells including CSCs. One of the issues that are still in progress is to increase bioavailability. Cur nanoparticles [73–77] and derivatives [78–80] are being tested to overcome the limitations of Cur regarding bioavailability.

References

1. Bray, F., et al. (2018). Global cancer statistics 2018: GLOBOCAN estimates of incidence and mortality worldwide for 36 cancers in 185 countries. *CA: a Cancer Journal for Clinicians, 68*(6), 394–424.
2. Siegel, R. L., Miller, K. D., & Jemal, A. (2020). Cancer statistics, 2020. *CA: a Cancer Journal for Clinicians, 70*(1), 7–30.
3. Bond, J. H. (2002). Fecal occult blood test screening for colorectal cancer. *Gastrointestinal Endoscopy Clinics of North America, 12*(1), 11–21.
4. Carroll, M. R., Seaman, H. E., & Halloran, S. P. (2014). Tests and investigations for colorectal cancer screening. *Clinical Biochemistry, 47*(10–11), 921–939.
5. Force, U. S. P. S. T., et al. (2016). Screening for colorectal cancer: US preventive services task force recommendation statement. *JAMA, 315*(23), 2564–2575.
6. Issa, I. A., & Noureddine, M. (2017). Colorectal cancer screening: An updated review of the available options. *World Journal of Gastroenterology, 23*(28), 5086–5096.
7. Levin, B., et al. (2008). Screening and surveillance for the early detection of colorectal cancer and adenomatous polyps, 2008: A joint guideline from the American Cancer Society, the US multi-society task force on colorectal cancer, and the American College of Radiology. *CA: a Cancer Journal for Clinicians, 58*(3), 130–160.
8. Siegel, R. L., et al. (2017). Colorectal cancer statistics, 2017. *CA: a Cancer Journal for Clinicians, 67*(3), 177–193.
9. Arnold, M., et al. (2017). Global patterns and trends in colorectal cancer incidence and mortality. *Gut, 66*(4), 683–691.
10. Aggarwal, B. B., Kumar, A., & Bharti, A. C. (2003). Anticancer potential of curcumin: preclinical and clinical studies. *Anticancer Research, 23*(1A), 363–398.
11. Deguchi, A. (2015). Curcumin targets in inflammation and cancer. *Endocrine, Metabolic & Immune Disorders Drug Targets, 15*(2), 88–96.
12. Devassy, J. G., Nwachukwu, I. D., & Jones, P. J. (2015). Curcumin and cancer: Barriers to obtaining a health claim. *Nutrition Reviews, 73*(3), 155–165.
13. Hossain, D. M., et al. (2012). Curcumin: The multi-targeted therapy for cancer regression. *Frontiers in Bioscience (Scholar Edition), 4*, 335–355.
14. Tong, W., et al. (2016). Curcumin suppresses colon cancer cell invasion via AMPK-induced inhibition of NF-kappaB, uPA activator and MMP9. *Oncology Letters, 12*(5), 4139–4146.
15. Park, J., & Conteas, C. N. (2010). Anti-carcinogenic properties of curcumin on colorectal cancer. *World Journal of Gastrointestinal Oncology, 2*(4), 169–176.
16. Jobin, C., et al. (1999). Curcumin blocks cytokine-mediated NF-kappa B activation and proinflammatory gene expression by inhibiting inhibitory factor I-kappa B kinase activity. *Journal of Immunology, 163*(6), 3474–3483.
17. Li, N., et al. (2019). Curcumin and curcumol inhibit NF-kappaB and TGF-beta 1/Smads signaling pathways in CSE-treated RAW246.7 cells. *Evidence-based Complementary and Alternative Medicine, 2019*, 3035125.
18. Ogiwara, H., et al. (2013). Curcumin suppresses multiple DNA damage response pathways and has potency as a sensitizer to PARP inhibitor. *Carcinogenesis, 34*(11), 2486–2497.
19. Milacic, V., et al. (2008). Curcumin inhibits the proteasome activity in human colon cancer cells in vitro and in vivo. *Cancer Research, 68*(18), 7283–7292.
20. Kim, K. C., & Lee, C. (2010). Curcumin induces downregulation of E2F4 expression and apoptotic cell death in HCT116 human colon cancer cells; involvement of reactive oxygen species. *The Korean Journal of Physiology & Pharmacology, 14*(6), 391–397.
21. Goel, A., Boland, C. R., & Chauhan, D. P. (2001). Specific inhibition of cyclooxygenase-2 (COX-2) expression by dietary curcumin in HT-29 human colon cancer cells. *Cancer Letters, 172*(2), 111–118.
22. Lev-Ari, S., et al. (2005). Celecoxib and curcumin synergistically inhibit the growth of colorectal cancer cells. *Clinical Cancer Research, 11*(18), 6738–6744.

23. Rao, C. V. (2007). Regulation of COX and LOX by curcumin. *Advances in Experimental Medicine and Biology, 595*, 213–226.
24. Kunnumakkara, A. B., et al. (2009). Curcumin sensitizes human colorectal cancer to capecitabine by modulation of cyclin D1, COX-2, MMP-9, VEGF and CXCR4 expression in an orthotopic mouse model. *International Journal of Cancer, 125*(9), 2187–2197.
25. Hanahan, D., & Weinberg, R. A. (2011). Hallmarks of cancer: The next generation. *Cell, 144* (5), 646–674.
26. Sever, R., & Brugge, J. S. (2015). Signal transduction in cancer. *Cold Spring Harbor Perspectives in Medicine, 5*(4), a006098.
27. Hurtado, M., et al. (2018). Novel survivin inhibitor for suppressing pancreatic cancer cells growth via downregulating Sp1 and Sp3 transcription factors. *Cellular Physiology and Biochemistry, 51*(4), 1894–1907.
28. Hurtado, M., et al. (2018). Investigational agents to enhance the efficacy of chemotherapy or radiation in pancreatic cancer. *Critical Reviews in Oncology/Hematology, 126*, 201–207.
29. Ravindranathan, P., et al. (2018). A combination of curcumin and oligomeric proanthocyanidins offer superior anti-tumorigenic properties in colorectal cancer. *Scientific Reports, 8*(1), 13869.
30. Yin, J., et al. (2019). Curcumin reverses oxaliplatin resistance in human colorectal cancer via regulation of TGF-beta/Smad2/3 signaling pathway. *Oncotargets and Therapy, 12*, 3893–3903.
31. Ruiz de Porras, V., et al. (2016). Curcumin mediates oxaliplatin-acquired resistance reversion in colorectal cancer cell lines through modulation of CXC-chemokine/NF-kappaB signalling pathway. *Scientific Reports, 6*, 24675.
32. Longley, D. B., & Johnston, P. G. (2005). Molecular mechanisms of drug resistance. *The Journal of Pathology, 205*(2), 275–292.
33. Torgovnick, A., & Schumacher, B. (2015). DNA repair mechanisms in cancer development and therapy. *Frontiers in Genetics, 6*, 157.
34. Zaal, E. A., & Berkers, C. R. (2018). The influence of metabolism on drug response in cancer. *Frontiers in Oncology, 8*, 500.
35. Henderson, M. J., et al. (2011). ABCC multidrug transporters in childhood neuroblastoma: Clinical and biological effects independent of cytotoxic drug efflux. *Journal of the National Cancer Institute, 103*(16), 1236–1251.
36. Sodani, K., et al. (2012). Multidrug resistance associated proteins in multidrug resistance. *Chinese Journal of Cancer, 31*(2), 58–72.
37. Cao, D., et al. (2017). The role of MRP1 in the multidrug resistance of colorectal cancer. *Oncology Letters, 13*(4), 2471–2476.
38. Zhang, L. H., et al. (2019). LINC00957 acted as prognostic marker was associated with fluorouracil resistance in human colorectal cancer. *Frontiers in Oncology, 9*(776).
39. Wang, Z. K., et al. (2018). Long non-coding RNA LINC00261 sensitizes human colon cancer cells to cisplatin therapy. *Brazilian Journal of Medical and Biological Research, 51*.
40. Allgayer, H., et al. (2002). Activation of Src kinase in primary colorectal carcinoma. *Cancer, 94* (2), 344–351.
41. Cassidy, J., et al. (2004). XELOX (capecitabine plus oxaliplatin): Active first-line therapy for patients with metastatic colorectal cancer. *Journal of Clinical Oncology : Official Journal of the American Society of Clinical Oncology, 22*, 2084–2091.
42. Fellner, C. (2017). Promising drugs in clinical development to treat advanced colorectal cancer. *P & T : A Peer-Reviewed Journal for Formulary Management, 42*(4), 262–265.
43. Li, Q., et al. (2015). Hedyotis diffusa Willd overcomes 5-fluorouracil resistance in human colorectal cancer HCT-8/5-FU cells by downregulating the expression of P-glycoprotein and ATP-binding cassette subfamily G member 2. *Experimental and Therapeutic Medicine, 10*(5), 1845–1850.
44. Valverde, A., et al. (2017). The addition of celecoxib improves the antitumor effect of cetuximab in colorectal cancer: Role of EGFR-RAS-FOXM1-β-catenin signaling axis. *Oncotarget, 8*(13), 21754–21769.

45. Zahreddine, H., & Borden, K. L. (2013). Mechanisms and insights into drug resistance in cancer. *Frontiers in Pharmacology, 4*, 28.
46. van der Mijn, J. C., et al. (2014). Predictive biomarkers in renal cell cancer: Insights in drug resistance mechanisms. *Drug Resistance Updates, 17*(4–6), 77–88.
47. Lau, M. T., et al. (2020). Systematic functional identification of cancer multi-drug resistance genes. *Genome Biology, 21*(1), 27.
48. Lu, W. D., et al. (2013). Effect of curcumin on human colon cancer multidrug resistance in vitro and in vivo. *Clinics (São Paulo, Brazil), 68*(5), 694–701.
49. Zhang, C., et al. (2018). Curcumin reverses irinotecan resistance in colon cancer cell by regulation of epithelial-mesenchymal transition. *Anti-Cancer Drugs, 29*(4), 334–340.
50. Shakibaei, M., et al. (2014). Curcumin chemosensitizes 5-fluorouracil resistant MMR-deficient human colon cancer cells in high density cultures. *PLoS One, 9*(1), e85397.
51. Shakibaei, M., et al. (2013). Curcumin enhances the effect of chemotherapy against colorectal cancer cells by inhibition of NF-κB and Src protein kinase signaling pathways. *PLoS One, 8*(2), e57218–e57218.
52. Montgomery, A., et al. (2016). Curcumin sensitizes silymarin to exert synergistic anticancer activity in colon cancer cells. *Journal of Cancer, 7*(10), 1250–1257.
53. Eo, H. J., Park, G. H., & Jeong, J. B. (2016). Inhibition of Wnt signaling by silymarin in human colorectal cancer cells. *Biomolecules & Therapeutics, 24*(4), 380–386.
54. Clarke, M. F., et al. (2006). Cancer stem cells--perspectives on current status and future directions: AACR workshop on cancer stem cells. *Cancer Research, 66*(19), 9339–9344.
55. Kitamura, H., et al. (2009). Cancer stem cell: Implications in cancer biology and therapy with special reference to lung cancer. *Lung Cancer, 66*(3), 275–281.
56. Li, L., Borodyansky, L., & Yang, Y. (2009). Genomic instability en route to and from cancer stem cells. *Cell Cycle, 8*(7), 1000–1002.
57. Rapp, U. R., Ceteci, F., & Schreck, R. (2008). Oncogene-induced plasticity and cancer stem cells. *Cell Cycle, 7*(1), 45–51.
58. Dick, J. E. (2008). Stem cell concepts renew cancer research. *Blood, 112*(13), 4793–4807.
59. Hatano, Y., et al. (2017). Multifaceted interpretation of colon cancer stem cells. *International Journal of Molecular Sciences, 18*(7).
60. Ahmed, M., et al. (2019). Repurposing antibacterial AM404 as a potential anticancer drug for targeting colorectal cancer stem-like cells. *Cancers (Basel), 12*(1).
61. Bao, B., et al. (2013). Overview of cancer stem cells (CSCs) and mechanisms of their regulation: Implications for cancer therapy. *Current Protocols in Pharmacology, Chapter 14: p. Unit 14*, 25.
62. Ramasamy, T. S., et al. (2015). Targeting colorectal cancer stem cells using curcumin and curcumin analogues: Insights into the mechanism of the therapeutic efficacy. *Cancer Cell International, 15*, 96.
63. Reya, T., et al. (2001). Stem cells, cancer, and cancer stem cells. *Nature, 414*(6859), 105–111.
64. Wicha, M. S., Liu, S., & Dontu, G. (2006). Cancer stem cells: An old idea--a paradigm shift. *Cancer Research, 66*(4), 1883–1890. discussion 1895-6.
65. Sachlos, E., et al. (2012). Identification of drugs including a dopamine receptor antagonist that selectively target cancer stem cells. *Cell, 149*(6), 1284–1297.
66. Dashzeveg, N. K., et al. (2017). New advances and challenges of targeting cancer stem cells. *Cancer Research, 77*(19), 5222–5227.
67. Ricci-Vitiani, L., et al. (2007). Identification and expansion of human colon-cancer-initiating cells. *Nature, 445*(7123), 111–115.
68. Zang, S., et al. (2014). Curcumin: A promising agent targeting cancer stem cells. *Anti-Cancer Agents in Medicinal Chemistry, 14*(6), 787–792.
69. Li, Y., et al. (2018). Evaluation of curcumin, a natural product in turmeric, on Burkitt lymphoma and acute myeloid leukemia cancer stem cell markers. *Future Oncology, 14*(23), 2353–2360.
70. Huang, Y. T., et al. (2016). Curcumin induces apoptosis of colorectal cancer stem cells by coupling with CD44 marker. *Journal of Agricultural and Food Chemistry, 64*(11), 2247–2253.

71. Sordillo, P. P., & Helson, L. (2015). Curcumin and cancer stem cells: Curcumin has asymmetrical effects on cancer and normal stem cells. *Anticancer Research, 35*(2), 599–614.
72. Bighetti-Trevisan, R. L., et al. (2019). Cancer stem cells: Powerful targets to improve current anticancer therapeutics. *Stem Cells International, 2019*, 9618065.
73. Chaurasia, S., et al. (2016). Curcumin-polymeric nanoparticles against colon-26 tumor-bearing mice: Cytotoxicity, pharmacokinetic and anticancer efficacy studies. *Drug Development and Industrial Pharmacy, 42*(5), 694–700.
74. Li, L., et al. (2007). Liposomal curcumin with and without oxaliplatin: Effects on cell growth, apoptosis, and angiogenesis in colorectal cancer. *Molecular Cancer Therapeutics, 6*(4), 1276–1282.
75. Li, L., et al. (2014). Epithelial cell adhesion molecule aptamer functionalized PLGA-lecithin-curcumin-PEG nanoparticles for targeted drug delivery to human colorectal adenocarcinoma cells. *International Journal of Nanomedicine, 9*, 1083–1096.
76. Lotfi-Attari, J., et al. (2017). Co-delivery of curcumin and chrysin by polymeric nanoparticles inhibit synergistically growth and hTERT gene expression in human colorectal cancer cells. *Nutrition and Cancer, 69*(8), 1290–1299.
77. Wong, K. E., et al. (2019). Curcumin nanoformulations for colorectal cancer: A review. *Frontiers in Pharmacology, 10*, 152.
78. Basile, V., et al. (2009). Curcumin derivatives: Molecular basis of their anti-cancer activity. *Biochemical Pharmacology, 78*(10), 1305–1315.
79. Mbese, Z., Khwaza, V., & Aderibigbe, B. A. (2019). Curcumin and its derivatives as potential therapeutic agents in prostate, colon and breast cancers. *Molecules, 24*(23).
80. Cen, L., et al. (2009). New structural analogues of curcumin exhibit potent growth suppressive activity in human colorectal carcinoma cells. *BMC Cancer, 9*, 99.

Chapter 11
Molecular Pathways Involved in the Pathogenesis of Pancreatic Cancer: Role of Phytochemicals in Targeting the Clinical Outcomes

Bayarmaa Mandzhieva, Rima Shobar, Anum Jalil, Hammad Zafar, Mamoon Ur Rashid, Ranjeet Kumar, Akash Khetpal, and Sarfraz Ahmad

Abstract Pancreatic cancer is the fourth leading cause of cancer-related deaths in the United States. Its high mortality is due to delayed diagnosis as it often produces minimal symptoms early in the disease. Surgical resection, radiation therapy, and chemotherapy are essential treatment components. It is well known that chemotherapy options include gemcitabine monotherapy, 5-fluorouracil, leucovorin, irinotecan, and oxaliplatin (FOLFIRINOX) combination and the combination of gemcitabine plus albumin-bound (nab) paclitaxel. Despite these therapeutic options, the average 5-year survival rate continues to be less than 5%; therefore more efficacious approaches need to be explored. There are novel potential therapies under investigation such as immunotherapy and compounds from natural sources. Many recently published epidemiological studies have shown a strong association between phytochemicals and reduced incidence of cancers. This chapter is an overview of the current knowledge and the potential anticancer properties of various natural products, such as curcumin, benzyl isothiocyanate, capsaicin, resveratrol,

B. Mandzhieva (✉) · R. Shobar · A. Jalil · M. U. Rashid · R. Kumar
Department of Internal Medicine, AdventHealth, Orlando, FL, USA
e-mail: bayarmaa.mandzhieva.MD@adventhealth.com; rima.shobar.MD@adventhealth.com; anum.jalil.MD@adventhealth.com; mamoon.rashid.MD@adventhealth.com; ranjeet.kumar.MD@adventhealth.com

H. Zafar
Department of Internal Medicine, AdventHealth, Orlando, FL, USA

Department of Internal Medicine, AdventHealth, Orlando, FL, USA
e-mail: hammad.zafar.MD@adventhealth.com

A. Khetpal
Dow University of Health Sciences, Karachi, Sindh, Pakistan

S. Ahmad (✉)
AdventHealth Cancer Institute, FSU and UCF Colleges of Medicine, Orlando, FL, USA
e-mail: sarfraz.ahmad@adventhealth.com

G. P. Nagaraju (ed.), *Phytochemicals Targeting Tumor Microenvironment in Gastrointestinal Cancers*, https://doi.org/10.1007/978-3-030-48405-7_11

and tea polyphenols. These findings lay the groundwork to support that there exist some association of anticancer properties of phytochemicals in the management of pancreatic malignancy.

Keywords Pancreatic cancer · Pathobiology · Molecular pathways · Phytochemicals · Curcumin · Resveratrol · Quercetin · Isothiocyanates · Capsaicin · Tea polyphenols · Clinical outcomes

Abbreviations

ATM/Chk1	Ataxia-telangiectasia mutated/checkpoint kinase 1
ASK1	Apoptosis signal-regulating kinase 1
BITC	Benzyl isothiocyanate
Blc2	B-cell lymphoma 2
CCND1	Cyclin D1
COX-2	Cyclooxygenase-2
CXCR4	C-X-C motif chemokine receptor 4
DNMTs	DNA methyltransferases
ERK	Extracellular signal-regulated kinase
FAK	Focal adhesion kinase
FOXO	Forkhead box O
Gli1	Glioma-associated oncogene homolog 1
HDACs	Histone deacetylases
HATs	Histone acetyltransferases
HIF-1α	Hypoxia-inducible factor-1α
HSP	Heat-shock protein
ICAM-1	Intercellular adhesion molecule-1
IL-8	Interleukin-8
JAK2	Janus kinase 2
MAPK	Mitogen-activated protein kinase
MEK	MAPK/ERK kinase
MMP-9	Matrix metallopeptidase 9
MKK	MAP kinase kinase
NF-κB	Nuclear factor κB
PGE2	Prostaglandin E_2
PI3K/AKT	Phosphoinositide 3 kinase/AKT
Res-AuNPs	Resveratrol-conjugated gold nanoparticles
Src Rous	Sarcoma oncogene cellular homolog
STAT3	Signal transducer activator transcription 3
VEGF	Vascular endothelial growth factor
WT1	Wilms tumor-suppressor gene-1
XIAP	Inhibitor of apoptosis, X-linked

1 Introduction/Background

In 2020, it is expected that in the United States there will be approximately 57,600 new cases of pancreatic cancer and about 47,050 related deaths [1, 2]. The understanding of pancreatic cancer (PC) carcinogenesis will help us identify better targets for more effective therapies. Previous studies have suggested that there is an association between the development of PC and type 2 diabetes and obesity influenced by a complex interaction of genetic background and environmental factors. It has been established that smoking has the strongest environmental influence on this disease.

In a study conducted by Jones et al., it was found that PC was associated with 63 core genetic mutations in 12 common pathways [3]. Pancreatic cancer originates from the precursor lesions called pancreatic intraepithelial neoplasias (PanINs), as a consequence of the sequential accumulation of mutations in key oncogenes and tumor-suppressor genes. PC carcinogenesis stems from four major molecular mutations involving TP53, SMAD4, KRAS, and CDKN2A. Other associated pathways include activation of RTKs, PI3K/AKT, EGFR, and STAT3 and deactivation of tumor-suppressor protein pathways, namely p16INK4/Rb.

The treatment options of pancreatic malignancy depend on the stage at diagnosis. Surgery is an option for early stages and may improve the 5-year survival rate. Adjuvant therapy which includes chemotherapy and radiotherapy is commonly used after surgical resection. The following chemo-agents are used for the management of pancreatic cancer: gemcitabine, 5-fluorouracil (5-FU), oxaliplatin, cisplatin, docetaxel, paclitaxel, capecitabine, and irinotecan including liposomal form. Notably, gemcitabine and 5-FU have been the standard of care for the treatment of PC. Over the recent years, there has been minimal progress in the development of novel treatments for metastatic PC.

Postsurgical relapse and emergence of the intrinsic resistance to chemotherapy represent barriers to the success of available treatments. Due to high mortality rate associated with PC, the research for newer management strategies is a high priority. Phytochemicals are a new and appealing treatment strategy for PC. Multiple epidemiological studies published in the peer-reviewed literature over the past few decades, although with severe limitations, have shown a strong association between fruit and vegetable consumption and decreased incidence of pancreatic cancer [4].

Phytochemicals are derived from natural plants and target multiple molecular pathways involved in PC oncogenesis. They alter epigenomic compounds, cell signaling pathways, and tumor-suppressing miRNAs. These natural bioactive products can reduce and scavenge free radicals as well as considerably sensitize neoplastic cells to chemotherapy, and as a result of that potentiate the chemo-drugs [5]. It has been shown that the advantages of phytochemicals are increased cost-effectiveness and safety profiles.

This chapter reviews potential antineoplastic effects of various phytochemicals and emphasizes the need for better designed clinical studies to further characterize

Table 11.1 Natural sources, chemical structures, and potential anticarcinogenic effects (targets) of various phytochemicals

Phytochemicals	Natural source	Chemical structure	Signaling pathways	Targets
Isothiocyanates	Cruciferous vegetable (watercress, cabbage, cauliflower, mustard, and horseradish) 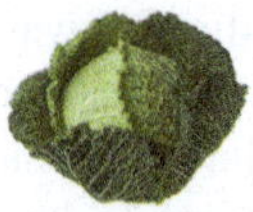 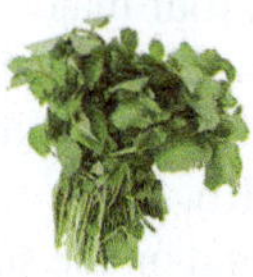	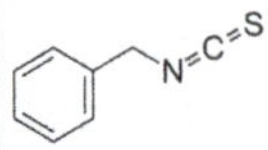	AKT, STAT3, HDAC, NFkB [82–84]	• Inactivation of NF-kappaB/p65 could be the underlying mechanism of BITC-induced apoptosis via inhibition of HDAC1/HDAC3 [82] • Reduced levels of activated and total STAT-3 protein [83] • Neovascularization through suppression of STAT-3 as well as STAT-3-induced HIF-1α and VEGF [86] • Downregulates the activation of AKT • Inhibition of FOXO phosphorylation [84] • ROS generation, G2/M cell cycle arrest, and apoptosis [89]
Curcumin	*Curcuma longa* (turmeric) 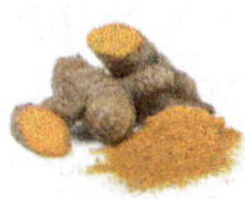 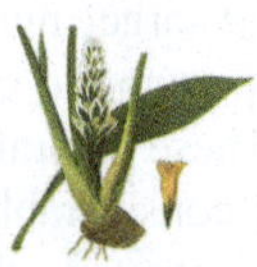	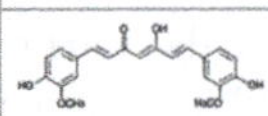	NFkB, STAT3, Notch-1, SP1, WT1, COX-II, ATM/Chk1, PI3K/Akt [66–73]	• Inhibits NF-kB and its downstream effectors COX-2, PGE2, and IL-8 [68] • G2/M cell cycle arrest and apoptosis [73] • Downregulates the expression of p50, p65, and specificity proteins (Sp1, Sp3, and Sp4) [67] • Inhibited STAT3 signaling in pancreatic cancer [66] • Effect on epigenetic modulators:

(continued)

Table 11.1 (continued)

Phytochemicals	Natural source	Chemical structure	Signaling pathways	Targets
				Histone deacetylases (HDACs) and acetyltransferases (HATs), DNA methyltransferases (DNMTs) [79–81]
Capsaicin	Chili peppers 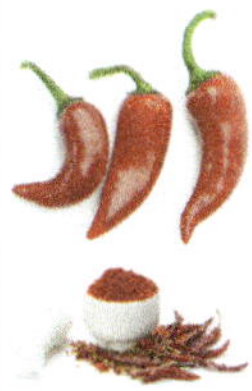	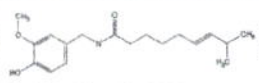 8-Methyl-*N*-vanillyl-6-nonenamide	Mitochondrial complex I and complex III activity ASK1, MKK4/MKK7-c-Jun NH2-terminal kinase (JNK)- and MKK3/MKK6-p-38 MAPK-signaling cascade	• Apoptosis in pancreatic cancer cells via ROS generation and mitochondrial disruption [43] • Disturbs the cellular redox homeostasis via depletion of GSH level and inhibition of superoxide dismutase, catalase, and glutathione peroxidase [44] • Reduces Trx expression and dissociates Trx-ASK1 complex resulting in the activation of ASK leading to apoptosis [47]
Green tea	*Camellia sinensis* var. sinensis 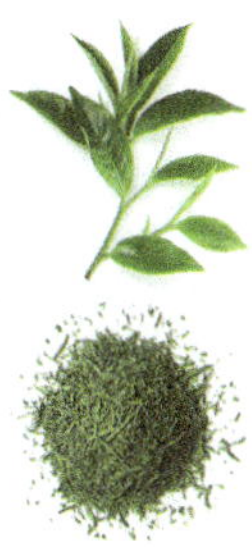	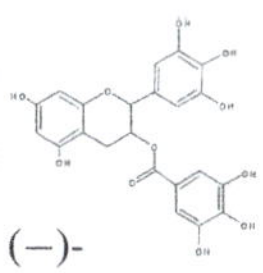 (−)-Epigallocatechin-3-gallate (EGCG) (−)-Epigallocatechin (EGC) (−)-Epicatechin-3-gallate (ECG) (−)-Epicatechin (EC)	HSP90, FAK, and STAT3	• Inhibits the expression of the Hsp90, Hsp75, and Hsp27 [50] • Induced apoptosis through caspase-3 and caspase-9 activation; induced proapoptotic Bax, Bak, and Bcl-Xs; and inhibited antiapoptotic Bcl-2 and Bcl-XL [55]. • Decreases the expression of the K-ras gene [56] • Inhibition of angiogenesis (vWF, VEGF, and

(continued)

Table 11.1 (continued)

Phytochemicals	Natural source	Chemical structure	Signaling pathways	Targets
				CD31) and metastasis (MMP-2, -7, -9, and -12) [57] • Inhibits phosphorylations of both FAK and IGF-1R [61] • Inhibits the STAT3 signaling pathway [62]
Resveratrol	Red grapes, peanuts, berries, and pines 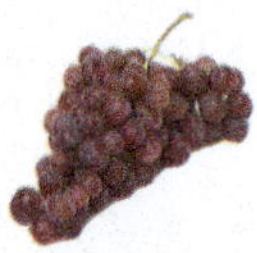 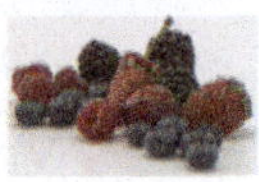 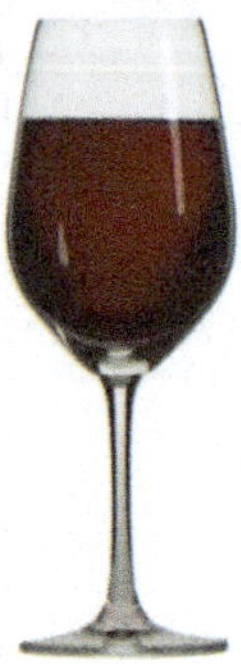	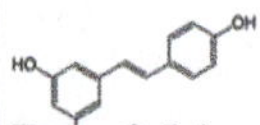 Trans-3,5,4-'-trihydroxy-trans-stilbene 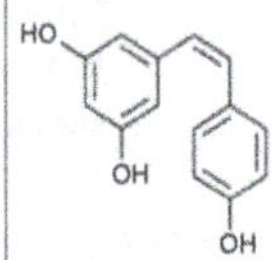 *cis*-resveratrol	Hedgehog, Src, STAT3, FOXO, leukotriene A4 hydrolase, and macrophage inhibitory cytokine-1	• Induces apoptosis in pancreatic cancer cells by targeting hedgehog pathway by decreasing the expression of Blc2, CCND1, Gli1, and Ptc1 [32] • Inhibits Src tyrosine kinase activity, thereby inhibiting the constitutive activation of STAT3 [33] • Inhibits phosphorylation of FOXOs through the inhibition of PI3K/AKT and MEK/ERK signaling [34] • Inhibits LTB4 production and expression of the LTB4 receptor 1 (BLT1) [37] • Downregulation of constitutive NF-κB activation and NF-κB-regulated gene products [39]
Soy isoflavone (genistein)	Lupin, fava beans, soybeans, kudzu 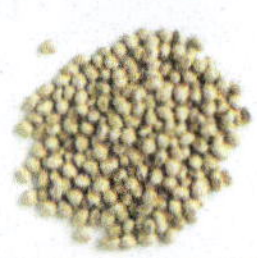	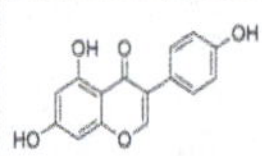	NF-kB	• Inhibits an oncogenic microRNA, miR-27a, inducing apoptosis [92]

(continued)

Table 11.1 (continued)

Phytochemicals	Natural source	Chemical structure	Signaling pathways	Targets
Quercetin	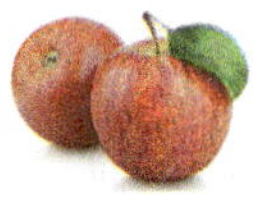 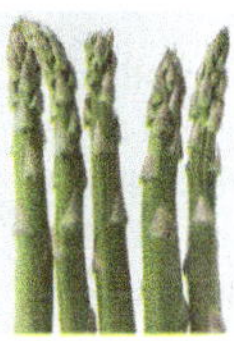	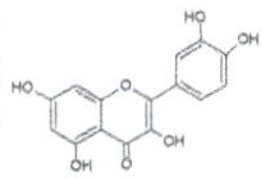	Sonic hedgehog pathway proteins β-Catenin	• Decreases aldehyde dehydrogenase-1 activity and inhibits epithelial-mesenchymal transition [93] • Upregulation of miR-let7-a and inhibition of K-ras with combination of quercetin, sulforaphane, and catechins [95]

the potential of these agents in targeting clinical outcomes of pancreatic malignancy (Tables 11.1, 11.2, 11.3, 11.4, 11.5, 11.6, and 11.7).

2 Gene Mutations and Molecular Pathways Associated with the PC Pathogenesis

KRAS, p53, CDKN2A, and SMAD4 are the most frequently mutated genes associated with PC oncogenesis. Out of these, KRAS is the most associated gene and is mutated in more than 95% of pancreatic cancers [6]. Below we describe these genes with better scope and perspectives of the disease.

2.1 KRAS

KRAS is an oncogene, based on chromosome 12, and encodes a GTPase molecule. Activating KRAS mutations impair the GTPase activity, which leads to a cascade of events [7]. KRAS mediates several different molecular pathways and participates in every step of tumorigenesis, i.e., from initiation to cellular proliferation, and metabolism to drug resistance patterns [8]. Several different downstream molecular pathways are also involved in tumorigenesis as a result of KRAS activation, including Raf/mitogen-activated protein kinase (MAPK), phosphoinositide 3-kinase (PI3K)/AKT/mammalian target of rapamycin (mTOR) signaling pathway, and nuclear

Table 11.2 Selective curcumin in vitro studies in pancreatic cancer

Plant/ phytochemical component	Animal/human cell line	Anticancer/chemoprevention mechanism	Reference
Curcumin	PANC-1 pancreatic cancer cell line	Induction of quinone oxidoreductase 1 (NQO1) and promoting its interaction with P53, increasing P53 stability	Patiño-Morales et al., 2019 [96]
L48H37 (curcumin analog)	Primary (PANC-1 and MIA PaCa-2), metastatic (SW1990 and ASPC-1)	L48H37 inhibits proliferation by inducing cell cycle arrest and promotes apoptosis, L48H37 alters MMP, increases ROS production, induces cell cycle arrest, and activates the ER stress pathway	Li et al., 2019 [97]
Curcumin and garcinol	PaCa cells (BxPC-3 and Panc-1)	Dose-dependent reduction in cell viability and increase in apoptosis were observed in both cell lines. High level of synergism with a potency (Dm) of the combination of garcinol and curcumin of two- to tenfold that of the individual agents	Parasramka et al., 2012 [98]
Curcumin	PANC-1 pancreatic cancer cell line	Curcumin induces the apoptosis of PANC-1 cells by activating the miR-340/ XIAP signaling pathway causing decreased XIAP expression in a dose-dependent manner	Yang et al., 2017 [99]
Curcumin	Five human pancreatic cancer cell lines (BxPC-3, Capan-1, Capan-2, ASPC-1, and HS766-T)	Inhibition of activation of nuclear factor-kB transcription factor, suppression of IkB kinase activity, reduction in interleukin-8, cyclooxygenase, and PGE-2; induction of apoptosis	Li et al., 2004 [68]
Curcumin	BxPC-3 and AsPC-1 pancreatic cancer cell lines	Suppressed cell growth and invasion, and induced cell apoptosis, increased miR-7 expression, and decreased SET8 expression	Ma et al., 2014 [100]
Curcumin and liposomal curcumin	BxPC-3 human pancreatic cancer cell line	Alters miRNA expression in human pancreatic cells, upregulating miRNA-22 and downregulating miRNA-199a	Sun et al., 2008 [101]

(continued)

Table 11.2 (continued)

Plant/ phytochemical component	Animal/human cell line	Anticancer/chemoprevention mechanism	Reference
Curcumin	BxPC-3 human pancreatic cancer cell line	Inhibits high glucose and EGF-induced proliferation in pancreatic cancer cells; by downregulating high glucose-induced activation of EGF/ERK and EGF/Akt pathways, and inhibition of EGF-induced invasive ability of pancreatic cancer cells, EGF-induced wound closure of pancreatic cancer cells and EGF-modulated expression of metastatic related factors	Li et al., 2019 [102]
Curcumin	Panc-1 human pancreatic carcinoma cell lines	Inhibits cell viability and cell proliferation, induces apoptosis by increased activation of caspase-9 and caspase-3, induces the expression of FOXO1 through the PI3K/Akt pathway, causes cell cycle arrest by increasing the expression levels of p21/WAF1/CIP1 and p27/KIP1, and decreases the expression of cyclin D1	Zhao et al., 2015 [70]
Curcumin	BxPC-3, MIA PaCa-2, Panc-1, MPanc-96	Potentiates the apoptotic effects of gemcitabine, and inhibits constitutive NF-κB activation	Kunnumakkara et al., 2007 [74]
Curcumin	MiaPaCa-2	Inhibits proliferation, enhances apoptosis, and downregulates NF-kB	Bimonte et al., 2013 [103]
Curcumin	BxPC-3	Antiproliferative effect, activation of ATM/Chk1, G2/M cell cycle arrest, causes DNA damage, and induces apoptosis, modulates expression of G2/M cell cycle regulatory proteins	Sahu et al., 2009 [73]
Curcumin	Panc28 cell line (gemcitabine resistant), L3.6pL cells (gemcitabine nonresistant)	Inhibits pancreatic cancer cell proliferation, inhibits constitutive NF-κB, decreases Sp transcription factors (Sp-1, Sp-3, Sp-4) and Sp-dependent responses (decreased expression of multiple Sp-dependent proteins including VEGF, VEGFR1, cyclin D1, and survivin)	Jutooru et al., 2010 [67]

(continued)

Table 11.2 (continued)

Plant/ phytochemical component	Animal/human cell line	Anticancer/chemoprevention mechanism	Reference
Curcumin	PANC-1 cells	Decreases IAP protein and mRNA expression, reduces cell viability, and induces morphological changes characteristic of cell death	Osterman et al., 2015 [104]
Curcumin + Tolfenamic acid (TA)	L3.6pl and MIA PaCa-2 cells	Synergistic effect on cell growth inhibition; inhibits Sp1, Sp3, and survivin expression; induces apoptosis; increases ROS level; suppresses NF-kB translocation to nucleus	Basha et al., 2016 [71]
Curcumin	PANC-1	Inhibits TGF-β1-stimulated PANC-1 cell proliferation, induces apoptosis, reverses EMT possibly through inhibition of the Shh-GLI1 signaling pathway, decreases expression of Shh, GLI1 and vimentin, increases expression of E-cadherin, decreases cell invasion, inhibits the invasion and migration of TGF-β1-stimulated PANC-1 cells	Sun et al., 2013 [105]
CDF (synthetic curcumin analogue)	MiaPaCa-2 and Panc-1 cells	Downregulates the expression of miR-221 and consequently upregulates the expression of PTEN, p27 (kip1), p57 (kip2), and PUMA, leading to the inhibition of cell proliferation and migration	Sarkar et al., 2013 [106]
Curcumin	AsPC-1, MiaPaCa-2, Panc-1, BxPC-3 human, and Pan02 mouse pancreatic cancer cells	Inhibits pancreatic cancer cell growth, induces G2-M cell cycle arrest inducing mitotic catastrophe, inhibits COX-2 and VEGF expression and translation, and induces CUGBP2 and TIA-1	Subramaniam et al., 2011 [107]
Curcumin	PANC-1	Inhibition of cellular proliferation, downregulation of expression of WT1 on mRNA and protein level	Glienke et al., 2010 [69]

(continued)

Table 11.2 (continued)

Plant/ phytochemical component	Animal/human cell line	Anticancer/chemoprevention mechanism	Reference
Curcumin	PANC-1, AsCP	Inhibits cell proliferation, inhibits constitutive STAT3 phosphorylation, and downregulates survivin/ BIRC5 gene expression	Glienke et al., 2010 [66]
Curcumin	Panc-1, BxPC-3, and MIA PaCa-2	Inhibits both constitutive and RT-induced NF-κB, inhibits FIR/SDR-induced gene, confers RT-inhibited cell viability/survival, activates caspase-3/7 activity, and subsequent cell death	Veeraraghava et al., 2011 [108]
Difluorinated curcumin (CDF)	AsPC-1 and MiaPaCa-2	Inhibits cell survival; inhibits the expression of MMP-9, EZH2, Shh, and cleaved Notch-1 in AsPC-1 and MiaPaCa-2 cell; inhibits the expression of EpCAM in AsPC-1 cells; inhibits the expression of ABCG2 and Hes-1 in MiaPaCa-2 cells	Bao et al., 2012 [109]
Liposomal curcumin	Human MiaPaCa	Antiproliferative effects	Ranjan et al., 2013 [110]
Curcumin	Gemcitabine-resistant PDAC cell lines	Resensitization of chemoresistant PDAC cells through the inhibition of the PRC2-PVT1-c-Myc axis; curcumin sensitized chemoresistant cancer cells by inhibiting the expression of the PRC2 subunit EZH2 and its related lncRNA PVT1	Yoshida et al., 2017 [111]

factor kappa B (NF-κB) signaling cascades. These cascades are the sites of action for various phytochemicals, which act to inhibit them that can potentially lead to the development of treatment options for PDAC [9, 10].

Table 11.3 Selective curcumin in vivo studies in pancreatic cancer

Plant/ phytochemical component(s)	Animal test model	Anticancer/chemoprevention mechanism(s)	Reference
L48H37 (curcumin analog)	Male BALB/c nude mice injected with control and KMT2D knockdown PDAC cells	Tumor weight and volume were significantly decreased in the KMT2D knockout group compared to the CTRL group; KMT2D depletion inhibited tumor growth synergistically with L48H37	Li et al., 2019 [97]
Curcumin	Male athymic *nu/nu* mice	Potentiates the antitumor, antiproliferative, and antiangiogenic effects of gemcitabine; inhibits NF-κB activation; potentiates the effect of gemcitabine in downregulating the expression of NF-κB-regulated gene products COX-2, ICAM, MMP, VEGF, cyclin-D, c-myc, survivin, Bcl-2, Bcl-xL, and IAP-1; decreases the expression of procaspase-3 and procaspase-9	Kunnumakkara et al., 2007 [74]
Curcumin	Female upstream to Foxn1 mice injected by MIA PaCa-2-RFP cells	Inhibits the tumor growth, inhibits NF-*κ*B activation, and downregulates NF-*κ*B-regulated gene products	Bimonte et al., 2013 [103]
Curcumin	Male athymic nude mice (injected with MiaPaCa)	Inhibits the growth of tumor xenografts, lowers CD31 staining, and obliterates the tumor vessels suggesting decreased angiogenesis	Subramaniam et al., 2011 [107]
Curcumin	Xenograft mouse model (L36pL cells)	Tumor growth and tumor weight inhibition	Jutooru et al., 2010 [67]
Difluorinated curcumin (CDF)	Female CB17 severe combined immunodeficient (SCID) mice (MIA PaCa-2 cells)	Tumor growth inhibition, reduced expression of EZH2	Bao et al., 2012 [109]
Liposomal curcumin	Female athymic *nu/nu* mice	Inhibits pancreatic tumor xenograft growth	Ranjan et al., 2013 [110]
Curcumin metformin	Nonobese diabetic/severe combined immunodeficiency disease (NOD/SCID) mice	Inhibition of cell growth of Panc1 adherent cells and sphere cells; Panc1 sphere cells were more sensitive to the two compounds than Panc1 adherent cells	Ning et al., 2016 [112]

Table 11.4 Selective curcumin clinical trials in pancreatic cancer

Plant/ phytochemical component(s)	Clinical trial type/ phase	N	Population study/cancer type	Results	Reference
Curcumin	Phase I	25	5 High-risk conditions/ premalignant	Not toxic to humans up to 8000 mg/day when taken by mouth for 3 months	Cheng et al., 2001 [113]
"C3" curcuminoid capsules	Phase I	15	Colon and rectal cancers	First report of the systemic parameters of pharmacokinetics and activity of curcumin that are likely to be of value in phase II chemoprevention/anticancer trials; consumption of 3.6 g of curcumin daily is linked with inhibition of PGE_2 induction in blood; dose-limiting toxicity was not observed	Sharma et al., 2004 [114]
Curcumin	Phase II	25	Pancreatic cancer	Poor oral bioavailability; two patients showed clinical biological activity (one showed ongoing stable disease for >18 months and the other showed brief but marked tumor regression) (73%); no toxicities were observed; expression of NF-kappaB, cyclooxygenase-2, and phosphorylated STAT3 was downregulated in peripheral blood mononuclear cells	Dhillon et al., 2008 [115]
Curcumin	Phase I/II	21	Pancreatic cancer	No dose-limiting toxicities observed in the phase I study; median survival time was 161 days and 1-year survival rate was 19%; combination therapy using 8 g oral curcumin daily with gemcitabine-based chemotherapy was safe and feasible in patients with pancreatic cancer	Kanai et al., 2011 [116]
Curcumin	Phase II	17	Pancreatic cancer	Low compliance at a dose of 8000 mg/day (dose reduced to 4000 mg/day) due to GI side effects, when taken together with systemic gemcitabine; 1 of 11 evaluable patients (9%) had partial response, 4 (36%) had stable disease, and 6 (55%) had tumor progression	Epelbaum et al., 2010 [117]

Table 11.5 Selective in vitro studies of resveratrol in pancreatic cancer

Parent compound/ phytochemical constituents	Animal/human cell line	Anticancer/chemoprevention mechanism(s)	Reference
Resveratrol	CD133+ and CD133− PANC-1 cells	Decreased N-cadherin and TNF-α immunoreactivities	Hoca et al. (2019) [118]
Resveratrol	PANC-1, MIA PaCa-2, HS766T, and AsPC-1 cell	Antiproliferative effects, induces apoptosis through activation of caspase-3 (PANC-1 and MIA PaCa-2 most sensitive), induced cell cycle arrest by inhibiting the FOXO transcription factors by shRNA (inhibited the expression of cyclin D1 and induced the expression of cell cycle inhibitors (p21/CIP1 and p27/KIP1) and Bim), inhibits cell proliferation by regulating PI3K/AKT pathway; inhibits AKT kinase activity	Roy et al. (2011) [34]
Resveratrol	Hamster (HPD1NR and HPD2NR) and human (AsPC1 and BxPC3) pancreatic cancer cell lines	Suppressed cell proliferation in human and hamster pancreatic cancer cells by inhibiting the G1 phase of the cell cycle with cyclin D1 downregulation and inactivation of AKT-GSK3β and ERK1/2 signaling	Kato et al. (2015) [119]
Resveratrol	Panc-1, Mia paca-2, human pancreatic cell lines	Inhibits cell proliferation and induces apoptosis in pancreatic cancer cells, suppresses the level of NAF-1 and enhances the expression of Nrf2 by inducing the accumulation of ROS; enhances the sensitivity of pancreatic cancer cells to gemcitabine through inhibition of NAF-1	Cheng et al. (2018) [120]
Resveratrol	PANC-1 and AsPC-1 human pancreatic cell lines	Inhibition of cell proliferation and induced apoptosis in pancreatic cancer cell lines; increases the fraction of sub-G0/G1-phase cells	Ding et al. (2002) [121]
Triacetyl resveratrol	AsPC1 and PANC1 human pancreatic cell line	Inhibited colony formation and induced apoptosis through caspase-3 activation and through suppression of the Sonic hedgehog (Shh) pathway,	Fu et al. (2019) [122]

(continued)

Table 11.5 (continued)

Parent compound/ phytochemical constituents	Animal/human cell line	Anticancer/chemoprevention mechanism(s)	Reference
		and through the modulation of cyclin D1 and Bcl2 expression, also inhibited epithelial mesenchymal transition (EMT) by upregulating the expression of E-cadherin and suppressing the expression of N-cadherin and transcription factors, snail, slug, and Zeb1, also inhibited Zeb1 3'UTR luciferase activity through the upregulation of microRNA (miR)200 family members	

2.2 *TP53*

TP53 gene encodes p53 protein and is found on chromosome 17 [6]. p53 is a tumor-suppressor gene which is involved in maintaining a check-and-balance on cellular proliferation by initiating cellular arrest, apoptosis, and cell death. Normally, cellular stress or DNA damage leads to higher p53 activity, which results in apoptosis of the impaired cells, thereby preventing the development of neoplasm. Loss-of-function mutations in p53 lead to uncontrolled cellular proliferation, ultimately leading to cancer formation [11].

2.3 *CDKN2A*

CDKN2A is located on chromosome 9. Two tumor-suppressor proteins p14 and p16 are encoded by this gene [6]. Loss-of-function mutation of this gene leads to unchecked cellular growth and proliferation [11]. Like p53, p16 is also a tumor-suppressor gene and works at the G1/S checkpoint in cell cycle where it leads to cell cycle arrest via the pRb-E2F pathway [12].

2.4 *SMAD4*

SMAD4 gene is found on chromosome 18 and is inactivated in 55% of PC. SMAD4 has a significant role in transforming growth factor-β (TGF-β)-mediated signaling pathway [6]. TGF-β is responsible for controlling many crucial cellular pathways

Table 11.6 Selective in vivo studies of resveratrol in pancreatic cancer

Parent compound/ phytochemical constituents	Animal species/tumor model inhibited	Molecular mechanism(s)/target (s)	Reference
Resveratrol	Syrian hamsters/N-nitrosobis (2-oxopropyl) amine (BOP)	No effect/tumor unchanged	Kuroiwa et al. (2006) [123]
Resveratrol	Athymic nude mice/MIA PaCa-2 cells	Inhibition of cancer cell growth/proliferation, synergistic apoptosis when combined with gemcitabine; inhibition of NF-κB activation in a dose-dependent manner, downregulates the NF-κB-regulated gene products, suppressed the constitutive expression of antiapoptotic (Bcl-2, Bcl-xL), proliferative (COX-2, cyclin D1), metastatic (MMP-9), and angiogenic (VEGF) protein expression in a dose-dependent manner, induced the cleavage of PARP	Harikumar et al. (2010) [39]
Resveratrol	Athymic nude mice/human MIA PaCa-2 cells	Inhibits proliferation and anchorage-independent cell growth by inhibiting LTA_4H (leukotriene A4 hydrolase) activity leading to inhibition of tumor formation in xenograft mouse models for pancreatic cancer	Oi et al. (2010) [37]
Resveratrol	Balb C nude mice/human PANC-1	Suppression of PANC1 tumor growth associated with inhibition of ERK, PI3K, AKT, FOXO1, and FOXO3a phosphorylation, and induction of apoptosis in tumor cells	Roy et al. (2011) [34]
Resveratrol	$Kras^{G12}D$ mice/spontaneous tumors	Resveratrol inhibits the growth and development of pancreatic cancer in Kras(G12D) mice. It inhibits the self-renewal capacity of pancreatic CSCs derived from human primary tumors and Kras(G12D) mice; induces apoptosis by activating caspase-3/7 and inhibiting the expression of Bcl-2 and XIAP in human CSCs. Resveratrol inhibits pluripotency-	Shankar et al. (2011) [124]

(continued)

Table 11.6 (continued)

Parent compound/ phytochemical constituents	Animal species/tumor model inhibited	Molecular mechanism(s)/target (s)	Reference
		maintaining factors (Nanog, Sox-2, c-Myc, and Oct-4) and drug resistance gene ABCG2 in CSCs. Inhibition of Nanog by shRNA enhances the inhibitory effects of resveratrol on self-renewal capacity of CSCs; inhibits CSC migration and invasion and markers of epithelial-mesenchymal transition (Zeb-1, slug, and snail)	
Resveratrol	*N*-Nitrosobis (2-oxopropyl) amine (BOP)-treated Syrian golden hamster model	Inhibits progression of pancreatic tumorigenesis (Ki-67 labeling index in ductal dysplasia was significantly decreased)	Kato et al. (2015) [119]

including cellular survival and differentiation and has inhibitory effects on cellular growth. Inactivation of TGF-β pathway leads to unchecked cellular proliferation and is one of the key mechanisms of cancer formation [13, 14].

3 Pathways

It is imperative to understand signaling pathways to better recognize the anticancer therapeutic agents. Below we describe some of the key pathways that are involved in the PDAC disease process.

3.1 Phosphoinositide 3-Kinase (PI3K)/AKT/Mammalian Target of Rapamycin (mTOR) Signaling Pathway

PI3K pathway involves a series of different protein kinases that activate in a sequential manner and are associated with advanced stages of pancreatic tumor. When PI3K is activated, it triggers AKT, which in turn activates mammalian target of rapamycin (mTOR). Oncogenic mutations of KRAS induce activation of this pathway, which results in cellular proliferation and is known to correspond with a relatively bad outcome. *PTEN* is a tumor-suppressor gene that regulates this pathway and loss of *PTEN* can lead to its unchecked activation [15, 16].

Table 11.7 Selective resveratrol clinical trials

Plant/ phytochemical component	Clinical trial type/phase	N	Population study/cancer type	Results	Reference
Plant-derived resveratrol formulation and resveratrol-containing freeze-dried grape powder (GP)	Phase 1 pilot clinical trial	8	Colon cancer	Resveratrol/GP had no effect on the Wnt pathway in colon cancer but significantly ($p < 0.03$) inhibited the Wnt target gene expression in normal colonic mucosa	Nguyen et al., 2009 [125]
SRT501 (micronized resveratrol)	Phase I randomized, double-blind pilot study	6	Colorectal cancer and hepatic metastases scheduled to undergo hepatectomy	SRT501 increases the cleavage of caspase-3 in malignant hepatic tissue	Howells et al., 2011 [126]
Resveratrol	Clinical trial, noncontrolled	20	Colorectal cancer	Decreases expression of Ki-67	Patel et al., 2010 [127]
Trans-resveratrol	Randomized, double-blind, placebo-controlled trial	39	Adult women with increased risk for breast cancer	Reduces the methylation of *RASSF-1α*	Zhu et al., 2012 [128]
SRT501 (micronized resveratrol) with or without bortezomib	Phase 2 clinical trial	24	Relapsed/ refractory multiple myeloma	Unacceptable safety profile and minimal efficacy in patients with relapsed/refractory multiple myeloma	Popat et al., 2002 [129]
Resveratrol (uncoated immediate-release tablets)	Phase 1 clinical trial	40 subjects	Healthy adults	Pharmacokinetic and metabolite profile; resveratrol had low bioavailability; but sulfate and glucuronide metabolites were abundant which have unknown efficacy; resveratrol did not cause any serious side effects	Boocock et al., 2007 [130]

(continued)

Table 11.7 (continued)

Plant/ phytochemical component	Clinical trial type/phase	N	Population study/cancer type	Results	Reference
Trans-resveratrol	Phase 1 clinical trial	9	Healthy adults	Pharmacokinetic and metabolite profile. Resveratrol metabolites have high affinity for protein binding (up to 50% protein bound)	Burkon et al., 2008 [131]
Trans-resveratrol	Phase 1 clinical trial	24	Healthy adults	Pharmacokinetic and metabolite profile. Resveratrol was well tolerated by young and elderly subjects	Nunes et al., 2013 [132]
Resveratrol	Phase 1 clinical trial	42	Healthy adults	Resveratrol modulates enzyme systems involved in carcinogen activation and detoxification; resveratrol was well tolerated	Chow et al., 2017 [133]
Resveratrol	Phase 1 clinical trial	40	Healthy adults	Safety profile, pharmacokinetics/ metabolite profile; resveratrol caused a reduction in IGF-1 and IGFBP-3 plasma levels. 2.5 and 5.0 g caused mild-to-moderate gastrointestinal symptoms	Brown et al., 2010 [134]

3.2 *Wnt/β-Catenin Signaling*

Wnt binding to its ligand receptor inhibits the breakdown of β-catenin intracellular protein, which is then transferred into the cell nucleus and interacts with transcription factors belonging to TCF/LEF (T-cell factor/lymphoid enhancer factor) family. This complex Wnt pathway affects cancer stem cells (CSCs), thus leading to tumorigenesis. Frizzled and LRP5/6 receptors play a major role in the Wnt signaling pathway and they mediate their effects through two cytoplasmic proteins, dishevelled (DVL) and axin [17–19].

3.3 *Janus Kinase/Signal Transducer and Transcription*

Constitutive activation of JAK/STAT pathway is involved in the pathogenesis of multiple neoplasms, including PC. JAK is a member of tyrosine kinase family, which interacts with transcription factors called STAT inside the nucleus, thus affecting many aspects of tumorigenesis, including cellular growth, survival, and apoptosis [20, 21].

3.4 *Raf/Mitogen-Activated Protein Kinase (MAPK)*

MAPK is another pathway that is turned on by mutations in KRAS. Similar to other pathways, persistent activation of MAPK plays vital roles in pancreatic cancer development. This cascade consists of many serine/threonine kinases that are activated by extracellular molecules like growth factors and hormones, including RAS, ERK (extracellular signal-regulated kinase), MEK, and RAF [22, 23].

3.5 *Nuclear Factor Kappa-B (NF-κB) Signaling Cascade*

NF-κB is persistently active in PC, mainly as a consequence of the KRAS mutation. This signaling cascade involves overexpression of interleukin-1α (IL-1α), leading to intranuclear translocation of NF-κB, which promotes inflammatory pathways involved in chronic pancreatitis, ultimately leading to the initiation and progression of pancreatic cancer [24, 25].

3.6 *ATM*

Ataxia telangiectasia-mutated (*ATM*) gene is another tumor-suppressor gene, which codes for the ATM protein that is involved in maintaining a balance between cellular activation and repair of the damaged cells. Alterations in this gene are also involved in many types of malignancies, including PC [26].

3.7 *Hedgehog*

Hedgehog signaling is a major pathway involved in the activation of pancreatic stem cells (Fig. 11.1). It includes three ligands for transmembrane proteins [Sonic hedgehog (Shh), Indian hedgehog (Ihh), and Desert hedgehog (Dhh)], two receptors

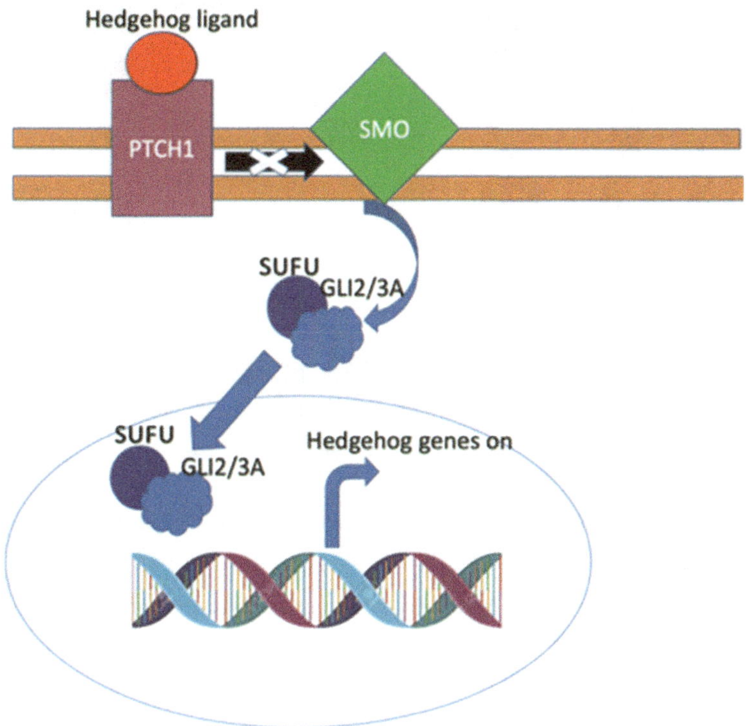

Fig. 11.1 The hedgehog pathway

(Ptch1 and Ptch2), a signal transducer Smoothened (Smo), and three transcription factors (Gli1, Gli2, and Gli3) which get upregulated and transferred into the cell nucleus, thus regulating downstream gene expressions [27, 28]. In the absence of ligand, Ptch1 suppresses the 7-(pass) transmembrane G-protein-coupled receptor (GPCR)-like protein Smoothened (SMO). Ligand binding eliminates this inhibition and allows the SMO to regulate a cytoplasmic complex containing suppressor of fused (SUFU) that alters the three glioma-associated (Gli) transcriptional regulators, which modulates target genes including Gli1, cyclin D1, Ptch1, Bcl-2, and c-Myc [29].

3.8 *Notch*

The Notch signaling pathway includes four NOTCH transmembrane receptors that are turned on when a Notch ligand binds to the designating receptor and goes

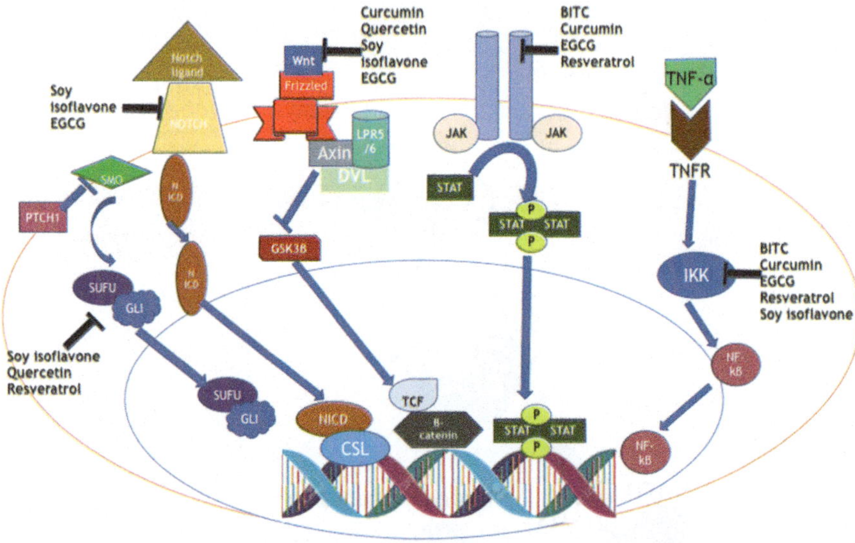

Fig. 11.2 Schematic representation of the mechanisms of actions of different phytochemicals

through multiple cleavages by various enzymes, thus mediating its effects by modulating target genes [30].

4 Role of Phytochemicals in Pancreatic Cancer

Figure 11.2 summarizes the schematic representation of the mechanisms of actions of different phytochemicals. Table 11.1 demonstrates natural sources and chemical structures and briefly summarizes targets of phytochemicals mentioned below.

4.1 Resveratrol

Resveratrol is a naturally occurring polyphenol, found in red wine, grape skin, peanuts, and berries, which possess anti-inflammatory and antioxidant properties [31]. Multiple studies have demonstrated the beneficial effects of resveratrol on many biological processes, including PC chemoprevention. This bioactive compound interferes with various stages of tumor initiation and proliferation and has been found to aim different signaling pathways in pancreatic malignancy such as hedgehog, STAT3, Src, macrophage inhibitory cytokine-1 (MAC-1), leukotriene A4 hydrolase (LTA4H), and FOXO. Specifically, resveratrol can induce apoptosis in PC cells by targeting the hedgehog pathway by decreasing the expression of pathway members such as Blc2, CCND1, Gli1, and Ptc1 [32]. Kotha et al. [33] established that resveratrol inhibits the constitutive activation of STAT3 in PC cells by suppressing the activity of Src tyrosine kinase. Resveratrol particularly targets PC cells that carry constitutively active *STAT3* oncogene and induces irreversible cell cycle arrest in these cells [33].

FOXO transcription factors play an important role in resveratrol-mediated PC growth inhibition. Resveratrol inhibits phosphorylation of FOXOs via inhibition of PI3K/AKT and MEK/ERK signaling, thus enhancing their translocation to the nucleus, binding to DNA and transcriptional activities, which induces apoptosis via activation of caspase-3 leading to growth arrest by inducing p21/CIP1 and p27/KIP1 and inhibiting cyclin D1, which are the downstream targets of FOXO [34].

The LTA4H is a bifunctional zinc metalloenzyme, which is overexpressed in pancreatic cancer [35]. It enhances the hydrolysis of the epoxide leukotriene A4 (LTA4) to leukotriene B4 (LTB4), which promotes cancer cell proliferation [36]. Oi et al. [37] showed that LTA4H is an important target for resveratrol-mediated anticancer effects. Their report strongly supports that resveratrol directly binds to LTA4H in vitro and inhibits proliferation and anchorage-independent growth of PC by suppressing LTB4 production and expression of the LTB4 receptor 1 (BLT1) [37].

Resveratrol showed insignificant toxicity to normal pancreatic cells [38]. Resveratrol also sensitizes pancreatic cancer cells to the antineoplastic effect of gemcitabine via downregulation of constitutive NF-κB activation and NF-κB-regulated gene products, which are the markers of proliferation, invasion, angiogenesis, and metastasis. Harikumar et al. [39] found that resveratrol significantly inhibits pancreatic tumor growth in an orthotopic model of human PC cells ($p < 0.001$) and that gemcitabine further enhanced this effect ($p < 0.001$). It suppressed the constitutive activation of NF-κB and expression of gene products responsible for proliferation (c-myc, cyclin-D1, COX-2), invasion (ICAM-1, MMP-9, CXCR4), angiogenesis (VEGF), and survival (Bcl-2, Bcl-xL, survivin, XIAP) [39].

In humans, the oral absorption of resveratrol is about 75% and occurs primarily by transepithelial diffusion. The oral bioavailability of resveratrol is considerably low (less than 1%) due to extensive metabolism in the intestine and liver resulting in decreased protective effects [40]. Therefore, efforts have been made to increase the bioavailability of resveratrol by synthesizing its derivatives. Various polymethoxylated resveratrol analogues exhibited stronger antiproliferative effects than resveratrol in tumor cell lines [41].

Thipe et al. [42] reported a novel green nanotechnology method to produce biocompatible resveratrol-conjugated gold nanoparticles (Res-AuNPs) to improve bioavailability. The investigators explored the in vitro stability of Res-AuNPs in pancreatic (PANC-1), breast (MDAMB-231), and prostate (PC-3) cancers. It has been shown that Res-AuNPs increase the bioavailability of resveratrol in vivo to optimize potential applications in cancer therapy [42]. Tables 11.5, 11.6, and 11.7 summarize selective in vitro studies, in vivo studies, and clinical trials of resveratrol in pancreatic cancer, available in the medical field nowadays.

4.2 Capsaicin

Capsaicin (8-methyl-*N*-vanillyl-6-nonenamide) is a phenolic compound found in chili peppers and is responsible for their burning and irritant effects. It has been demonstrated that capsaicin induces apoptosis in PC cells via the generation of reactive oxygen species (ROS) and mitochondrial disruption [43]. ROS are generated in cells mainly by mitochondrial electron transport chain complexes (ETC) and mediate apoptotic signaling pathway.

Pramanik et al. [44] demonstrated that capsaicin produces ROS (superoxide radical and hydrogen peroxide) by inhibiting mitochondrial complex I and complex III activity and through depletion of ATP levels in BxPC-3 and AsPC-1 human pancreatic cancer cell lines. Interestingly, capsaicin failed to induce apoptosis in normal pancreatic epithelial (HPDE-6) cells, which implies that capsaicin is selective towards malignant cells [44].

Cells maintain redox homeostasis through the balance between the generation of intracellular ROS and ROS-scavenging antioxidants. Under normal physiological circumstances, mitochondria carry adequate levels of antioxidants that prevent ROS production and oxidative injury. Reduced glutathione (GSH) is an intracellular antioxidant necessary to maintain intracellular redox balance. Capsaicin reduces the intracellular levels of GSH and suppresses superoxide dismutase, catalase, and glutathione peroxidase causing imbalanced redox homeostasis resulting in increased oxidative stress [44]. Capsaicin causes mitochondrial damage and induces apoptosis of pancreatic cells through mitochondrial ROS generation and depletion of intracellular antioxidants. However, normal pancreatic epithelial cells are resistant to these effects.

Apoptosis signal-regulating kinase 1 (ASK1), a member of the mitogen-activated protein kinase kinase kinase family, is activated primarily by ROS. Activated ASK1 activates both MKK4/MKK7-c-Jun NH2-terminal kinase (JNK)- and MKK3/MKK6-p-38 MAPK-signaling cascade [45]. ASK1 plays a major role in apoptosis, specifically via oxidative stress. Thioredoxin (Trx) is a cellular redox enzyme that directly inhibits ASK1. Trx overexpression has been found in several malignancies, including PC [46]. It has been shown that capsaicin suppresses Trx expression and causes dissociation of Trx-ASK1 complex leading to activation of ASK1 and downstream effectors resulting in apoptosis in tumor cells *in both* in vitro and in vivo *models* [47].

4.3 Green Tea

Green tea has been a famous beverage worldwide since ancient times. It is rich in catechin polyphenols such as epigallocatechin-3-gallate (EGCG), epicatechin (EC), and epicatechin-3-gallate (ECG), which have robust antioxidant activity and have been investigated in cancer chemoprevention [48]. Tea polyphenols directly inhibit tumor cell growth through apoptotic properties, inhibition of angiogenesis, and modulation of gene expression of heat-shock proteins. Among all catechins, EGCG received the most attention as an anticancer agent. Some of them target such molecules as STAT3, HSP90, and FAK that have been studied in PC.

HPAF-II is a well-differentiated human pancreatic ductal adenocarcinoma cell line which carries a TP53 mutation with unlimited replicative capability and a high metastatic potential [49]. Zhang et al. [50] treated HPAF-II cells with a green tea extract (GTE) and identified that it altered 32 protein expressions, which were involved in gene regulation, detoxification, metabolism, drug resistance, motility, and molecular chaperones of cancer cells [50].

Heat-shock proteins are molecular chaperones that are constitutively expressed in cells and control the normal folding, intracellular disposition, and proteolytic turnover of many of the main regulators of cell growth and survival. Hsp90 modulates the maturation of different oncogenic proteins to maintain proliferation, metastasis, and survival in pancreatic cancer [51]. Hsp75, the mitochondrial localized homologue tumor necrosis factor receptor-associated protein 1 (Trap1), is the member of the family of Hsp90 molecular chaperones whose role is to protect mitochondria from the effects of oxidative stress. Tumor mitochondria have increased expression of Trap1 compared to normal cells [52]. Hsp27 interacts with the main constituents of the apoptotic signaling pathway, specifically those involved in caspase activation [53]. The antiapoptotic effects of Hsp27 are responsible for the development of resistance to chemotherapy in tumor cells [54].

It has been reported by using a proteomic approach that GTE simultaneously suppressed the expression of Hsp90, Hsp75, and Hsp27. In addition, Zhang et al. revealed that GTE suppressed Hsp90 target Akt activation and mutant p53 levels, and caused PC cell apoptosis and growth suppression [50]. In vitro studies have shown that EGCG inhibits cell proliferation; induces apoptosis via activation of caspase-3 and caspase-9; induces proapoptotic Bax, Bak, and Bcl-Xs; and inhibits antiapoptotic Bcl-2 and Bcl-X_L [55]. Lyn-Cook et al. reported that EGCG suppresses the K-*ras* gene expression [56].

The AsPC-1 epithelial cell line is isolated from pancreatic tissue of a 62-year-old Caucasian female patient with metastatic pancreatic adenocarcinoma. Through in vivo studies, Shankar et al. [57] have demonstrated that EGCG inhibited the growth of AsPC-1 xenografts in nude mice treated with ECCG at 60 mg/kg dose for 6 weeks via various mechanisms, such as decrease in neoplastic cell proliferation, activation of caspase-3 and apoptosis, growth arrest (induction of $p21^{WAF1}$), and inhibition of angiogenesis (vWF, VEGF, and CD31) and metastasis (MMP-2, -7, -9, and -12). The doses of EGCG (60 mg/kg) used are quite pertinent to those in human studies [57]. Li et al. [58] recently reported that in human pancreatic cancer cell line Mia Paca-2 EGCG binding to the C-terminal region of Hsp90 impairs Hsp90 superchaperone complex causing downregulation of its client oncogenic proteins Akt, Her2, Cdk4, pERK, and Raf-1 [58].

Focal adhesion kinase (FAK) is a cytoplasmic tyrosine kinase that is overexpressed in cancers and it has been shown that the inhibition of FAK activity sensitizes malignant cells to apoptosis [59]. Not long ago, Liu et al. have determined that FAK and insulin-like growth factor 1 receptor (IGF-1R) interact to produce survival signals in PC cells [60]. Vu et al. [61] have proved for the first time that EGCG efficaciously suppressed phosphorylations of both FAK and IGF-1R in human PC cell lines BxPC-3 and AsPC-1, associated with inhibition of cell adhesion and proliferation [61]. Moreover, EGCG causes growth suppression and metastasis of PC cells and leads to apoptosis by inhibiting the STAT3 signaling pathway. It in addition enhances the therapeutic properties of gemcitabine [62].

Qanungo et al. have shown that EGCG dose-dependently generates stress signals by injuring mitochondria and ROS-mediated JNK activation in MIA PaCa-2 PC cells [63]. Other studies also demonstrated that EGCG interferes with the self-renewal capability of PC stem cells by the inhibition of pluripotency maintenance transcription factors (c-Myc, Nanog, and Oct-4) and the constitutes of sonic Hedgehog pathway. EGCG is useful in the PC prevention due to its antiproliferative, antiangiogenic, antimetastatic, and proapoptotic abilities in vitro and in vivo but further clinical studies are necessary to strengthen these findings in humans.

Not enough information is available regarding bioavailability and metabolism of catechin polyphenols in humans. A recent pharmacokinetics study of tea polyphenols in humans revealed that only a small percentage of the orally ingested catechins appears in the blood. The relatively poor bioavailability of tea catechins needs to be studied more extensively [64].

4.4 Curcumin

Curcumin, a natural polyphenolic compound, is derived from turmeric (*Curcuma longa*), which has been generally used as a natural food pigment, and in traditional health practice as an anti-inflammatory and antioxidant agent [65]. Curcumin targets various molecular pathways in PC cells such as Notch-1, PI3K/Akt, NF-kB, Sp1, WT1, COX-II, STAT3, and ATM/Chk1 [66–73]. Results from multiple studies demonstrated that the anticarcinogenic effects of curcumin are primarily due to its antiangiogenic properties, suppression of oxidative stress, and induction of apoptosis (Tables 11.2, 11.3, 11.4, 11.5, and 11.6).

Studies have also reported NF-kB as a prime target of curcumin in different PC models. The first report was presented by Li et al. [68], who determined that curcumin downregulated NF-κB and its downstream effectors such as PGE_2, COX-2, and IL-8 in human PC cells in a dose- and time-dependent manner with marked growth suppression and apoptosis [68].

Jutooru et al. [67] described that curcumin suppresses Panc28 and L3.6pL PC cells and cancer growth in nude mice bearing L3.6pL cells as xenografts by decreasing the expression of specificity protein (Sp) and Sp-dependent gene products. The *p65* and *p50* subunits of NF-κB are Sp-regulated genes and curcumin-induced suppression of the constitutive and induced NF-κB expression is partially because of downregulation of Sp transcription factors. The authors demonstrated that curcumin reduced the expression of p50, p65 proteins, and NF-κB, and also decreased Sp1, Sp3, and Sp4 transcription factors, which are known to be constitutively active in PC. The Sp transcription factors and NF-kB regulate several common genes such as vascular endothelial growth factor, cyclin D1, and survivin. Furthermore, the mitochondrial toxicity of curcumin and the subsequent induction of ROS in PC cells are the primary mechanisms of Sp downregulation [67].

Results from the study by Kunnumakkara et al. [74] showed that curcumin potentiates the antitumor effects of gemcitabine in PC by inhibiting NF-kB and NF-kB-regulated gene products, proliferation, and angiogenesis [74]. The constitutive activation of STAT3 plays a major role in the neoplastic activities, such as resistance to apoptosis, cell proliferation, angiogenesis, metastasis, and host immune evasion [75].

Survivin, the member of the inhibitor of apoptosis protein family (IAPs), is encoded by BIRC5 gene and occupies a key position because of its overexpression in cancer cells [76]. Glienke et al. determined that the expression of survivin/BIRC5 on the mRNA and protein levels was significantly suppressed, and the phosphorylation of STAT3 was inhibited in PC cell lines which led to induction of apoptosis [66].

Various derivatives of curcumin have been found to interfere with STAT3 signaling in PC. Lin et al. [77] demonstrated that diketone analogues of curcumin, FLLL31 and FLLL32, effectively suppressed the STAT3 signaling in PC. They were formulated to prefer interaction with both the Src homology 2 (SH2) domain of STAT3 and its upstream activator, the JAK2 kinase, which serves important roles in the STAT3 dimerization and signal transduction. The authors revealed that FLLL31 and FLLL32 derivatives of curcumin can effectively inhibit the constitutive signaling of STAT3 in vitro, inducing apoptosis in PC cell lines. The authors also reported that FLLL32 inhibits the processes of angiogenesis and tumor growth in vivo [77].

Hutzen et al. demonstrated that GO-Y030, which is a more potent synthetic analogue of curcumin, inhibits the STAT3 phosphorylation and transcriptional activity at considerably lower doses [78]. Sahu et al. [73] have shown that curcumin can inhibit the proliferation of BxPC-3 human PC cell line through the DNA damage-mediated G2/M cell cycle arrest and the induction of apoptosis via the activation of ATM/Chk1/Cdc25C, and inhibition of the expression of cyclin B1/Cdk1. Notably, curcumin had no effect on normal human pancreatic duct epithelial cells (HPDE-6). The results of this study demonstrate that Chk1 is a novel molecular target for curcumin in PC cells [73]. Recent data also suggests that curcumin can profoundly alter cellular epigenetics, including histone deacetylases (HDACs), histone acetyltransferases (HATs), and DNA methyltransferases (DNMTs) [79–81]. Tables 11.2, 11.3, and 11.4 further summarize selected preclinical and clinical studies related to curcumin in pancreatic cancer.

4.5 Isothiocyanates

Isothiocyanates are derived from glucosinolates (abundant in cruciferous vegetables) by hydrolysis via myrosinase enzyme (found in plants and bowel microflora). Benzyl isothiocyanate (BITC) has been found to inhibit multiple key signaling pathways, such as STAT3, NF-kB, AKT, and HDAC leading to PC growth suppression [82–84].

NF-kappaB/p65 is constitutively expressed in PC, where it acts as an important activator of transcription of multiple survival genes. Batra et al. [82] proposed that BITC-induced apoptosis is caused by inactivation of NF-kappaB/p65 via in vivo and in vitro inhibition of HDAC1/HDAC3. Researchers have evaluated the effect of BITC on normal HPDE-6 cells, NF-kappaB/p65, BxPC-3, and Capan-2 cells and revealed that exposure to BITC profoundly reduced NF-kappaB DNA-binding ability and transcriptional activity, as well as the expression and activation of cyclin D1, in both Capan-2 and BxPC-3 cells. Furthermore, BITC also caused a significant reduction in the expression of HDAC3 in Capan-2 and HDAC1 and HDAC3 in BxPC-3 cells [82].

STAT3 transcription factor is aberrantly activated in PC and promotes tumor survival. Sahu et al. [83] demonstrated that BITC targets STAT3 signaling and induces apoptosis leading to decreased survival of BxPC-3, Capan-2, AsPC-1, and MiaPaCa-2 cells. It has been shown that BITC treatment reduces STAT-3 protein levels (both total and activated), thus resulting in decreased STAT-3 DNA binding and transcriptional activities [83].

Angiogenesis is primarily activated during hypoxia by neoplasm-derived vascular endothelial growth factor (VEGF) and hypoxia-inducible factor (HIF-1α). STAT3 is essential for both the growth signal-induced and basal expression of HIF-1α and presents a compelling target for inhibition of VEGF expression in tumor cells [85]. Boreddy et al. [86] demonstrated that BITC substantially decreases tumor neovascularization through the suppression of STAT-3, STAT-3-induced HIF-1α, and VEGF expression. MMP-2 also plays a crucial role in tumor metastasis and angiogenesis. BITC significantly suppresses MMP-2 secretion in both hypoxic and normoxic BxPC-3 and PanC-1 cells [86].

Dysregulation of PI3K/AKT pathway causes uncontrolled proliferation in tumor cells. When activated, the serine/threonine kinase AKT mediates an antiapoptotic signal [87]. AKT regulates STAT3 and NF-kB, and therefore may represent a promising target for BITC. It has been reported that BITC markedly reduces the activation of AKT at Ser-308 and Ser-475, as well as inhibits the phosphorylation of many key molecules of the PI3K/AKT pathway including mTOR, PI3K, and PDK1, which leads to apoptosis in PC cells [84].

The FOXO family of transcription factors are important regulators of cell death that function downstream of PI3K signaling pathway and they promote tumor resistance and cell survival [88]. BITC inhibits FOXO phosphorylation and thus leads to the accumulation of FOXO proteins in the nucleus, causing upregulation of the FOXO transactivated pro-apoptotic protein Bim [84]. Furthermore, it has been reported that BITC promotes ROS generation. Sahu et al. revealed that ROS generation can lead to the activation of various members of MAP kinase family, such as P38, ERK, and JNK, causing apoptosis through G2/M cell cycle arrest [89]. Nevertheless, further research is needed to better comprehend the mechanism of BITC action in pancreatic cancer.

4.6 Soy Isoflavone (Genistein)

Genistein, a natural NF-kB inhibitor, has been demonstrated to enhance the effectiveness of chemotherapeutic drugs in pancreatic BxPC-3 cells [90]. Cancer stem cells (CSC) typically constitute a small fraction of total tumor cells and have the capacity for self-renewal and multipotency and as a result contribute to tumor growth, metastasis, resistance to treatment, and recurrence [91]. Also, genistein has been found to inhibit miR-27a, which is an oncogenic microRNA, and hence inhibits PC cell growth and induces apoptosis [92]. Therefore, isoflavones are considered promising agents for the treatment of PC by targeting multiple signaling pathways, such as the EMT and CSC phenotypes.

4.7 Quercetin

Quercetin is a flavonoid found mainly in fruits and vegetables. Zhou et al. reported that quercetin decreases the self-renewal properties of PC stem cells in vitro and in vivo via inhibition of aldehyde dehydrogenase-1 activity and suppression of epithelial-mesenchymal transition [93]. Tang et al. [62] found that quercetin enhances the inhibitory effects of EGCG on the self-renewal ability of PC stem cells through modulation of the Sonic hedgehog pathway. Cao et al. discovered that quercetin also downregulates the β-catenin in PC stem cells, impeding their capacity for self-renewal [94]. Furthermore, Appari et al. [95] described the complementary effects of quercetin, sulforaphane, and EGCG in decreasing the ability for self-renewal in PC stem cells, compared with individual dietary agents, and showed that they upregulate miR-let7-a and inhibit K-ras [95].

4.8 Conclusions, Limitations, and Future Perspectives

Pancreatic malignancy is a major cause of cancer death in the United States. The average 5-year survival rate for PC remains extremely low despite current therapeutic options. There is a dire need for research to develop novel and effective treatments. Phytochemicals are an emerging source for the discovery of new antineoplastic agents, which have shown many promising antineoplastic effects and have demonstrated success in in vitro and preclinical studies. Among the phytochemicals that show promise in pancreatic cancer are curcumin, resveratrol, quercetin, soy isoflavone (genistein), isothiocyanate, green tea, and capsaicin. In vitro research has advanced our comprehension of the molecular pathways that underlie the anticancer effects of these agents. However, there is a remaining gap in preclinical studies that compromises the use of phytochemicals in clinical practice. The inability to reproduce similar effectiveness of these agents in in vivo models including animal and human studies has been limited by numerous factors such as solubility, stability, lack of selectivity, and mostly poor bioavailability which would require higher and more frequent doses in in vivo studies that may lead to side effects. Moreover, the activity of these agents gets compromised further by the methods of their extraction and purification processes. Another aspect of using phytochemicals that has been considered a limitation is the lack of target specificity, but it has been more and more realized that such lack of specificity and multitargeted/pleiotropic effects of phytochemicals underline the indispensable quality of these anticancer agents. Additionally, combinations of the anticancer phytochemicals should be explored as they may be more effective than single agents alone.

Given the promises that these phytochemicals offer as anticancer agents, we must conduct more studies including clinical trials to further explore the pharmacokinetics, ideal dosages, adverse effects, drug interactions, and long-term safety of these agents. We also need to improve study designs to overcome methodological flaws such as the lack of appropriate control or placebo, small sample sizes, and short duration of trials. Future endeavors should also focus on improving methods of extraction/purification of these substances, improving drug delivery and bioavailability, and improving target selectivity. Continued efforts must be made towards the synthesis of novel analogues of phytochemicals to increase their bioavailability and efficacy, creation of formulations to selectively and more effectively deliver phytochemicals to their intended target organ/tissue, and lastly formulation of innovative delivery systems that can improve the pharmacokinetics of anticancer agents. The emergence of nanotechnology has expanded the horizon of anticancer therapy including phytochemicals' use as anticancer agents. The utilization of biocompatible and biodegradable nanoparticles represents novel delivery strategies to improve solubility, stability, and bioavailability of phytochemicals in pancreatic cancer.

Acknowledgements *Author Contributions*: All the authors have diligently contributed to the development and preparation of this research manuscript (book chapter), including the literature search, concept organization, data interpretation, and writings. All the authors have read and approved the final draft for publication.

Conflict of Interest: The authors declare that they have no conflicts of interest associated with this research manuscript.

Financial Disclosures: None to disclose.

References

1. Jemal, A., Siegel, R., Ward, E., et al. (2006). Cancer statistics, 2006. *CA: a Cancer Journal for Clinicians, 56*(2), 106–130. https://doi.org/10.3322/canjclin.56.2.106.
2. Siegel, R. L., Miller, K. D., & Jemal, A. (2020). Cancer statistics, 2020. *CA: a Cancer Journal for Clinicians, 70*(1), 7–30. https://doi.org/10.3322/caac.21590.
3. Jones, S., Zhang, X., Parsons, D. W., et al. (2008). Core signaling pathways in human pancreatic cancers revealed by global genomic analyses. *Science, 321*(5897), 1801–1806. https://doi.org/10.1126/science.1164368.
4. Block, G., Patterson, B., & Subar, A. (1992). Fruit, vegetables, and cancer prevention: A review of the epidemiological evidence. *Nutrition and Cancer, 18*(1), 1–29. https://doi.org/10.1080/01635589209514201.
5. Pietta, P. G. (2000). Flavonoids as antioxidants. *Journal of Natural Products, 63*(7), 1035–1042. https://doi.org/10.1021/np9904509.
6. Saiki, Y., & Horii, A. (2014). Molecular pathology of pancreatic cancer. *Pathology International, 64*(1), 10–19. https://doi.org/10.1111/pin.12114.
7. Grant, T. J., Hua, K., & Singh, A. (2016). Molecular pathogenesis of pancreatic cancer. *Progress in Molecular Biology and Translational Science, 144*, 241–275. https://doi.org/10.1016/bs.pmbts.2016.09.008.
8. Mann, K. M., Ying, H., Juan, J., Jenkins, N. A., & Copeland, N. G. (2016). KRAS-related proteins in pancreatic cancer. *Pharmacology & Therapeutics, 168*, 29–42. https://doi.org/10.1016/j.pharmthera.2016.09.003.
9. di Magliano, M. P., & Logsdon, C. D. (2013). Roles for KRAS in pancreatic tumor development and progression. *Gastroenterology, 144*(6), 1220–1229. https://doi.org/10.1053/j.gastro.2013.01.071.
10. Abramson, M. A., Jazag, A., van der Zee, J. A., & Whang, E. E. (2007). The molecular biology of pancreatic cancer. *Gastrointestinal Cancer Research, 1*(4 Suppl 2), S7–S12.
11. Gharibi, A., Adamian, Y., & Kelber, J. A. (2016). Cellular and molecular aspects of pancreatic cancer. *Acta Histochemica, 118*(3), 305–316. https://doi.org/10.1016/j.acthis.2016.01.009.
12. Serra, S., & Chetty, R. (2018). p16. *Journal of Clinical Pathology, 71*(10), 853–858. https://doi.org/10.1136/jclinpath-2018-205216.
13. Shi, Y., & Massagué, J. (2003). Mechanisms of TGF-beta signaling from cell membrane to the nucleus. *Cell, 113*(6), 685–700. https://doi.org/10.1016/s0092-8674(03)00432-x.
14. Siegel, P. M., & Massagué, J. (2003). Cytostatic and apoptotic actions of TGF-beta in homeostasis and cancer. *Nature Reviews. Cancer, 3*(11), 807–821. https://doi.org/10.1038/nrc1208.
15. Mohammed, A., Janakiram, N. B., Pant, S., & Rao, C. V. (2015). Molecular targeted intervention for pancreatic cancer. *Cancers, 7*(3), 1499–1542. https://doi.org/10.3390/cancers7030850.
16. Yin, Y., & Shen, W. H. (2008). PTEN: A new guardian of the genome. *Oncogene, 27*(41), 5443–5453. https://doi.org/10.1038/onc.2008.241.
17. Subramaniam, D., Kaushik, G., Dandawate, P., & Anant, S. (2018). Targeting cancer stem cells for chemoprevention of pancreatic cancer. *Current Medicinal Chemistry, 25*(22), 2585–2594. https://doi.org/10.2174/0929867324666170127095832.
18. Duchartre, Y., Kim, Y.-M., & Kahn, M. (2016). The Wnt signaling pathway in cancer. *Critical Reviews in Oncology/Hematology, 99*, 141–149. https://doi.org/10.1016/j.critrevonc.2015.12.005.
19. MacDonald, B. T., & He, X. (2012). Frizzled and LRP5/6 receptors for Wnt/β-catenin signaling. *Cold Spring Harbor Perspectives in Biology, 4*(12). https://doi.org/10.1101/cshperspect.a007880.
20. Matsuoka, T., & Yashiro, M. (2016). Molecular targets for the treatment of pancreatic cancer: Clinical and experimental studies. *World Journal of Gastroenterology, 22*(2), 776–789. https://doi.org/10.3748/wjg.v22.i2.776.

21. Pencik, J., Pham, H. T. T., Schmoellerl, J., et al. (2016). JAK-STAT signaling in cancer: From cytokines to non-coding genome. *Cytokine, 87*, 26–36. https://doi.org/10.1016/j.cyto.2016.06.017.
22. Furukawa, T. (2015). Impacts of activation of the mitogen-activated protein kinase pathway in pancreatic cancer. *Frontiers in Oncology, 5*, 23. https://doi.org/10.3389/fonc.2015.00023.
23. Kolch, W. (2000). Meaningful relationships: The regulation of the Ras/Raf/MEK/ERK pathway by protein interactions. *The Biochemical Journal, 351*(Pt 2), 289–305.
24. Prabhu, L., Mundade, R., Korc, M., Loehrer, P. J., & Lu, T. (2014). Critical role of NF-κB in pancreatic cancer. *Oncotarget, 5*(22), 10969–10975.
25. Pramanik, K. C., Makena, M. R., Bhowmick, K., & Pandey, M. K. (2018). Advancement of NF-κB signaling pathway: A novel target in pancreatic cancer. *International Journal of Molecular Sciences, 19*(12). https://doi.org/10.3390/ijms19123890.
26. Kim, H., Saka, B., Knight, S., et al. (2014). Having pancreatic cancer with tumoral loss of ATM and normal TP53 protein expression is associated with a poorer prognosis. *Clinical Cancer Research: An Official Journal of the American Association for Cancer Research, 20* (7), 1865–1872. https://doi.org/10.1158/1078-0432.CCR-13-1239.
27. Merchant, A. A., & Matsui, W. (2010). Targeting hedgehog: A cancer stem cell pathway. *Clinical Cancer Research, 16*(12), 3130–3140. https://doi.org/10.1158/1078-0432.CCR-09-2846.
28. Ng, J. M. Y., & Curran, T. (2011). The Hedgehog's tale: Developing strategies for targeting cancer. *Nature Reviews. Cancer, 11*(7), 493–501. https://doi.org/10.1038/nrc3079.
29. McMillan, R., & Matsui, W. (2012). Molecular pathways: The hedgehog signaling pathway in cancer. *Clinical Cancer Research, 18*(18), 4883–4888. https://doi.org/10.1158/1078-0432.CCR-11-2509.
30. Ranganathan, P., Weaver, K. L., & Capobianco, A. J. (2011). Notch signalling in solid tumours: A little bit of everything but not all the time. *Nature Reviews. Cancer, 11*(5), 338–351. https://doi.org/10.1038/nrc3035.
31. Keylor, M. H., Matsuura, B. S., & Stephenson, C. R. J. (2015). Chemistry and biology of resveratrol-derived natural products. *Chemical Reviews, 115*(17), 8976–9027. https://doi.org/10.1021/cr500689b.
32. Mo, W., Xu, X., Xu, L., et al. (2011). Resveratrol inhibits proliferation and induces apoptosis through the hedgehog signaling pathway in pancreatic cancer cell. *Pancreatology, 11*(6), 601–609. https://doi.org/10.1159/000333542.
33. Kotha, A., Sekharam, M., Cilenti, L., et al. (2006). Resveratrol inhibits Src and Stat3 signaling and induces the apoptosis of malignant cells containing activated Stat3 protein. *Molecular Cancer Therapeutics, 5*(3), 621–629. https://doi.org/10.1158/1535-7163.MCT-05-0268.
34. Roy, S. K., Chen, Q., Fu, J., Shankar, S., & Srivastava, R. K. (2011). Resveratrol inhibits growth of orthotopic pancreatic tumors through activation of FOXO transcription factors. *PLoS One, 6*(9), e25166. https://doi.org/10.1371/journal.pone.0025166.
35. Chen, X., Wang, S., Yang, N. W., & CS. Leukotriene A4 hydrolase as a target for cancer prevention and therapy. *Current Cancer Drug Targets.* http://www.eurekaselect.com/62181/article. Published May 1, 2004.
36. Tong, W.-G., Ding, X.-Z., Hennig, R., et al. (2002). Leukotriene B4 receptor antagonist LY293111 inhibits proliferation and induces apoptosis in human pancreatic cancer cells. *Clinical Cancer Research, 8*(10), 3232–3242.
37. Oi, N., Jeong, C.-H., Nadas, J., et al. (2010). Resveratrol, a red wine polyphenol, suppresses pancreatic cancer by inhibiting leukotriene A4hydrolase. *Cancer Research, 70*(23), 9755–9764. https://doi.org/10.1158/0008-5472.CAN-10-2858.
38. Zhou, J.-H., Cheng, H.-Y., Yu, Z.-Q., He, D.-W., Pan, Z., & Yang, D.-T. (2011). Resveratrol induces apoptosis in pancreatic cancer cells. *Chinese Medical Journal, 124*(11), 1695–1699.
39. Harikumar, K. B., Kunnumakkara, A. B., Sethi, G., et al. (2010). Resveratrol, a multitargeted agent, can enhance antitumor activity of gemcitabine in vitro and in orthotopic mouse model of

human pancreatic cancer. *International Journal of Cancer, 127*(2), 257–268. https://doi.org/10.1002/ijc.25041.

40. Walle, T. (2011). Bioavailability of resveratrol. *Annals of the New York Academy of Sciences, 1215*, 9–15. https://doi.org/10.1111/j.1749-6632.2010.05842.x.
41. Bernhaus, A., Ozsvar-Kozma, M., Saiko, P., et al. (2009). Antitumor effects of KITC, a new resveratrol derivative, in AsPC-1 and BxPC-3 human pancreatic carcinoma cells. *Investigational New Drugs, 27*(5), 393–401. https://doi.org/10.1007/s10637-008-9183-7.
42. Thipe, V. C., Panjtan Amiri, K., Bloebaum, P., et al. (2019). Development of resveratrol-conjugated gold nanoparticles: Interrelationship of increased resveratrol corona on anti-tumor efficacy against breast, pancreatic and prostate cancers. *International Journal of Nanomedicine, 14*, 4413–4428. https://doi.org/10.2147/IJN.S204443.
43. Zhang, R., Humphreys, I., Sahu, R. P., Shi, Y., & Srivastava, S. K. (2008). In vitro and in vivo induction of apoptosis by capsaicin in pancreatic cancer cells is mediated through ROS generation and mitochondrial death pathway. *Apoptosis : An International Journal on Programmed Cell Death, 13*(12), 1465–1478. https://doi.org/10.1007/s10495-008-0278-6.
44. Pramanik, K. C., Boreddy, S. R., & Srivastava, S. K. (2011). Role of mitochondrial electron transport chain complexes in capsaicin mediated oxidative stress leading to apoptosis in pancreatic cancer cells. *PLoS One, 6*(5), e20151. https://doi.org/10.1371/journal.pone.0020151.
45. Ichijo, H., Nishida, E., Irie, K., et al. (1997). Induction of apoptosis by ASK1, a mammalian MAPKKK that activates SAPK/JNK and p38 signaling pathways. *Science, 275*(5296), 90–94. https://doi.org/10.1126/science.275.5296.90.
46. Ohashi, S., Nishio, A., Nakamura, H., et al. (2006). Overexpression of redox-active protein thioredoxin-1 prevents development of chronic pancreatitis in mice. *Antioxidants & Redox Signaling, 8*(9–10), 1835–1845. https://doi.org/10.1089/ars.2006.8.1835.
47. Pramanik, K. C., & Srivastava, S. K. (2012). Apoptosis signal-regulating kinase 1–thioredoxin complex dissociation by capsaicin causes pancreatic tumor growth suppression by inducing apoptosis. *Antioxidants & Redox Signaling, 17*(10), 1417–1432. https://doi.org/10.1089/ars.2011.4369.
48. Seeram, N. P., Henning, S. M., Niu, Y., Lee, R., Scheuller, H. S., & Heber, D. (2006). Catechin and caffeine content of green tea dietary supplements and correlation with antioxidant capacity. *Journal of Agricultural and Food Chemistry, 54*(5), 1599–1603. https://doi.org/10.1021/jf052857r.
49. Deer, E. L., González-Hernández, J., Coursen, J. D., et al. (2010). Phenotype and genotype of pancreatic cancer cell lines. *Pancreas, 39*(4), 425–435. https://doi.org/10.1097/MPA.0b013e3181c15963.
50. Zhang, L., Pang, E., Loo, R. R. O., et al. (2011). Concomitant inhibition of HSP90, its mitochondrial localized homologue TRAP1 and HSP27 by green tea in pancreatic cancer HPAF-II cells. *Proteomics, 11*(24), 4638–4647. https://doi.org/10.1002/pmic.201100242.
51. Whitesell, L., & Lindquist, S. L. (2005). HSP90 and the chaperoning of cancer. *Nature Reviews. Cancer, 5*(10), 761–772. https://doi.org/10.1038/nrc1716.
52. Kang, B. H., Plescia, J., Song, H. Y., et al. (2009). Combinatorial drug design targeting multiple cancer signaling networks controlled by mitochondrial Hsp90. *The Journal of Clinical Investigation, 119*(3), 454–464. https://doi.org/10.1172/JCI37613.
53. Garrido, C., Brunet, M., Didelot, C., Zermati, Y., Schmitt, E., & Kroemer, G. (2006). Heat shock proteins 27 and 70: Anti-apoptotic proteins with tumorigenic properties. *Cell Cycle Georget Tex., 5*(22), 2592–2601. https://doi.org/10.4161/cc.5.22.3448.
54. Garrido, C., Gurbuxani, S., Ravagnan, L., & Kroemer, G. (2001). Heat shock proteins: Endogenous modulators of apoptotic cell death. *Biochemical and Biophysical Research Communications, 286*(3), 433–442. https://doi.org/10.1006/bbrc.2001.5427.
55. Shankar, S., Suthakar, G., & Srivastava, R. K. (2007). Epigallocatechin-3-gallate inhibits cell cycle and induces apoptosis in pancreatic cancer. *Frontiers in Bioscience: A Virtual Library of Medicine, 12*, 5039–5051. https://doi.org/10.2741/2446.

56. Lyn-Cook, B. D., Rogers, T., Yan, Y., Blann, E. B., Kadlubar, F. F., & Hammons, G. J. (1999). Chemopreventive effects of tea extracts and various components on human pancreatic and prostate tumor cells in vitro. *Nutrition and Cancer, 35*(1), 80–86. https://doi.org/10.1207/S1532791480-86.
57. Shankar, S., Ganapathy, S., Hingorani, S. R., & Srivastava, R. K. (2008). EGCG inhibits growth, invasion, angiogenesis and metastasis of pancreatic cancer. *Frontiers in Bioscience: A Virtual Library of Medicine, 13*, 440–452. https://doi.org/10.2741/2691.
58. Li, Y., Zhang, T., Jiang, Y., Lee, H.-F., Schwartz, S. J., & Sun, D. (2009). (−)-Epigallocatechin-3-gallate inhibits Hsp90 function by impairing Hsp90 association with cochaperones in pancreatic cancer cell line Mia Paca-2. *Molecular Pharmaceutics, 6*(4), 1152–1159. https://doi.org/10.1021/mp900037p.
59. Golubovskaya, V. M., Gross, S., Kaur, A. S., et al. (2003). Simultaneous inhibition of focal adhesion kinase and SRC enhances detachment and apoptosis in colon cancer cell lines. *Molecular Cancer Research, 1*(10), 755–764.
60. Liu, W., Bloom, D. A., Cance, W. G., Kurenova, E. V., Golubovskaya, V. M., & Hochwald, S. N. (2008). FAK and IGF-IR interact to provide survival signals in human pancreatic adenocarcinoma cells. *Carcinogenesis, 29*(6), 1096–1107. https://doi.org/10.1093/carcin/bgn026.
61. Vu, H. A., Beppu, Y., Chi, H. T., et al. (2010). Green tea epigallocatechin gallate exhibits anticancer effect in human pancreatic carcinoma cells via the inhibition of both focal adhesion kinase and insulin-like growth factor-I receptor. *Journal of Biomedicine & Biotechnology, 2010*, 290516. https://doi.org/10.1155/2010/290516.
62. Tang, S.-N., Fu, J., Shankar, S., & Srivastava, R. K. (2012). EGCG enhances the therapeutic potential of gemcitabine and CP690550 by inhibiting STAT3 signaling pathway in human pancreatic cancer. *PLoS One, 7*(2), e31067. https://doi.org/10.1371/journal.pone.0031067.
63. Qanungo, S., Das, M., Haldar, S., & Basu, A. (2005). Epigallocatechin-3-gallate induces mitochondrial membrane depolarization and caspase-dependent apoptosis in pancreatic cancer cells. *Carcinogenesis, 26*(5), 958–967. https://doi.org/10.1093/carcin/bgi040.
64. Lee, M. J., Maliakal, P., Chen, L., Meng, X., Bondoc, F. Y., Prabhu, S., Lambert, G., Mohr, S., & Yang, C. S. (2002). Pharmacokinetics of tea catechins after ingestion of green tea and (−)-epigallocatechin-3-gallate by humans: Formation of different metabolites and individual variability. *Cancer Epidemiology, Biomarkers & Prevention, 11*(10 Pt 1), 1025–1032. https://cebp.aacrjournals.org/content/11/10/1025.
65. Aggarwal, B. B., Sundaram, C., Malani, N., & Ichikawa, H. (2007). Curcumin: The Indian solid gold. *Advances in Experimental Medicine and Biology, 595*, 1–75. https://doi.org/10.1007/978-0-387-46401-5_1.
66. Glienke, W., Maute, L., Wicht, J., & Bergmann, L. (2010). Curcumin inhibits constitutive STAT3 phosphorylation in human pancreatic cancer cell lines and downregulation of survivin/BIRC5 gene expression. *Cancer Investigation, 28*(2), 166–171. https://doi.org/10.3109/07357900903287006.
67. Jutooru, I., Chadalapaka, G., Lei, P., & Safe, S. (2010). Inhibition of NFkappaB and pancreatic cancer cell and tumor growth by curcumin is dependent on specificity protein down-regulation. *The Journal of Biological Chemistry, 285*(33), 25332–25344. https://doi.org/10.1074/jbc.M109.095240.
68. Li, L., Aggarwal, B. B., Shishodia, S., Abbruzzese, J., & Kurzrock, R. (2004). Nuclear factor-kappaB and IkappaB kinase are constitutively active in human pancreatic cells, and their down-regulation by curcumin (diferuloylmethane) is associated with the suppression of proliferation and the induction of apoptosis. *Cancer, 101*(10), 2351–2362. https://doi.org/10.1002/cncr.20605.
69. Glienke, W., Maute, L., Wicht, J., & Bergmann, L. (2009). Wilms' tumour gene 1 (WT1) as a target in curcumin treatment of pancreatic cancer cells. *European Journal of Cancer 1990, 45*(5), 874–880. https://doi.org/10.1016/j.ejca.2008.12.030.

70. Zhao, Z., Li, C., Xi, H., Gao, Y., & Xu, D. (2015). Curcumin induces apoptosis in pancreatic cancer cells through the induction of forkhead box O1 and inhibition of the PI3K/Akt pathway. *Molecular Medicine Reports, 12*(4), 5415–5422. https://doi.org/10.3892/mmr.2015.4060.
71. Basha, R., Connelly, S. F., Sankpal, U. T., et al. (2016). Small molecule tolfenamic acid and dietary spice curcumin treatment enhances antiproliferative effect in pancreatic cancer cells via suppressing Sp1, disrupting NF-kB translocation to nucleus and cell cycle phase distribution. *The Journal of Nutritional Biochemistry, 31*, 77–87. https://doi.org/10.1016/j.jnutbio.2016.01.003.
72. Padhye, S., Banerjee, S., Chavan, D., et al. (2009). Fluorocurcumins as cyclooxygenase-2 inhibitor: Molecular docking, pharmacokinetics and tissue distribution in mice. *Pharmaceutical Research, 26*(11), 2438–2445. https://doi.org/10.1007/s11095-009-9955-6.
73. Sahu, R. P., Batra, S., & Srivastava, S. K. (2009). Activation of ATM/Chk1 by curcumin causes cell cycle arrest and apoptosis in human pancreatic cancer cells. *British Journal of Cancer, 100*(9), 1425–1433. https://doi.org/10.1038/sj.bjc.6605039.
74. Kunnumakkara, A. B., Guha, S., Krishnan, S., Diagaradjane, P., Gelovani, J., & Aggarwal, B. B. (2007). Curcumin potentiates antitumor activity of gemcitabine in an orthotopic model of pancreatic cancer through suppression of proliferation, angiogenesis, and inhibition of nuclear factor-kappaB-regulated gene products. *Cancer Research, 67*(8), 3853–3861. https://doi.org/10.1158/0008-5472.CAN-06-4257.
75. Wang, T., Niu, G., Kortylewski, M., et al. (2004). Regulation of the innate and adaptive immune responses by Stat-3 signaling in tumor cells. *Nature Medicine, 10*(1), 48–54. https://doi.org/10.1038/nm976.
76. Garg, H., Suri, P., Gupta, J. C., Talwar, G. P., & Dubey, S. (2016). Survivin: A unique target for tumor therapy. *Cancer Cell International, 16*, 49. https://doi.org/10.1186/s12935-016-0326-1.
77. Lin, L., Hutzen, B., Zuo, M., et al. (2010). Novel STAT3 phosphorylation inhibitors exhibit potent growth suppressive activity in pancreatic and breast cancer cells. *Cancer Research, 70*(6), 2445–2454. https://doi.org/10.1158/0008-5472.CAN-09-2468.
78. Hutzen, B., Friedman, L., Sobo, M., et al. (2009). Curcumin analogue GO-Y030 inhibits STAT3 activity and cell growth in breast and pancreatic carcinomas. *International Journal of Oncology, 35*(4), 867–872. https://doi.org/10.3892/ijo_00000401.
79. Bora-Tatar, G., Dayangaç-Erden, D., Demir, A. S., Dalkara, S., Yelekçi, K., & Erdem-Yurter, H. (2009). Molecular modifications on carboxylic acid derivatives as potent histone deacetylase inhibitors: Activity and docking studies. *Bioorganic & Medicinal Chemistry, 17*(14), 5219–5228. https://doi.org/10.1016/j.bmc.2009.05.042.
80. Liu, H., Chen, Y., Cui, G., & Zhou, J. (2005). Curcumin, a potent anti-tumor reagent, is a novel histone deacetylase inhibitor regulating B-NHL cell line Raji proliferation. *Acta Pharmacologica Sinica, 26*(5), 603–609. https://doi.org/10.1111/j.1745-7254.2005.00081.x.
81. Medina-Franco, J. L., López-Vallejo, F., Kuck, D., & Lyko, F. (2011). Natural products as DNA methyltransferase inhibitors: A computer-aided discovery approach. *Molecular Diversity, 15*(2), 293–304. https://doi.org/10.1007/s11030-010-9262-5.
82. Batra, S., Sahu, R. P., Kandala, P. K., & Srivastava, S. K. (2010). Benzyl isothiocyanate-mediated inhibition of histone deacetylase leads to NF-kappaB turnoff in human pancreatic carcinoma cells. *Molecular Cancer Therapeutics, 9*(6), 1596–1608. https://doi.org/10.1158/1535-7163.MCT-09-1146.
83. Sahu, R. P., & Srivastava, S. K. (2009). The role of STAT-3 in the induction of apoptosis in pancreatic cancer cells by benzyl isothiocyanate. *Journal of the National Cancer Institute, 101*(3), 176–193. https://doi.org/10.1093/jnci/djn470.
84. Boreddy, S. R., Pramanik, K. C., & Srivastava, S. K. (2011). Pancreatic tumor suppression by benzyl isothiocyanate is associated with inhibition of PI3K/AKT/FOXO pathway. *Clinical Cancer Research, 17*(7), 1784–1795. https://doi.org/10.1158/1078-0432.CCR-10-1891.

85. Xu, Q., Briggs, J., Park, S., et al. (2005). Targeting Stat3 blocks both HIF-1 and VEGF expression induced by multiple oncogenic growth signaling pathways. *Oncogene, 24*(36), 5552–5560. https://doi.org/10.1038/sj.onc.1208719.
86. Boreddy, S. R., Sahu, R. P., & Srivastava, S. K. (2011). Benzyl isothiocyanate suppresses pancreatic tumor angiogenesis and invasion by inhibiting HIF-α/VEGF/rho-GTPases: Pivotal role of STAT-3. *PLoS One, 6*(10), e25799. https://doi.org/10.1371/journal.pone.0025799.
87. Schlieman, M. G., Fahy, B. N., Ramsamooj, R., Beckett, L., & Bold, R. J. (2003). Incidence, mechanism and prognostic value of activated AKT in pancreas cancer. *British Journal of Cancer, 89*(11), 2110–2115. https://doi.org/10.1038/sj.bjc.6601396.
88. Gomes, A. R., Brosens, J. J., & Lam, E. W.-F. (2008). Resist or die: FOXO transcription factors determine the cellular response to chemotherapy. *Cell Cycle Georget Tex., 7*(20), 3133–3136. https://doi.org/10.4161/cc.7.20.6920.
89. Sahu, R. P., Zhang, R., Batra, S., Shi, Y., & Srivastava, S. K. (2009). Benzyl isothiocyanate-mediated generation of reactive oxygen species causes cell cycle arrest and induces apoptosis via activation of MAPK in human pancreatic cancer cells. *Carcinogenesis, 30*(10), 1744–1753. https://doi.org/10.1093/carcin/bgp157.
90. Kumar, G., Farooqui, M., & Rao, C. V. (2018). Role of dietary cancer-preventive phytochemicals in pancreatic cancer stem cells. *Current Pharmacology Reports, 4*(4), 326–335. https://doi.org/10.1007/s40495-018-0145-2.
91. Chang, J. C. (2016). Cancer stem cells: Role in tumor growth, recurrence, metastasis, and treatment resistance. *Medicine (Baltimore), 95*(1 Suppl 1), S20–S25. https://doi.org/10.1097/MD.0000000000004766.
92. Xia, J., Cheng, L., Mei, C., et al. (2014). Genistein inhibits cell growth and invasion through regulation of miR-27a in pancreatic cancer cells. *Current Pharmaceutical Design, 20*(33), 5348–5353. https://doi.org/10.2174/1381612820666140128215756.
93. Zhou, W., Kallifatidis, G., Baumann, B., et al. (2010). Dietary polyphenol quercetin targets pancreatic cancer stem cells. *International Journal of Oncology, 37*(3), 551–561. https://doi.org/10.3892/ijo_00000704.
94. Cao, C., Sun, L., Mo, W., Sun, L., Luo, J., Yang, Z., & Ran, Y. (2015). Quercetin mediates β-catenin in pancreatic cancer stem-like cells. *Pancreas, 44*(8), 1334–1339. https://doi.org/10.1097/MPA.0000000000000400.
95. Appari, M., Babu, K. R., Kaczorowski, A., Gross, W., & Herr, I. (2014). Sulforaphane, quercetin and catechins complement each other in elimination of advanced pancreatic cancer by miR-let-7 induction and K-ras inhibition. *International Journal of Oncology, 45*(4), 1391–1400. https://doi.org/10.3892/ijo.2014.2539.
96. Patiño-Morales, C. C., Soto-Reyes, E., Arechaga-Ocampo, E., et al. (2020). Curcumin stabilizes p53 by interaction with NAD(P)H:quinone oxidoreductase 1 in tumor-derived cell lines. *Redox Biology, 28*, 101320. https://doi.org/10.1016/j.redox.2019.101320.
97. Li, S.-S., Jiang, W.-L., Xiao, W.-Q., et al. (2019). KMT2D deficiency enhances the anti-cancer activity of L48H37 in pancreatic ductal adenocarcinoma. *World Journal of Gastrointestinal Oncology, 11*(8), 599–621. https://doi.org/10.4251/wjgo.v11.i8.599.
98. Parasramka, M. A., & Gupta, S. V. (2012). Synergistic effect of garcinol and curcumin on antiproliferative and apoptotic activity in pancreatic cancer cells. *Journal of Oncology, 2012*, 709739. https://doi.org/10.1155/2012/709739.
99. Yang, D., Li, Y., & Zhao, D. (2017). Curcumin induces apoptotic cell death in human pancreatic cancer cells via the miR-340/XIAP signaling pathway. *Oncology Letters, 14*(2), 1811–1816. https://doi.org/10.3892/ol.2017.6321.
100. Ma, J., Fang, B., Zeng, F., et al. (2014). Curcumin inhibits cell growth and invasion through up-regulation of miR-7 in pancreatic cancer cells. *Toxicology Letters, 231*(1), 82–91. https://doi.org/10.1016/j.toxlet.2014.09.014.
101. Sun, M., Estrov, Z., Ji, Y., Coombes, K. R., Harris, D. H., & Kurzrock, R. (2008). Curcumin (diferuloylmethane) alters the expression profiles of microRNAs in human pancreatic cancer

cells. *Molecular Cancer Therapeutics, 7*(3), 464–473. https://doi.org/10.1158/1535-7163.MCT-07-2272.
102. Li, W., Wang, Z., Xiao, X., et al. (2019). Curcumin attenuates hyperglycemia-driven EGF-induced invasive and migratory abilities of pancreatic cancer via suppression of the ERK and AKT pathways. *Oncology Reports, 41*(1), 650–658. https://doi.org/10.3892/or.2018.6833.
103. Bimonte, S., Barbieri, A., Palma, G., Luciano, A., Rea, D., & Arra, C. (2013). Curcumin inhibits tumor growth and angiogenesis in an orthotopic mouse model of human pancreatic cancer. *BioMed Research International, 2013*, 810423. https://doi.org/10.1155/2013/810423.
104. Osterman, C. J. D., Lynch, J. C., Leaf, P., et al. (2015). Curcumin modulates pancreatic adenocarcinoma cell-derived exosomal function. *PLoS One, 10*(7), e0132845. https://doi.org/10.1371/journal.pone.0132845.
105. Sun, X.-D., Liu, X.-E., & Huang, D.-S. (2013). Curcumin reverses the epithelial-mesenchymal transition of pancreatic cancer cells by inhibiting the hedgehog signaling pathway. *Oncology Reports, 29*(6), 2401–2407. https://doi.org/10.3892/or.2013.2385.
106. Sarkar, S., Dubaybo, H., Ali, S., et al. (2013). Down-regulation of miR-221 inhibits proliferation of pancreatic cancer cells through up-regulation of PTEN, p27(kip1), p57(kip2), and PUMA. *American Journal of Cancer Research, 3*(5), 465–477.
107. Subramaniam, D., Ramalingam, S., Linehan, D. C., et al. (2011). RNA binding protein CUGBP2/CELF2 mediates curcumin-induced mitotic catastrophe of pancreatic cancer cells. *PLoS One, 6*(2), e16958. https://doi.org/10.1371/journal.pone.0016958.
108. Veeraraghavan, J., Natarajan, M., Lagisetty, P., Awasthi, V., Herman, T. S., & Aravindan, N. (2011). Impact of curcumin, raspberry extract, and neem leaf extract on rel protein-regulated cell death/radiosensitization in pancreatic cancer cells. *Pancreas, 40*(7), 1107–1119. https://doi.org/10.1097/MPA.0b013e31821f677d.
109. Bao, B., Ali, S., Banerjee, S., et al. (2012). Curcumin analogue CDF inhibits pancreatic tumor growth by switching on suppressor microRNAs and attenuating EZH2 expression. *Cancer Research, 72*(1), 335–345. https://doi.org/10.1158/0008-5472.CAN-11-2182.
110. Ranjan, A. P., Mukerjee, A., Helson, L., Gupta, R., & Vishwanatha, J. K. (2013). Efficacy of liposomal curcumin in a human pancreatic tumor xenograft model: Inhibition of tumor growth and angiogenesis. *Anticancer Research, 33*(9), 3603–3609.
111. Yoshida, K., Toden, S., Ravindranathan, P., Han, H., & Goel, A. (2017). Curcumin sensitizes pancreatic cancer cells to gemcitabine by attenuating PRC2 subunit EZH2, and the lncRNA PVT1 expression. *Carcinogenesis, 38*(10), 1036–1046. https://doi.org/10.1093/carcin/bgx065.
112. Ning, X., Du, Y., Ben, Q., et al. (2016). Bulk pancreatic cancer cells can convert into cancer stem cells (CSCs) in vitro and 2 compounds can target these CSCs. *Cell Cycle Georget Tex., 15*(3), 403–412. https://doi.org/10.1080/15384101.2015.1127471.
113. Cheng, A. L., Hsu, C. H., Lin, J. K., et al. (2001). Phase I clinical trial of curcumin, a chemopreventive agent, in patients with high-risk or pre-malignant lesions. *Anticancer Research, 21*(4B), 2895–2900.
114. Sharma, R. A., Euden, S. A., Platton, S. L., et al. (2004). Phase I clinical trial of oral curcumin: Biomarkers of systemic activity and compliance. *Clinical Cancer Research, 10*(20), 6847–6854. https://doi.org/10.1158/1078-0432.CCR-04-0744.
115. Dhillon, N., Aggarwal, B. B., Newman, R. A., et al. (2008). Phase II trial of curcumin in patients with advanced pancreatic cancer. *Clinical Cancer Research, 14*(14), 4491–4499. https://doi.org/10.1158/1078-0432.CCR-08-0024.
116. Kanai, M., Yoshimura, K., Asada, M., et al. (2011). A phase I/II study of gemcitabine-based chemotherapy plus curcumin for patients with gemcitabine-resistant pancreatic cancer. *Cancer Chemotherapy and Pharmacology, 68*(1), 157–164. https://doi.org/10.1007/s00280-010-1470-2.

117. Epelbaum, R., Schaffer, M., Vizel, B., Badmaev, V., & Bar-Sela, G. (2010). Curcumin and gemcitabine in patients with advanced pancreatic cancer. *Nutrition and Cancer, 62*(8), 1137–1141. https://doi.org/10.1080/01635581.2010.513802.
118. Hoca, M., Becer, E., Kabadayı, H., Yücecan, S., & Vatansever, H. S. (2019). The effect of resveratrol and quercetin on epithelial-mesenchymal transition in pancreatic cancer stem cell. *Nutrition and Cancer*, 1–12. https://doi.org/10.1080/01635581.2019.1670853.
119. Kato, A., Naiki-Ito, A., Nakazawa, T., et al. (2015). Chemopreventive effect of resveratrol and apocynin on pancreatic carcinogenesis via modulation of nuclear phosphorylated GSK3β and ERK1/2. *Oncotarget, 6*(40), 42963–42975. https://doi.org/10.18632/oncotarget.5981.
120. Cheng, L., Yan, B., Chen, K., et al. (2018). Resveratrol-induced downregulation of NAF-1 enhances the sensitivity of pancreatic cancer cells to gemcitabine via the ROS/Nrf2 signaling pathways. *Oxidative Medicine and Cellular Longevity*. https://doi.org/10.1155/2018/9482018.
121. Ding, X.-Z., & Adrian, T. E. (2002). Resveratrol inhibits proliferation and induces apoptosis in human pancreatic cancer cells. *Pancreas, 25*(4), e71.
122. Fu, J., Shrivastava, A., Shrivastava, S. K., Srivastava, R. K., & Shankar, S. (2019). Triacetyl resveratrol upregulates miRNA-200 and suppresses the Shh pathway in pancreatic cancer: A potential therapeutic agent. *International Journal of Oncology, 54*(4), 1306–1316. https://doi.org/10.3892/ijo.2019.4700.
123. Kuroiwa, Y., Nishikawa, A., Kitamura, Y., et al. (2006). Protective effects of benzyl isothiocyanate and sulforaphane but not resveratrol against initiation of pancreatic carcinogenesis in hamsters. *Cancer Letters, 241*(2), 275–280. https://doi.org/10.1016/j.canlet.2005.10.028.
124. Shankar, S., Nall, D., Tang, S.-N., et al. (2011). Resveratrol inhibits pancreatic cancer stem cell characteristics in human and KrasG12D transgenic mice by inhibiting pluripotency maintaining factors and epithelial-mesenchymal transition. *PLoS One, 6*(1). https://doi.org/10.1371/journal.pone.0016530.
125. Nguyen, A. V., et al. (2009). Results of a phase I pilot clinical trial examining the effect of plant-derived resveratrol and grape powder on Wnt pathway target gene expression in colonic mucosa and colon cancer. *Cancer Management and Research, 1*, 25–37.
126. Howells, L. M., et al. (2011). Phase I randomized, double-blind pilot study of micronized resveratrol (SRT501) in patients with hepatic metastases—Safety, pharmacokinetics, and pharmacodynamics. *Cancer Prevention Research (Philadelphia, PA.), 4*, 1419–1425.
127. Patel, K. R., et al. (2010). Clinical pharmacology of resveratrol and its metabolites in colorectal cancer patients. *Cancer Research, 70*, 7392–7399.
128. Zhu, W., et al. (2012). Trans-resveratrol alters mammary promoter hypermethylation in women at increased risk for breast cancer. *Nutrition and Cancer, 64*, 393–400.
129. Popat, R., et al. (2013). A phase 2 study of SRT501 (resveratrol) with bortezomib for patients with relapsed and or refractory multiple myeloma. *British Journal of Haematology, 160*, 714–717.
130. Boocock, D. J., et al. (2007). Phase I dose escalation pharmacokinetic study in healthy volunteers of resveratrol, a potential cancer chemopreventive agent. *Cancer Epidemiology, Biomarkers & Prevention, 16*, 1246–1252.
131. Burkon, A., & Somoza, V. (2008). Quantification of free and protein-bound trans-resveratrol metabolites and identification of trans-resveratrol-C/O-conjugated diglucuronides – Two novel resveratrol metabolites in human plasma. *Molecular Nutrition & Food Research, 52*, 549–557.
132. Nunes, T., et al. (2009). Pharmacokinetics of trans-resveratrol following repeated administration in healthy elderly and young subjects. *Journal of Clinical Pharmacology, 49*, 1477–1482.
133. Chow, H.-H. S., et al. (2010). Resveratrol modulates drug and carcinogen metabolizing enzymes in a healthy volunteer study. *Cancer Prevention Research (Philadelphia, PA.), 3*, 1168–1175.
134. Brown, V. A., et al. (2010). Repeat dose study of the cancer chemopreventive agent resveratrol in healthy volunteers: Safety, pharmacokinetics, and effect on the insulin-like growth factor axis. *Cancer Research, 70*, 9003–9011.

Chapter 12
Role of Dietary Supplementation of Natural Products in the Prevention and Treatment of Liver Diseases

Sathish Kumar Mungamuri and Yamini Javvadi

Abstract The practice of medicine using either natural agents as they are or derivatives of natural products for treating the human diseases is commonly referred to as "natural medicine" or "naturotherapy." The usage of naturotherapy has been there for thousands of years for many human diseases. Naturopathy medication, by definition, must exist in the nature, and is generally used without addition of any chemicals, without or with marginal processing. Herbs, diet supplements, plant derivatives, nutrient supplementation, etc. generally fall into the category of natural medication. Liver, being the most important in detoxification of chemicals and major regulator of body energy storage and expenditure as well as the central hub of metabolic activity, is constantly under the pressure of getting damaged. Humans encounter many liver diseases like alcoholic liver disease, nonalcoholic fatty liver disease, nonalcoholic steatohepatitis, cirrhosis, hepatitis, and cancer. The prevalence of liver diseases is increasing each year, demanding the high need for developing effective therapies. Although, over the years, we have achieved a considerable advance in liver disease prevention, screening, diagnostic, and treatment methodologies, the rate of liver diseases is in continuous rise. In addition, because targeted therapy for liver diseases is not much successful till now, the appreciation related to traditional herbal medicine is constantly increasing. In this chapter, we discuss briefly few of the herbal plants, which showed efficacy in in vitro studies. We also highlight the preclinical evaluation undertaken for each of these plants towards the goal for healing a variety of liver diseases.

Keywords Naturopathy · Natural medicine · Herbal medicine · Herbal plants · Liver disease · Hepatocellular carcinoma · Liver cirrhosis

S. K. Mungamuri (✉)
Division of Food Safety, Indian Council of Medical Research - National Institute of Nutrition, Hyderabad, Telangana, India

Y. Javvadi
Department of Biotechnology, Sri Padmavathi Mahila Visvavidyalayam, Tirupati, Andhra Pradesh, India

G. P. Nagaraju (ed.), *Phytochemicals Targeting Tumor Microenvironment in Gastrointestinal Cancers*, https://doi.org/10.1007/978-3-030-48405-7_12

Abbreviations

ACP	Acid phosphatase
ALD	Alcoholic liver disease
ALP	Alkaline phosphatase
ALT	Alanine transaminase
AST/SGOT	Serum glutamic-oxaloacetic transaminase
HBV	Hepatitis B virus
HCC	Hepatocellular carcinoma
HCV	Hepatitis C virus
LC	Liver cirrhosis
LP	Liquid paraffin
LPS	Lipopolysaccharide
NAFLD	Nonalcoholic fatty liver disease
NASH	Nonalcoholic steatohepatitis
PPARα	Peroxisome proliferator-activated receptor-alpha
SREBP-1	Sterol-regulatory element-binding protein-1

1 Introduction

Liver is the largest gland of the body weighing about 1.4 kg in average adult. The most impressive fact about liver is its potency to regenerate completely even with a minimum of $1/4^{th}$ of the tissue remaining, without interruption of its functions. It has both secretary and excretory functions such as (1) metabolism of carbohydrates, proteins, and lipids; (2) storage of vitamins and minerals; (3) processing of drugs and hormones; (4) synthesis of bile salts; (6) supporting blood clot formation; (7) phagocytosis; (8) hematopoietic function; (9) hemolysis; (10) activation of vitamin D; and (11) excretion of bilirubin. It is not of much surprise that liver is more prone to diseases, as it performs many multidimensional functions. Intake of high-fat diet, high alcohol consumption, and exposure to harmful pollutants/carcinogens often lead to various chronic liver diseases like hepatitis (HBV or HCV related), ALD, NAFLD, NASH, LC, and HCC in humans. With each passing year, there has been increasing evidence supporting a very high prevalence of these liver diseases; among that HCC is the sixth most commonly diagnosed cancer and fourth leading cause of cancer deaths worldwide and it alone contributes to 782,000 deaths in 2018. According to the GLOBOCAN reports 841,000 new cases were reported with HCC in 2018 [1]. In a meta-analysis, the global prevalence of NAFLD is 25.2% and NASH is between 1.5% and 6.5% [2]. A modeling study conducted in the United States estimated that the prevalence of NASH will increase up to 63% by 2030, which ultimately leads to increased incidence of NASH-related diseases like cirrhosis, HCC, and deaths [3]. Although there are great advances in the prevention, screening, and novel technologies in the diagnosis and treatment, the survival rate remains low. The efficiency of current synthetic therapeutic agents like cisplatin, 5-fluorouracil, doxorubicin, orlistat, sibutramine, and rimonabant in treating chronic liver disease is not satisfactory and these chemicals have undesirable side effects. Moreover, some diseases like NAFLD and NASH have no FDA-approved therapy till date [4]. Thus, in order to prevent and treat these liver diseases, effective medications and treatment strategies need to be developed. In that scenario, plants and plant derivatives seem like torchbearer to the modern research. There is a constant increase in the research investment in traditional herbal medicine, which was previously underappreciated. In this chapter, we briefly discuss various herbal plants, which showed efficacy in in vitro studies, as well as highlight their preclinical evaluation for treating various liver diseases (Table 12.1).

1.1 Andrographis paniculata *(Burm. f.) Nees* *(*A. paniculata*)*

Andrographis paniculata (Acanthaceae), commonly known as the "king of bitters," is a renowned hepatoprotective and hepatostimulant agent [5]. Along with its hepatoprotective activity, this plant is also traditionally used for curing diabetes [6], malaria [7], and snake bite. Protective effects of this plant are credited to the presence of major phytoconstituents "andrographolide and arabinogalactan" [8].

Preclinical Studies Preclinical studies by Singha et al. proved that intraperitoneal administration of andrographolide and arabinogalactan protein of *A. paniculata* is responsible for hepatoprotective effects. Reduction in the levels of biochemical parameters (AST, ALT, ACP, ALP, and LP) in the liver and kidneys is indicative of its benefit [8]. There are studies reporting that *A. paniculata* exhibits hepatoprotective effects against thioacetamide (TAA)-induced hepatic fibrogenesis and cirrhosis in rats by decreasing collagen production and inflammation response in the mice [9, 10]. It was reported that, in adult male rats, ethanol extracts of *A. paniculata* inhibit intrahepatic cholestasis by regulating the NF-κB signaling [11]. The treatment with andrographolide protects the liver from H_2O_2 and LPS/D-GalN-induced liver damage [12, 13].

1.2 Amaranthus spinosus *Linn*

Amaranthus spinosus L. (Amaranthaceae) commonly known as "chaulai" is an annual herb distributed all over the world. The leaves of *A. spinosus* have high medicinal value. It is used to ward off swelling around stomach and to cure hepatic disorders, jaundice, scanty urine, and wounds [14, 15]. *A. spinosus* is well known for its antimalarial [16] and antioxidant properties [17]. *A. spinosus* comprises a number of bioactive components like kaempferol, diglycosides, quercetin, amaranthine, isoamaranthine, betanin, isobetanin, and hydroxycinnamates [18].

Preclinical Studies In an in vivo study by Hussain et al., alcoholic extract of *A. spinosus* showed potential hepatoprotective activity [19]. Results of yet another finding revealed that 50% of ethanolic whole-plant extract of *A. spinosus* protects the liver against D-galactosamine/LPS-induced liver injury in rats [20]. All these results signify the potential application of this herb for treatment against liver problems.

1.3 Cynara cardunculus

Cynara cardunculus L. (Asteraceae), generally known as artichoke, is a perennial thistle. This plant is vastly distributed in Southern Europe, where it is consumed as vegetable and is also formulated in herbal tea. The extracts of *C. cardunculus* have been widely used since decades in folk medicine to treat hepatitis, diabetes, rheumatism, urinary stones, and various hepatobiliary diseases. It also has hypolipidemic and hypoglycemic effects [21]. Artichokes are classified as functional food [22], and the edible flower of artichoke is known to have a health protective potential and also strengthens the liver and gallbladder functions [23]. The major components of artichoke are naringenin, apigenin glycosides, luteolin-7-glucoside, and high levels of inulin [21, 22].

Preclinical and Clinical Studies Both in vitro and in vivo studies have reported the hepatoprotective, anticarcinogenic, and hypocholesterolemic functions of *Cynara cardunculus* [24, 25].

1.4 Cichorium intybus

Cichorium intybus (Asteraceae), commonly known as chicory, is a perennial herbaceous plant. In Ayurvedic medicine, chicory seeds are used in hepatobiliary disorders and in Persian folk medicine and the seeds and leaves of *C. intybus* are considered as hepatoprotective and antidiabetic [26]. The phytochemical esculetin is a phenolic compound of *C. intybus* [27].

Preclinical Studies In an in vivo study, it was reported that the extracts of *C. intybus* seeds, root, and root callus showed hepatoprotective activity against acetaminophen and CCl_4-induced hepatic damage [28, 29]. Pretreatment of rats with esculetin also prevented CCl_4 and paracetamol-induced hepatic injury [27]. Cichotyboside is a component isolated from the seeds of *C. intybus*, and exhibited hepatoprotective activity similar to silymarin against CCl_4-induced toxicity in Wistar rats [30]. Ziamajidi et al. showed that chicory seed extracts will have ameliorative affect against oleic acid-induced non-alcoholic fatty liver disease NAFLD/NASH via modulation of PPARα and SREBP-1 [31].

1.5 Curcuma longa *L.*

Curcuma longa L. (Zingiberaceae) is commonly known as turmeric, wherein curcumin is the main active ingredient. It has been used since ages in the Indian subcontinent to treat various illnesses such as rheumatism, body pains, skin diseases, intestinal worms, diarrhea, intermittent fevers, hepatic disorders, biliousness, urinary discharges, dyspepsia, inflammations, constipation, leukoderma, amenorrhea, and colic. This research is much focused on curcumin, because of its potentiality to treat many diseases without any side effects. Curcumin has the ability to treat a wide variety of inflammatory diseases, cancer, diabetes, cardiovascular diseases, arthritis, Alzheimer's disease, psoriasis, etc., through modulation of numerous molecular targets [32]. This provides a rational molecular basis to use Curcumin for treating hepatic disorders [33].

Preclinical Studies It was reported that curcumin protects from liver injury induced by ethanol, thioacetamide, iron overdose, cholestasis, and acute subchronic and chronic CCl_4 intoxication. Furthermore, it can reverse CCl_4-induced cirrhosis to some extent [33]. *Curcuma longa* extracts also reduced the visceral fat and delayed pathogenesis in HBV-X protein transgenic mice [34]. The administration of curcumin had also reduced the hyperplastic nodules, liver damage markers, body weight, and hypoproteinemia in the liver of diethyl-nitrosamine/phenobarbital-challenged Wistar rats. It also demonstrated anticancer activity against chemical-induced hepatocarcinogenesis [35].

1.6 Cassia occidentalis

Cassia occidentalis (Fabaceae) is also known as Senna coffee/Negro coffee and it is a communal wild plant. This plant is considered as an important ingredient of several polyherbal preparations marketed for liver diseases. This plant has several biological activities such as blood purification, anti-allergic, anti-inflammatory, antioxidant [36], antinociceptive, antifungal, antidiabetic, hepatoprotective, hypolipidemic, and anti-atherosclerogenic activities [37]. *C. occidentalis* is also traditionally used to cure hepato-myo-encephalopathy and skin diseases like psoriasis and leprosy [38]. Bioactive constituents are mainly achrosin, aloeemodin, cassia occidentanol I, cassia occidentanol II, emodin, anthraquinones, anthrones, apigenin, aurantiobtusin, campesterol, cassiollin, chryso-obtusin, chrysophanic acid, chrysarobin, chrysophanol, and chrysoeriol.

Preclinical Studies Jafri et al. demonstrated the hepatoprotective role of aqueous ethanolic extract of leaves of *C. occidentalis* against paracetamol-induced liver injury. The conclusive remark was in the favor of significant hepatoprotection [39].

1.7 Citrus paradise

The common name of *Citrus paradise* (Rutaceae) is grapefruit. Grapefruit is prized for its high content of vitamin C, folic acid, phenolic acid, potassium, calcium, iron, limonoids, terpenes, monoterpenes, and D-glucaric acid. It is an incredible source of many phytochemicals and nutrients that contribute to a healthy diet. Naringin is the flavonoid in greatest concentration in the grapefruit, and in humans it is metabolized into naringenin [40, 41]. β-Carotene and lycopene are present in red and pink grapefruit varieties. It has been used in traditional medicine for its antimicrobial, antifungal, anti-inflammatory, antioxidant, antiviral, anticarcinogenic, and anti-allergic properties [42, 43].

Preclinical Studies The study conducted by Lee et al. revealed so many interesting facts about naringenin and its future perspectives. Oral administration of naringenin notably diminished DMN-induced hepatic damage in rats. It also restored natural protein levels. Finally they concluded that naringenin had anti-fibrinogenic and hepatoprotective effects, suggesting that it could be useful in the treatment of hepatic fibrosis [44]. It was reported that the administration of naringenin to rats with ethanol-induced liver injury considerably decreased the levels of ALT, AST, and thiobarbituric acid-reactive substances and significantly increased the levels of antioxidant enzymes. Further, in their study these biochemical parameters correlated well with the histological changes [45]. In a similar study, it was proved that naringenin ameliorated the cadmium-induced oxidative damage in the rat liver [46]. Taken together these findings suggest that naringenin has a therapeutic potential to treat liver diseases.

1.8 Crocus sativus *L.*

Crocus sativus L. belongs to Iridaceae family and it is native to Asia. The dried stigmas of *C. sativus* are known as saffron, and have been used as flavoring agent since ancient times. It has been used to treat various diseases like insomnia, cognitive defects, cardiovascular diseases, and cancer. The therapeutic efficiency of saffron is mainly due to its major bioactive derivatives crocin, crocetin, picrocrocin, and safranal [47, 48]. The research over the past few years revealed that saffron plays a dominant role in the pathophysiology of some important pathological conditions like atherosclerosis, metabolic syndrome, liver cancer, neurodegenerative diseases, asthma, and allergy.

Preclinical Studies Recently, the results of an in vivo comparative study of anticancer activity between saffron extracts and its bioactive component crocetin demonstrated that crocetin was more potent in inducing cytotoxicity in cancer cells than saffron extracts. The overall highlight of this research is that crocetin is a potential anticancer agent that can be used for cancer prevention and treatment [49]. In an in vivo study, crocin showed hepatoprotective activity against the oxidative stress and inflammation caused by methotrexate [50]. It was reported that the pretreatment with *Crocus sativus* petals guards the liver from the damage caused by acetaminophen in animal models [51]. Crocin administration also showed hepatoprotective activity against the liver damage induced by morphine [52].

1.9 Daucus carota

Daucus carota (Apiaceae) is the scientific name of carrot. Carrot is called as vitaminized food due to the presence of numerous phytonutrients like phenolics, polyacetylenes, carotenoids, and ascorbic acid [53]. They are considered as a functional food with significant health-promoting properties. *D. carota* is the excellent source of vitamin A to treat night blindness. Besides its antioxidant property, it also has anticancer [54, 55], antimutagenic, chemopreventive, photoprotective, and immune-enhancing properties and is also able to activate the platelets [56].

Preclinical Studies The methanolic extracts of *Daucus carota* seeds had showed hepatoprotective and antioxidant activity against thioacetamide-induced oxidative stress in experimental rat models (Singh, [57]). Bishayee et al. demonstrated that carrot extract offers a significant hepatoprotective activity against CCl_4-induced liver damage in experimental animals [58].

1.10 Eclipta alba

Eclipta alba (Asteraceae) commonly known as bhringaraj is a perennial shrub mostly found in moist tropical countries. *E. alba* contains alkaloids, flavonoids, glycosides, polyacetylenes, and triterpenoids. Wedelolactone and demethyl wedelolactone are coumestan and are also mainly found in *Eclipta alba*. In traditional medicine, it is extensively used for treatments such as to grow hair, for gastrointestinal disorders, and also as hepatoprotective and neuroprotective agent [59, 60].

Preclinical Studies The coumestan constituents of *E. alba* showed potent antihepatotoxic activities in CCL_4-, galactosamine-, and phalloidin-induced liver damage in animal models [61]. In a recent study by Naik et al., *E. alba* showed protective activities against hyperlipidemia induced by high-fat diet in animal models [62].

1.11 Ficus carica

Ficus carica (Moraceae), commonly known as fig, is a small tree grown in many countries. It has many nutritive and medicinal properties and it was widely used in ancient systems of medicine as an antibacterial, antifungal, antioxidant, and antiviral agent. Every part of this plant has a unique medicinal value. Fig fruit and roots are used to cure indigestion, anorexia, cardiovascular problems, and cancers. In addition, fig leaf is also used against the anemia [63]. *F. carica* leaves are reported to have high phenolic substance, organic acid content, and antioxidant potential than fig pulp and crusts [64]. *F. carica* is useful in treating liver and spleen disorders, and gout and leaves are especially used for treating jaundice. Furanocoumarins, psoralen, and daidzein are the phytoconstituents of *F. carica* leaves [65].

Preclinical Studies Gond and Khadabadi had reported that the petroleum ether extracts of fig leaves provided promising results in the treatment of rifampicin-induced hepatic damage in rat models [66]. Recently, in an in vivo study, *F. carica* has been shown to play a modulatory protective role in the liver and kidney against γ-irradiation. These authors have recommended that *F. carica* should be included in everyday diet [67].

1.12 Fumaria indica

Fumaria indica (Fumariaceae) is commonly called as parpata. It is a small annual herb that widely grows in plain sand lower hills. It has been used as a liver-protective agent. However the limited evidence suggests that more research should be carried out. The active components of *Fumaria indica* are protopine and fumariline [68]. *F. indica* is used as a blood purifier in skin diseases, styptic and febrifuge, and is also used in the disorder of liver in folk medicine. However, overdose of *F. indica* may cause diarrhea [69].

Preclinical Studies Rathi et al. in their study showed that butanol extracts of *F. indica* lead to hepatoprotection [70]. The effect of methanolic extract of *Fumaria indica* was evaluated in albino rats and the results demonstrated the anti-hepatotoxic activity of monomethyl fumarate [71].

1.13 Ginkgo biloba *L.*

Ginkgo biloba L. (Ginkgoaceae) is also known as maidenhair tree. The leaves of *G. biloba* occupied a unique status in Chinese traditional medicine. Ginkgo is widely used to cure Alzheimer's and dementia, and this plant has cardioprotective, anti-asthmatic, antioxidant, antidiabetic, hepatoprotective, photoprotective, and anti-inflammatory activities [72–74]. Flavonol glycosides (quercetin, kaempferol, and isorhamnetin), shikimic acid, bilobanone, and ginkgolides are the phytoconstituents of *G. biloba*. Ginseng is a widely used drug derived from *Ginkgo biloba*. There are numerous studies showing the hepatoprotective activity of *G. biloba* [75]. However, in certain cases, it has been shown to cause skin allergic reactions [76].

Preclinical Studies Naik and Panda had reported that the oral administration of *Ginkgo biloba* phytosomes (GBP) showed remarkable hepatoprotection proportionate to silymarin [73]. In another finding, GBP exhibited hepatoprotective effects against CCl_4-induced oxidative damage [77].

1.14 Glycyrrhiza glabra

Glycyrrhiza glabra (Fabaceae) is commonly known as licorice. Glycyrrhiza species are the most important herbaceous plants in traditional Chinese medicine. *G. glabra* has diverse pharmacological activities [78]. Hippocrates prescribed *G. glabra* for the treatment of chest diseases, including dry cough and asthma. Glycyrrhizin is the major bioactive constituent and is mainly found in the *G. glabra* root. Glycyrrhizin is anti-inflammatory and antiviral by nature. It has been used for the treatment of chronic hepatitis and tumors and for the protection of liver functions. Glycyrrhizin had a protective effect against immunosuppression and an effect of reducing the incidence of sodium and water retention [79]. There are no obvious side effects reported.

Preclinical studies Intraperitoneal administration of glycyrrhizin and epidermal growth factor (EGF) has been shown to stimulate both liver regeneration and recovery of liver functions in rats after the surgical removal of 70% of the total liver [80]. Glycyrrhizin also protects the liver from LPS [81] and CCl_4-induced liver damage [82]. In an in vivo study, glycyrrhizin has been found to suppress the release of HCV particle, when it is used alone or combined with interferon [83]. In a similar study, glycyrrhizin inhibited the liver inflammation in concanavalin-A (Con A)-induced hepatitis mice model, which closely imitated the pathology of human autoimmune hepatitis [84]. In a clinical study, it was reported that lamivudine combined with glycyrrhizin is effective in controlling HBV replication in cancer patients [85]. Overall, it is noteworthy that glycyrrhizin has the therapeutic potential to prevent liver injury and hepatitis.

1.15 Phyllanthus emblica

Phyllanthus emblica (Phyllanthaceae) is commonly called as amla (Indian gooseberry). Amla is an Indian indigenous system of medicine and has eminent position in traditional medicine all over the world. Every part of this plant has significant medicinal value. The fruits have been widely used to treat liver disorders, diabetes, cancer, diarrhea, jaundice, inflammation, blood pressure, sore throat, dry mouth, indigestion, abdominal pain, and cough [86]. Tannins, flavonoids, vitamins, amino acids, and carbohydrates are the most important constituents of *P. emblica*. Among those, hydrolyzable tannins (e.g., gallic acid, ellagic acid, corilagin, chebulagic acid, and geraniin) are predominant active constituents of *P. emblica* [87].

Preclinical Studies In a recent study, it was reported that the water extract of *P. emblica* fruits shows a protective effect on high-fat diet-induced NAFLD in SD rats [88]. Further, it significantly decreased fat accumulation and ROS production in HepG2 cells and also inhibited hepatic fibrosis in HSC-T6 cells [88]. There are a number of studies reporting that gallic acid protects the liver from injuries induced by various hepatotoxic agents, including paracetamol, sodium fluoride, cyclophosphamide, and carbon tetrachloride in vivo [89–92]. Hsu and Yen proved that intake of gallic acid reduces dyslipidemia and hepatosteatosis in high-fat diet-induced rats [93]. In a similar study, Chao et al. found that gallic acid ameliorates the NAFLD pathogenesis [94]. Like gallic acid, ellagic acid also showed hepatoprotective activity against paracetamol-, CCl_4-, alcohol-, D-galactosamine-, and concanavalin-induced hepatocarcinogenesis as well as showed antiviral properties against HBV and HCV, in murine models [95]. Corilagin was also identified to be highly effective in retarding the growth of xenografted Hep3B hepatocellular carcinoma cells [96].

1.16 Picrorhiza kurroa

Picrorhiza kurroa (Plantaginaceae) is one of the oldest medicinal plants commonly known as kutki. The root extracts of *P. kurroa* possess strong hepatoprotective activity [97]. *P. kurroa* includes chemical components such as picroside I, picroside II, and iridoid glycosides D-mannitol, cucurbitacins, kutkiol, kutki sterol, and apocynin, which are powerful anti-inflammatory agents and platelet aggregation reducers. The mixture of kutkoside and picroside I is known as picroliv. Picroliv is a highly active component of root extracts and it is primarily involved in the regeneration of liver parenchyma cells, protein, and nucleic acid synthesis and stimulates immune response during acute and chronic toxicity [98]. Since decades *P. kurroa* has been used in the treatment of anemia, asthma, obesity, malaria, stomach ache, fever, immune disorders, skin diseases, bronchial asthma, as well as viral hepatitis. It is a powerful anti-inflammatory, a cathartic, and a cholagogue agent. Picroliv and vimlin are the commercially available herbal products of *P. kurroa*. No harmful side effects have been reported yet.

Preclinical Studies Picroliv exhibits a strong hepatoprotective activity against aflatoxin B1 (AFB1)-induced hepatotoxicity [99]. In an in vivo study picroliv ameliorated the effect of cadmium-induced hepatotoxicity [100].

1.17 Scutellaria baicalensis Georgi

Scutellaria baicalensis Georgi (Lamiaceae) is often referred to as golden herb/skull cap and Huang-Qin (Chinese) and it is native to East Asian countries with over 2000 years of history. The wide array of pharmacological activities of *Scutellaria baicalensis Georgi* made the plant to be named in two ancient books, namely (1) The Classic of Herbal Medicine (written between 200 and 250 AD) and (2) Compendium of Materia Medica (published in the year 1593). *Scutellaria baicalensis Georgi* is used in the treatment of cold, lung and liver problems [101], diarrhea, dysentery, hypertension, hemorrhaging, insomnia, and respiratory infections. It shows antiviral, anticarcinogenic, free radical scavenging, antioxidant, immunostimulatory, and antiproliferative effects on vascular smooth muscle cells and hepatic stellate cells [102, 103]. Baicalein, wogonin, and wogonoside are the known flavonoids of *S. baicalensis*. Baicalein is widely explored for its medicinal properties and it is the important component of Xiao Chai Hu Tang (Chinese) or Sho-saiko-to (SST, Japanese) herbal formulations prescribed for human liver diseases [104, 105].

Preclinical Studies In an in vitro study, baicalin was proved to be able to protect hepatocytes from oxidative stress [106]. A growing number of studies had confirmed that baicalin offers hepatoprotective activity against liver injury [107–110].

1.18 Silybum marianum

The common name of *Silybum marianum* (Asteraceae) is milk thistle. The fruit of *S. marianum* contains silymarin, which is responsible for its hepatoprotective activity. Silymarin is a complex mixture of silychristin, silybin, and silymarin [111]. Silymarin is well recognized for its four main functions: (1) free radical scavenging activity, (2) membrane permeability regulation, (3) stimulation of DNA polymerase I, and (4) regeneration of liver cells and protein synthesis [112]. The extracts of this plant are used as liver tonics in traditional medicine to prevent hepatotoxicity and to solubilize the gallstones. This plant is also used for treating alcoholic liver disease, acute and chronic viral hepatitis, diabetes, hay fever, inflammation, and constipation. Legalon is a commercially available product of *S. marianum* being used in liver ailments. Mild laxative effects are reported in patients with silymarin sensitivity (Table 12.1).

Preclinical Studies Salam et al. reported that the administration of silymarin in combination with MSP showed protective activity against the CCl_4-induced hepatocellular necrosis [113]. A similar study conducted by Kim et al. provided evidence that the mixture of aloe vera and *Silybum marianum*, and *Ginkgo biloba* and *Silybum marianum*, had hepatoprotective effects against chronic and acute lesions induced by the organochlorine (OC) compound and N-nitrosodiethyl-amine (NDEA), respectively [114]. Silymarin reduces the liver injury caused by acetaminophen, CCl_4,

Table 12.1 List of herbal plants showing promise towards treatment of various liver diseases

S. no.	Name of the plant	Part used	Chemical constituent/ active component	Animal model	Hepatotoxic agent
1	*Amaranthus spinosus* (Amaranthaceae)	Whole plant	Amaranthine, isoamaranthine kaempferol, diglycosides, quercetin, betanin, isobetanin, hydroxycinnamates	Rats	LPS/D-GalN
2	*Andrographis paniculata* (Acanthaceae)	Whole plant	Andrographolide and arabinogalactan	Rats	Thioacetamide (TAA), hydrogen peroxide, and LPS/D-GalN
3	*Cynara cardunculus* (Asteraceae)				
4	*Cichorium intybus* (Asteraceae)	Seeds and root	Esculetin, cichotyboside	Rats	Acetaminophen and CCl4. Oleic acid-induced NAFLD
5	*Curcuma longa* (Zingiberaceae)	Root	Curcumin	Rats and mice	Thioacetamide, iron, and CCl4
6	*Cassia occidentalis* (Fabaceae)	Leaves	Achrosin, aloeemodin, cassia occidentanol I, cassia occidentanol II, emodin, anthraquinones, anthrones, apigenin, aurantiobtusin, campesterol, cassiollin, chrysoobtusin, chrysophanic acid, chrysarobin, chrysophanol, chrysoeriol	Rats	Acetaminophen
7	*Citrus paradise* (Rutaceae)	Fruit peel	Naringin	Rats	DMN and cadmium
8	*Crocus sativus* (Iridaceae)	Dried stigmas of flower	Crocin, crocetin, picrocrocin, and safranal	Rats	Methotrexate, acetaminophen, and morphine
9	*Daucus carota* (Apiaceae)	Seeds and roots	Phenolics, polyacetylenes, carotenoids, and ascorbic acid	Rats	Thioacetamide and CCl4
10	*Eclipta alba* (Asteraceae)	Whole plant	Coumestan (wedelolactone and demethyl wedelolactone)	Rats	Carbon tetrachloride, galactosamine, and phalloidin

(continued)

Table 12.1 (continued)

S. no.	Name of the plant	Part used	Chemical constituent/ active component	Animal model	Hepatotoxic agent
11	*Ficus carica* (Moraceae)	Roots, leaves, and fruit	Furanocoumarins, psoralen, and daidzein	Rats	Rifampicin and gamma radiation
12	*Fumaria indica* (Fumariaceae)	Whole plant	Protopine and fumariline	Rats	Carbon tetrachloride, paracetamol, and rifampicin
13	*Ginkgo biloba* L (Ginkgoaceae)	Seeds and leaves	Shikimic acid, bilobanone, and ginkgolides	Rats	CCl4
14	*Glycyrrhiza glabra* (Fabaceae)	Roots	Glycyrrhizin	Rats and mice	LPS, CCl4, and concanavalin-A
15	*Phyllanthus emblica* (Phyllanthaceae)	Fruit	Gallic acid, ellagic acid, corilagin, chebulagic acid, and geraniin	Rats	Paracetamol, sodium fluoride, cyclophosphamide, carbon tetrachloride, and concanavalin
16	*Picrorhiza kurroa* (Plantaginaceae)	Root	Picroside I, picroside II, and iridoid glycoside d-mannitol, cucurbitacins, kutkiol, kutki sterol, and apocynin	Rats	Aflatoxin B1 and cadmium
17	*Scutellaria baicalensis Georgi* (Lamiaceae)	Aerial parts	Baicalein, wogonin, and wogonoside	Rats	Iron, CCl4, and LPS/D-GalN
18	*Silybum marianum* (Asteraceae)	Whole plant	Silymarin (silychristin, silybin, and silymarin)	Rats	CCl4, organochlorine N-nitrosodiethylamine (NDEA) acetaminophen, iron, and phenylhydrazine
19	*Salvia miltiorrhiza Bunge* (Lamiaceae)	Root	Tanshinones	Rats	Iron, CCl4, and LPS/D-GalN
20	*Vitis vinifera* (Vitaceae)	Fruit and seed	Catechins, epicatechins, anthocyanidins, proanthocyanidins, and resveratrol	Rats	Methotrexate, DMN, and CCl4
21	*Zanthoxylum armatum* (Rutaceae)	Bark	Alpha- and beta-amyrins, fargesin, dictamine, berberine, xanthoplanine, armatamid, asarinin, and lupeol	Rats	CCl4

(continued)

Table 12.1 (continued)

S. no.	Name of the plant	Part used	Chemical constituent/ active component	Animal model	Hepatotoxic agent
22	*Zingiber officinale* (Zingiberaceae)	Rhizome	Gingerol, paradols, zingerone, zingiberol, and shogaol	Rats	DMN and piroxicam

The table shows the list of various herbs (along with the family they belong to) and the part of the plant and the active chemical ingredient. Various agents used in animal models for inducing hepatotoxicity and the protection given by each of the herb are also highlighted

radiation, iron overload, phenylhydrazine, alcohol, cold ischemia, and *Amanita phalloides* in animals (Chen, [115]). Silybin also exhibits significant anti-inflammatory effect in cirrhotic rat liver [116].

1.19 Salvia miltiorrhiza Bunge

Salvia miltiorrhiza Bunge (Lamiaceae) is also known as red sage/Chinese sage/ Danshen. More than 70 active components have been isolated and structurally identified from *S. miltiorrhiza* [117], and are broadly categorized into two groups: (1) hydrophilic compounds such as salvianolic acids and (2) lipophilic chemicals, including diterpenoid and tanshinones. Tanshinones are unique components to *S. miltiorrhiza*, and are not yet found in other Chinese herbs. Among the tanshinones, tanshinone I, tanshinone IIA, and cryptotanshinone are the foremost bioactive constituents with various pharmacological effects including antibacterial, antioxidant, antitumor, antiplatelet, and hepatoprotection [118] activities. *S. miltiorrhiza* can increase blood flow into the liver to reduce the potential damage by clearing the harmful substance in the liver. The extracts of *S. miltiorrhiza* (tanshinones) are traditionally used in the treatment of cardiovascular and cerebrovascular diseases, cirrhosis [119, 120], and cancer [121, 122]. Its product, Fu fang Dan shen Di wan, is the first Chinese herbal medicine approved by the FDA for clinical tests in the United States.

Preclinical Studies It was reported that the active ingredients of *S. miltiorrhiza* showed hepatoprotective effect against CCl_4-induced liver injury in rats [123]. In an interesting study, treatment of chronic iron-overloaded mice with *S. miltiorrhiza* improved the hepatic morphology, and decreased the iron deposition [124]. Oral administration of cryptotanshinone from *S. miltiorrhiza* showed hepatoprotective effects against D-galactosamine (GalN)/lipopolysaccharide (LPS)-induced fulminant hepatic failure [125].

1.20 Vitis vinifera

Vitis vinifera is commonly called as grape vine. This plant is well known for its antioxidant, anticarcinogenic, immunomodulatory, anti-diabetes, anti-atherogenic, neuroprotective, anti-obesity, antiaging, and anti-infection properties. In addition, it has chemopreventive activity against cardiovascular disease and some cancers. Grape juice and grape seeds are rich sources of flavonoids such as catechins, epicatechins, anthocyanidins, proanthocyanidins, and resveratrol [126]. Resveratrol is a polyphenolic phytochemical and there are numerous studies signifying the hepatoprotective properties of resveratrol. Resveratrol can prevent hepatic damage caused by free radicals and inflammatory cytokines [127].

Preclinical Studies It was reported that the treatment with procyanidin in a liver cancer xenograft model exerted antiangiogenic activity in a dose-dependent manner [128]. The grape seed extracts from winery waste showed anticarcinogenic activity against HCC by promoting apoptosis in cancer cells [129]. Resveratrol showed hepatoprotective activity against methotrexate-induced hepatic injury [130], DMN-induced injury [131], and CCl_4-challenged liver tissue [132]. Resveratrol had been shown to activate the pro-apoptotic pathway in vivo [133]. These studies suggest that resveratrol can be used for treating liver injury, fibrosis, cirrhosis, and hepatocarcinogenesis.

1.21 Zanthoxylum armatum

Zanthoxylum armatum DC. (Rutaceae) is commonly called as Timur (or) Nepal pepper. *Z. armatum* is a sub-deciduous shrub and is being extensively used in the Indian System of Medicine over many years [134]. The phytochemical constituent's α- and β-amyrins, fargesin, dictamine, berberine, xanthoplanine, armatamid, asarinin, and lupeol have high pharmaceutical importance [135]. *Z. armatum* has anthelmintic, stomachic, and carminative properties [134]. The fruits and seed extracts are employed as an aromatic tonic in fever and dyspepsia, and for expelling roundworms [135]. No adverse effects have been reported yet for this natural product.

Preclinical Studies It was reported that the administration of ethanolic bark extracts of *Z. armatum* for 7 days shows hepatoprotective activity against CCl_4-induced liver injury in Wistar rats. *Z. armatum* extracts enhanced the level of antioxidants; reduced the level of AST, ALT, ALP, and serum enzymes; and led to the recovery of damaged cells [136].

1.22 Zingiber officinale

Zingiber officinale (Zingiberaceae), widely known as ginger, is a perennial plant and the rhizome is extensively used as a spice all over the world. It is very potent in treating arthritis, sore throat, indigestion, dementia, muscular aches, and fever [137–139]. Ginger is characterized as functional food to its nutritional and phytochemical composition. Gingerol, paradols, zingerone, zingiberol, and shogaol are the main phytochemicals of *Zingiber officinale* [140].

Preclinical Studies In an in vivo study, ginger essential oil (GEO) exhibited hepatoprotective activity through its antioxidant potential against alcoholic fatty liver disease [141]. Lai et al. reported that GEO exhibited protective effect against NAFLD induced by high-fat diet in mice [142]. Recent studies also highlighted that ginger also shows hepatoprotective activity against diethyl-nitrosamine- and piroxicam-induced liver hepatotoxicity [143, 144].

2 Conclusions

It is a known fact that liver is the vital organ of the body and it performs a minimum of 500 functions. So, it is more liable to diseases. To cure these diseases, many chemically synthesized drugs are invented. But their usage causes uncountable side effects than improving the pathogenesis condition. To overcome all these detriments, there is a continuous demand for alternative therapy. One of the holistic approaches to treat liver diseases is the use of "natural medicine." Natural therapy for liver diseases is increasing worldwide, mainly because of their safety and efficacy, but also because of their relative expediency. Having said that, there is a great lack of comprehensiveness and huge controversies, regarding the safety and the mechanisms of action of these natural medicines. Having said that, it should not be taken by any means that the natural therapy does not have side effects. The most common side effects of using natural compounds include injury to liver, intestinal pneumonia, and acute respiratory failure, of which the licensed naturopathic doctors are aware. Although the natural medication is beneficial therapeutically, utmost care needs to be taken while treating the side effects. To prevent the complications arising due to the natural medicine, it is strongly advised that these medicines should be prescribed only by the licensed and certified physicians.

In this communication, we presented a few of such plants. Some of these plants and plant derivatives show good and satisfactory results in basic experimental and preclinical studies. However, more studies are required to evaluate the effects of these compounds before clinical use. So, we should take a step forward to develop these phytoconstituents into medicines. As prevention is always better than cure, we should include these plants and their products in diet. The two reasons, (1) often people thinking that natural medicines have no side effects and (2) lack of regulations to oversee the utilization of natural medicine, are the major concerns that often lead to long-term and excess consumption of natural drugs that often bring undesirable reactions. Finally, both the doctor and the patient should be aware of the risks involved in taking the natural medicine and be careful while going for the natural therapy for liver diseases.

Conflict of Interest The authors declare no conflict of interest related to this book chapter.

References

1. Bray, F., Ferlay, J., Soerjomataram, I., Siegel, R. L., Torre, L. A., & Jemal, A. (2018). Global cancer statistics 2018: GLOBOCAN estimates of incidence and mortality worldwide for 36 cancers in 185 countries. *CA: a Cancer Journal for Clinicians, 68*(6), 394–424.
2. Younossi, Z., & Henry, L. (2016). Contribution of alcoholic and nonalcoholic fatty liver disease to the burden of liver-related morbidity and mortality. *Gastroenterology, 150*(8), 1778–1785.
3. Estes, C., Razavi, H., Loomba, R., Younossi, Z., & Sanyal, A. J. (2018). Modeling the epidemic of nonalcoholic fatty liver disease demonstrates an exponential increase in burden of disease. *Hepatology, 67*(1), 123–133.
4. Kleiner, D. E., & Makhlouf, H. R. (2016). Histology of nonalcoholic fatty liver disease and nonalcoholic steatohepatitis in adults and children. *Clinics in Liver Disease, 20*(2), 293–312.
5. Trivedi, N. P., & Rawal, U. M. (2001). Hepatoprotective and antioxidant property of Andrographis paniculata (Nees) in BHC induced liver damage in mice. *Indian Journal of Experimental Biology, 39*(1), 41–46.
6. Subramanian, R., Asmawi, M. Z., & Sadikun, A. (2008). In vitro alpha-glucosidase and alpha-amylase enzyme inhibitory effects of Andrographis paniculata extract and andrographolide. *Acta Biochimica Polonica, 55*(2), 391–398.
7. Mishra, K., Dash, A. P., Swain, B. K., & Dey, N. (2009). Anti-malarial activities of Andrographis paniculata and Hedyotis corymbosa extracts and their combination with curcumin. *Malaria Journal, 8*, 26.
8. Singha, P. K., Roy, S., & Dey, S. (2007). Protective activity of andrographolide and arabinogalactan proteins from Andrographis paniculata Nees against ethanol-induced toxicity in mice. *Journal of Ethnopharmacology, 111*(1), 13–21.
9. Abdulaziz Bardi, D., Halabi, M. F., Hassandarvish, P., Rouhollahi, E., Paydar, M., Moghadamtousi, S. Z., Al-Wajeeh, N. S., Ablat, A., Abdullah, N. A., & Abdulla, M. A. (2014). Andrographis paniculata leaf extract prevents thioacetamide-induced liver cirrhosis in rats. *PLoS One, 9*(10), e109424.
10. Lee, T. Y., Chang, H. H., Wen, C. K., Huang, T. H., & Chang, Y. S. (2014). Modulation of thioacetamide-induced hepatic inflammations, angiogenesis and fibrosis by andrographolide in mice. *Journal of Ethnopharmacology, 158 Pt A*, 423–430.
11. Khamphaya, T., Chansela, P., Piyachaturawat, P., Suksamrarn, A., Nathanson, M. H., & Weerachayaphorn, J. (2016). Effects of andrographolide on intrahepatic cholestasis induced by alpha-naphthylisothiocyanate in rats. *European Journal of Pharmacology, 789*, 254–264.
12. Mittal, S. P. K., Khole, S., Jagadish, N., Ghosh, D., Gadgil, V., Sinkar, V., & Ghaskadbi, S. S. (2016). Andrographolide protects liver cells from H2O2 induced cell death by upregulation of Nrf-2/HO-1 mediated via adenosine A2a receptor signalling. *Biochimica et Biophysica Acta, 1860*(11 Pt A), 2377–2390.
13. Pan, C. W., Yang, S. X., Pan, Z. Z., Zheng, B., Wang, J. Z., Lu, G. R., Xue, Z. X., & Xu, C. L. (2017). Andrographolide ameliorates d-galactosamine/lipopolysaccharide-induced acute liver injury by activating Nrf2 signaling pathway. *Oncotarget, 8*(25), 41202–41210.

14. Berghofer, E., & Schoenlechner, R. (2002). In P. S. Belton & J. R. N. Taylor (Eds.), *Grain Amaranth. Pseudocereals and less common cereals: Grain properties and utilization potential* (pp. 219–260). Berlin, Heidelberg: Springer.
15. Perumal Samy, R., Ignacimuthu, S., & Raja, D. P. (1999). Preliminary screening of ethnomedicinal plants from India. *Journal of Ethnopharmacology, 66*(2), 235–240.
16. Hilou, A., Nacoulma, O. G., & Guiguemde, T. R. (2006). In vivo antimalarial activities of extracts from Amaranthus spinosus L. and Boerhaavia erecta L. in mice. *Journal of Ethnopharmacology, 103*(2), 236–240.
17. Amin, I., Norazaidah, Y., & Hainida, K. I. E. (2006). Antioxidant activity and phenolic content of raw and blanched Amaranthus species. *Food Chemistry, 94*(1), 47–52.
18. Stintzing, F. C., Kammerer, D., Schieber, A., Adama, H., Nacoulma, O. G., & Carle, R. (2004). Betacyanins and phenolic compounds from Amaranthus spinosus L. and Boerhavia erecta L. *Z Naturforsch C J Biosci, 59*(1–2), 1–8.
19. Zeashan, H., Amresh, G., Singh, S., & Rao, C. V. (2008). Hepatoprotective activity of Amaranthus spinosus in experimental animals. *Food and Chemical Toxicology, 46*(11), 3417–3421.
20. Zeashan, H., Amresh, G., Singh, S., & Rao, C. V. (2010). Protective effect of Amaranthus spinosus against D-galactosamine/lipopolysaccharide-induced hepatic failure. *Pharmaceutical Biology, 48*(10), 1157–1163.
21. Colantuono, A., Ferracane, R., & Vitaglione, P. (2018). Potential bioaccessibility and functionality of polyphenols and cynaropicrin from breads enriched with artichoke stem. *Food Chemistry, 245*, 838–844.
22. Lattanzio, V., Kroon, P. A., Linsalata, V., & Cardinali, A. (2009). Globe artichoke: A functional food and source of nutraceutical ingredients. *Journal of Functional Foods, 1*(2), 131–144.
23. Shen, Q., Dai, Z., & Lu, Y. (2010). Rapid determination of caffeoylquinic acid derivatives in Cynara scolymus L. by ultra-fast liquid chromatography/tandem mass spectrometry based on a fused core C18 column. *Journal of Separation Science, 33*(20), 3152–3158.
24. Ferracane, R., Pellegrini, N., Visconti, A., Graziani, G., Chiavaro, E., Miglio, C., & Fogliano, V. (2008). Effects of different cooking methods on antioxidant profile, antioxidant capacity, and physical characteristics of artichoke. *Journal of Agricultural and Food Chemistry, 56*(18), 8601–8608.
25. Llorach, R., Espin, J. C., Tomas-Barberan, F. A., & Ferreres, F. (2002). Artichoke (Cynara scolymus L.) byproducts as a potential source of health-promoting antioxidant phenolics. *Journal of Agricultural and Food Chemistry, 50*(12), 3458–3464.
26. Pushparaj, P. N., Low, H. K., Manikandan, J., Tan, B. K., & Tan, C. H. (2007). Anti-diabetic effects of Cichorium intybus in streptozotocin-induced diabetic rats. *Journal of Ethnopharmacology, 111*(2), 430–434.
27. Gilani, A. H., Janbaz, K. H., & Shah, B. H. (1998). Esculetin prevents liver damage induced by paracetamol and CCL4. *Pharmacological Research, 37*(1), 31–35.
28. Gilani, A. H., & Janbaz, K. H. (1994). Evaluation of the liver protective potential of Cichorium intybus seed extract on acetaminophen and CCl4-induced damage. *Phytomedicine, 1*(3), 193–197.
29. Zafar, R., & Mujahid Ali, S. (1998). Anti-hepatotoxic effects of root and root callus extracts of Cichorium intybus L. *Journal of Ethnopharmacology, 63*(3), 227–231.
30. Ahmed, B., Khan, S., Masood, M. H., & Siddique, A. H. (2008). Anti-hepatotoxic activity of cichotyboside, a sesquiterpene glycoside from the seeds of Cichorium intybus. *Journal of Asian Natural Products Research, 10*(3–4), 223–231.
31. Ziamajidi, N., Khaghani, S., Hassanzadeh, G., Vardasbi, S., Ahmadian, S., Nowrouzi, A., Ghaffari, S. M., & Abdirad, A. (2013). Amelioration by chicory seed extract of diabetes- and oleic acid-induced non-alcoholic fatty liver disease (NAFLD)/non-alcoholic steatohepatitis (NASH) via modulation of PPARalpha and SREBP-1. *Food and Chemical Toxicology, 58*, 198–209.

32. Pari, L., Tewas, D., & Eckel, J. (2008). Role of curcumin in health and disease. *Archives of Physiology and Biochemistry, 114*(2), 127–149.
33. Rivera-Espinoza, Y., & Muriel, P. (2009). Pharmacological actions of curcumin in liver diseases or damage. *Liver International, 29*(10), 1457–1466.
34. Kim, J., Ha, H. L., Moon, H. B., Lee, Y. W., Cho, C. K., Yoo, H. S., & Yu, D. Y. (2011). Chemopreventive effect of Curcuma longa Linn on liver pathology in HBx transgenic mice. *Integrative Cancer Therapies, 10*(2), 168–177.
35. Sreepriya, M., & Bali, G. (2005). Chemopreventive effects of embelin and curcumin against N-nitrosodiethylamine/phenobarbital-induced hepatocarcinogenesis in Wistar rats. *Fitoterapia, 76*(6), 549–555.
36. Sreejith, G., Latha, P. G., Shine, V. J., Anuja, G. I., Suja, S. R., Sini, S., Shyama, S., Pradeep, S., Shikha, P., & Rajasekharan, S. (2010). Anti-allergic, anti-inflammatory and anti-lipid peroxidant effects of Cassia occidentalis Linn. *Indian Journal of Experimental Biology, 48* (5), 494–498.
37. Fidele, N., Joseph, B., Emmanuel, T., & Theophile, D. (2017). Hypolipidemic, antioxidant and anti-atherosclerogenic effect of aqueous extract leaves of Cassia. Occidentalis Linn (Caesalpiniaceae) in diet-induced hypercholesterolemic rats. *BMC Complementary and Alternative Medicine, 17*(1), 76.
38. Vashishtha, V. M., Kumar, A., John, T. J., & Nayak, N. C. (2007). Cassia occidentalis poisoning as the probable cause of hepatomyoencephalopathy in children in western Uttar Pradesh. *The Indian Journal of Medical Research, 125*(6), 756–762.
39. Jafri, M. A., Jalis Subhani, M., Javed, K., & Singh, S. (1999). Hepatoprotective activity of leaves of Cassia occidentalis against paracetamol and ethyl alcohol intoxication in rats. *Journal of Ethnopharmacology, 66*(3), 355–361.
40. Kumar, A., Dogra, S., & Prakash, A. (2010). Protective effect of naringin, a citrus flavonoid, against colchicine-induced cognitive dysfunction and oxidative damage in rats. *Journal of Medicinal Food, 13*(4), 976–984.
41. Pereira, R. M., Andrades, N. E., Paulino, N., Sawaya, A. C., Eberlin, M. N., Marcucci, M. C., Favero, G. M., Novak, E. M., & Bydlowski, S. P. (2007). Synthesis and characterization of a metal complex containing naringin and Cu, and its antioxidant, antimicrobial, anti-inflammatory and tumor cell cytotoxicity. *Molecules, 12*(7), 1352 1366.
42. Nogata, Y., Sakamoto, K., Shiratsuchi, H., Ishii, T., Yano, M., & Ohta, H. (2006). Flavonoid composition of fruit tissues of citrus species. *Bioscience, Biotechnology, and Biochemistry, 70* (1), 178–192.
43. Peterson, J. J., Dwyer, J. T., Beecher, G. R., Bhagwat, S. A., Gebhardt, S. E., Haytowitz, D. B., & Holden, J. M. (2006). Flavanones in oranges, tangerines (mandarins), tangors, and tangelos: A compilation and review of the data from the analytical literature. *Journal of Food Composition and Analysis, 19*, S66–S73.
44. Lee, M. H., Yoon, S., & Moon, J. O. (2004). The flavonoid naringenin inhibits dimethylnitrosamine-induced liver damage in rats. *Biological & Pharmaceutical Bulletin, 27* (1), 72–76.
45. Jayaraman, J., Veerappan, M., & Namasivayam, N. (2009). Potential beneficial effect of naringenin on lipid peroxidation and antioxidant status in rats with ethanol-induced hepatotoxicity. *The Journal of Pharmacy and Pharmacology, 61*(10), 1383–1390.
46. Renugadevi, J., & Prabu, S. M. (2010). Cadmium-induced hepatotoxicity in rats and the protective effect of naringenin. *Experimental and Toxicologic Pathology, 62*(2), 171–181.
47. Bathaie, S. Z., Farajzade, A., & Hoshyar, R. (2014). A review of the chemistry and uses of crocins and crocetin, the carotenoid natural dyes in saffron, with particular emphasis on applications as colorants including their use as biological stains. *Biotechnic & Histochemistry, 89*(6), 401–411.
48. Rameshrad, M., Razavi, B. M., & Hosseinzadeh, H. (2018). Saffron and its derivatives, crocin, crocetin and safranal: A patent review. *Expert Opinion on Therapeutic Patents, 28*(2), 147–165.

49. Gezici, S. J. (2019). Comparative anticancer activity analysis of saffron extracts and a principle component, crocetin for prevention and treatment of human malignancies. *Journal of Food Science and Technology, 56*(12), 5435–5443.
50. Kalantar, M., Kalantari, H., Goudarzi, M., Khorsandi, L., Bakhit, S., & Kalantar, H. (2019). Crocin ameliorates methotrexate-induced liver injury via inhibition of oxidative stress and inflammation in rats. *Pharmacological Reports, 71*(4), 746–752.
51. Bandegi, A. R., Rashidy-Pour, A., Vafaei, A. A., & Ghadrdoost, B. (2014). Protective effects of Crocus Sativus L. extract and crocin against chronic-stress induced oxidative damage of brain, liver and kidneys in rats. *Advanced Pharmaceutical Bulletin, 4*(Suppl 2), 493–499.
52. Salahshoor, M. R., Khashiadeh, M., Roshankhah, S., Kakabaraei, S., & Jalili, C. (2016). Protective effect of crocin on liver toxicity induced by morphine. *Research in Pharmaceutical Sciences, 11*(2), 120–129.
53. Ahmad, T., Cawood, M., Iqbal, Q., Arino, A., Batool, A., Tariq, R. M. S., Azam, M., & Akhtar, S. (2019). Phytochemicals in Daucus carota and their health benefits - review article. *Food, 8*(9).
54. Dreosti, I. E. (1993). Vitamins A, C, E and beta-carotene as protective factors for some cancers. *Asia Pacific Journal of Clinical Nutrition, 2*(Suppl 1), 21–25.
55. Speizer, F. E., Colditz, G. A., Hunter, D. J., Rosner, B., & Hennekens, C. (1999). Prospective study of smoking, antioxidant intake, and lung cancer in middle-aged women (USA). *Cancer Causes & Control, 10*(5), 475–482.
56. Rock, C. L. (1997). Carotenoids: Biology and treatment. *Pharmacology & Therapeutics, 75* (3), 185–197.
57. Singh, K., Singh, N., Chandy, A., & Manigauha, A. (2012). In vivo antioxidant and hepatoprotective activity of methanolic extracts of Daucus carota seeds in experimental animals. *Asian Pacific Journal of Tropical Biomedicine, 2*(5), 385–388.
58. Bishayee, A., Sarkar, A., & Chatterjee, M. (1995). Hepatoprotective activity of carrot (Daucus carota L.) against carbon tetrachloride intoxication in mouse liver. *Journal of Ethnopharmacology, 47*(2), 69–74.
59. Hall, J. D., Willis, D. W., Evatt, B. L., & Jackson, D. W. (1987). Using a monoclonal antibody to identify patients with type I and type II von Willebrand's disease. *Thrombosis and Haemostasis, 57*(3), 332–336.
60. Saxena, A. K., Singh, B., & Anand, K. K. (1993). Hepatoprotective effects of Eclipta alba on subcellular levels in rats. *Journal of Ethnopharmacology, 40*(3), 155–161.
61. Wagner, H., Geyer, B., Kiso, Y., Hikino, H., & Rao, G. S. (1986). Coumestans as the main active principles of the liver drugs Eclipta alba and Wedelia calendulacea. *Planta Medica, 5*, 370–374.
62. Satheesh Naik, K., Gurushanthaiah, M., Kavimani, M., Prabhu, K., & Lokanadham, S. (2018). Hepatoprotective role of Eclipta alba against high fatty diet treated experimental models - a histopathological study. *Maedica (Buchar), 13*(3), 217–222.
63. Mawa, S., Husain, K., & Jantan, I. (2013). Ficus carica L. (Moraceae): Phytochemistry, traditional uses and biological activities. *Evidence-based Complementary and Alternative Medicine, 2013*, 974256.
64. Solomon, A., Golubowicz, S., Yablowicz, Z., Grossman, S., Bergman, M., Gottlieb, H. E., Altman, A., Kerem, Z., & Flaishman, M. A. (2006). Antioxidant activities and anthocyanin content of fresh fruits of common fig (Ficus carica L.). *Journal of Agricultural and Food Chemistry, 54*(20), 7717–7723.
65. Ali, B., Mujeeb, M., Aeri, V., Mir, S. R., Faiyazuddin, M., & Shakeel, F. (2012). Anti-inflammatory and antioxidant activity of Ficus carica Linn. Leaves. *Natural Product Research, 26*(5), 460–465.
66. Gond, N. Y., & Khadabadi, S. S. (2008). Hepatoprotective activity of Ficus carica leaf extract on rifampicin-induced hepatic damage in rats. *Indian Journal of Pharmaceutical Sciences, 70* (3), 364–366.

67. Fouad, D., Alhatem, H., Abdel-Gaber, R., & Ataya, F. (2019). Hepatotoxicity and renal toxicity induced by gamma-radiation and the modulatory protective effect of Ficus carica in male albino rats. *Research in Veterinary Science, 125*, 24–35.
68. Pandey, V. B., Dasgupta, B., Bhattacharya, S. K., Lal, R., & Das, P. K. (1971). Chemistry and pharmacology of the major alkaloid of fumaria indica (Haussk) pugsley. *Current Science, 40* (17), 455–457.
69. Khare, C. P. (2004). *Indian Herbal Remedies* (p. 524). Berlin: Springer.
70. Rathi, A., Srivastava, A. K., Shirwaikar, A., Singh Rawat, A. K., & Mehrotra, S. (2008). Hepatoprotective potential of Fumaria indica Pugsley whole plant extracts, fractions and an isolated alkaloid protopine. *Phytomedicine, 15*(6–7), 470–477.
71. Rao, K. S., & Mishra, S. H. (1998). Antihepatotoxic activity of monomethyl fumarate isolated from Fumaria indica. *Journal of Ethnopharmacology, 60*(3), 207–213.
72. Mohanta, T. K., Tamboli, Y., & Zubaidha, P. K. (2014). Phytochemical and medicinal importance of Ginkgo biloba L. *Natural Product Research, 28*(10), 746–752.
73. Naik, S. R., & Panda, V. S. (2008). Hepatoprotective effect of Ginkgoselect Phytosome in rifampicin induced liver injury in rats: Evidence of antioxidant activity. *Fitoterapia, 79*(6), 439–445.
74. Shenoy, K. A., Somayaji, S. N., & Bairy, K. L. (2002). Evaluation of hepatoprotective activity of Ginkgo biloba in rats. *Indian Journal of Physiology and Pharmacology, 46*(2), 167–174.
75. Parimoo, H. A., Sharma, R., Patil, R. D., Sharma, O. P., Kumar, P., & Kumar, N. (2014). Hepatoprotective effect of Ginkgo biloba leaf extract on lantadenes-induced hepatotoxicity in guinea pigs. *Toxicon, 81*, 1–12.
76. Kleijnen, J., & Knipschild, P. (1992). Ginkgo biloba. *Lancet, 340*(8828), 1136–1139.
77. Naik, S. R., & Panda, V. S. (2007). Antioxidant and hepatoprotective effects of Ginkgo biloba phytosomes in carbon tetrachloride-induced liver injury in rodents. *Liver International, 27*(3), 393–399.
78. Hosseinzadeh, H., & Nassiri-Asl, M. (2015). Pharmacological effects of glycyrrhiza spp. and its bioactive constituents: Update and review. *Phytotherapy Research, 29*(12), 1868–1886.
79. Wan, X. Y., Luo, M., Li, X. D., & He, P. (2009). Hepatoprotective and anti-hepatocarcinogenic effects of glycyrrhizin and matrine. *Chemico-Biological Interactions, 181*(1), 15–19.
80. Kimura, M., Moro, T., Motegi, H., Maruyama, H., Sekine, M., Okamoto, H., Inoue, H., Sato, T., & Ogihara, M. (2008). In vivo glycyrrhizin accelerates liver regeneration and rapidly lowers serum transaminase activities in 70% partially hepatectomized rats. *European Journal of Pharmacology, 579*(1–3), 357–364.
81. Ogiku, M., Kono, H., Hara, M., Tsuchiya, M., & Fujii, H. (2011). Glycyrrhizin prevents liver injury by inhibition of high-mobility group box 1 production by Kupffer cells after ischemia-reperfusion in rats. *The Journal of Pharmacology and Experimental Therapeutics, 339*(1), 93–98.
82. Lee, C. H., Park, S. W., Kim, Y. S., Kang, S. S., Kim, J. A., Lee, S. H., & Lee, S. M. (2007). Protective mechanism of glycyrrhizin on acute liver injury induced by carbon tetrachloride in mice. *Biological & Pharmaceutical Bulletin, 30*(10), 1898–1904.
83. Fujisawa, Y., Sakamoto, M., Matsushita, M., Fujita, T., & Nishioka, K. (2000). Glycyrrhizin inhibits the lytic pathway of complement--possible mechanism of its anti-inflammatory effect on liver cells in viral hepatitis. *Microbiology and Immunology, 44*(9), 799–804.
84. Abe, M., Akbar, F., Hasebe, A., Horiike, N., & Onji, M. (2003). Glycyrrhizin enhances interleukin-10 production by liver dendritic cells in mice with hepatitis. *Journal of Gastroenterology, 38*(10), 962–967.
85. Matsuo, K., Takenaka, K., Shimomura, H., Fujii, N., Shinagawa, K., Kiura, K., & Harada, M. (2001). Lamivudine and glycyrrhizin for treatment of chemotherapy-induced hepatitis B virus (HBV) hepatitis in a chronic HBV carrier with non-Hodgkin lymphoma. *Leukemia & Lymphoma, 41*(1–2), 191–195.

86. Krishnaveni, M., & Mirunalini, S. (2010). Therapeutic potential of Phyllanthus emblica (amla): The ayurvedic wonder. *Journal of Basic and Clinical Physiology and Pharmacology, 21*(1), 93–105.
87. Yang, B., & Liu, P. (2014). Composition and biological activities of hydrolyzable tannins of fruits of Phyllanthus emblica. *Journal of Agricultural and Food Chemistry, 62*(3), 529–541.
88. Huang, C. Z., Tung, Y. T., Hsia, S. M., Wu, C. H., & Yen, G. C. (2017). The hepatoprotective effect of Phyllanthus emblica L. fruit on high fat diet-induced non-alcoholic fatty liver disease (NAFLD) in SD rats. *Food & Function, 8*(2), 842–850.
89. Jadon, A., Bhadauria, M., & Shukla, S. (2007). Protective effect of Terminalia belerica Roxb. and gallic acid against carbon tetrachloride induced damage in albino rats. *Journal of Ethnopharmacology, 109*(2), 214–218.
90. Nabavi, S. M., Habtemariam, S., Nabavi, S. F., Sureda, A., Daglia, M., Moghaddam, A. H., & Amani, M. A. (2013). Protective effect of gallic acid isolated from Peltiphyllum peltatum against sodium fluoride-induced oxidative stress in rat's kidney. *Molecular and Cellular Biochemistry, 372*(1–2), 233–239.
91. Oyagbemi, A. A., Omobowale, O. T., Asenuga, E. R., Akinleye, A. S., Ogunsanwo, R. O., & Saba, A. B. (2016). Cyclophosphamide-induced hepatotoxicity in Wistar rats: The modulatory role of gallic acid as a hepatoprotective and chemopreventive phytochemical. *International Journal of Preventive Medicine, 7*, 51.
92. Rasool, M. K., Sabina, E. P., Ramya, S. R., Preety, P., Patel, S., Mandal, N., Mishra, P. P., & Samuel, J. (2010). Hepatoprotective and antioxidant effects of gallic acid in paracetamol-induced liver damage in mice. *The Journal of Pharmacy and Pharmacology, 62*(5), 638–643.
93. Hsu, C. L., & Yen, G. C. (2007). Effect of gallic acid on high fat diet-induced dyslipidaemia, hepatosteatosis and oxidative stress in rats. *The British Journal of Nutrition, 98*(4), 727–735.
94. Chao, J., Huo, T. I., Cheng, H. Y., Tsai, J. C., Liao, J. W., Lee, M. S., Qin, X. M., Hsieh, M. T., Pao, L. H., & Peng, W. H. (2014). Gallic acid ameliorated impaired glucose and lipid homeostasis in high fat diet-induced NAFLD mice. *PLoS One, 9*(2), e96969.
95. Garcia-Nino, W. R., & Zazueta, C. (2015). Ellagic acid: Pharmacological activities and molecular mechanisms involved in liver protection. *Pharmacological Research, 97*, 84–103.
96. Hau, D. K., Zhu, G. Y., Leung, A. K., Wong, R. S., Cheng, G. Y., Lai, P. B., Tong, S. W., Lau, F. Y., Chan, K. W., Wong, W. Y., Lam, K. H., Cheng, C. H., Cheung, F., Chui, C. H., Gambari, R., & Fong, D. W. (2010). In vivo anti-tumour activity of corilagin on Hep3B hepatocellular carcinoma. *Phytomedicine, 18*(1), 11–15.
97. Girish, C., Koner, B. C., Jayanthi, S., Ramachandra Rao, K., Rajesh, B., & Pradhan, S. C. (2009). Hepatoprotective activity of picroliv, curcumin and ellagic acid compared to silymarin on paracetamol induced liver toxicity in mice. *Fundamental & Clinical Pharmacology, 23*(6), 735–745.
98. Tiwari, S. S., Pandey, M. M., Srivastava, S., & Rawat, A. K. (2012). TLC densitometric quantification of picrosides (picroside-I and picroside-II) in Picrorhiza kurroa and its substitute Picrorhiza scrophulariiflora and their antioxidant studies. *Biomedical Chromatography, 26*(1), 61–68.
99. Rastogi, R., Srivastava, A. K., & Rastogi, A. K. (2001). Biochemical changes induced in liver and serum of aflatoxin B1-treated male Wistar rats: Preventive effect of picroliv. *Pharmacology & Toxicology, 88*(2), 53–58.
100. Yadav, N., & Khandelwal, S. (2006). Effect of Picroliv on cadmium-induced hepatic and renal damage in the rat. *Human & Experimental Toxicology, 25*(10), 581–591.
101. Zhao, Q., Chen, X. Y., & Martin, C. (2016). Scutellaria baicalensis, the golden herb from the garden of Chinese medicinal plants. *Science Bulletin (Beijing), 61*(18), 1391–1398.
102. Gao, Z., Huang, K., Yang, X., & Xu, H. (1999). Free radical scavenging and antioxidant activities of flavonoids extracted from the radix of Scutellaria baicalensis Georgi. *Biochimica et Biophysica Acta, 1472*(3), 643–650.
103. Inoue, T., & Jackson, E. K. (1999). Strong antiproliferative effects of baicalein in cultured rat hepatic stellate cells. *European Journal of Pharmacology, 378*(1), 129–135.

104. Shimizu, I. (2000). Sho-saiko-to: Japanese herbal medicine for protection against hepatic fibrosis and carcinoma. *Journal of Gastroenterology and Hepatology, 15*(Suppl), D84–D90.
105. Shimizu, I., Ma, Y. R., Mizobuchi, Y., Liu, F., Miura, T., Nakai, Y., Yasuda, M., Shiba, M., Horie, T., Amagaya, S., Kawada, N., Hori, H., & Ito, S. (1999). Effects of Sho-saiko-to, a Japanese herbal medicine, on hepatic fibrosis in rats. *Hepatology, 29*(1), 149–160.
106. Ai, Z. L., Zhang, W. S., Yao, S. K., Xie, B. S., & Gao, C. (2011). Effect of baicalin on liver fatty acid binding protein in oxidative stress model in vitro. *Zhonghua Gan Zang Bing Za Zhi, 19*(12), 927–931.
107. Huang, H. L., Wang, Y. J., Zhang, Q. Y., Liu, B., Wang, F. Y., Li, J. J., & Zhu, R. Z. (2012). Hepatoprotective effects of baicalein against CCl(4)-induced acute liver injury in mice. *World Journal of Gastroenterology, 18*(45), 6605–6613.
108. Kim, S. J., Moon, Y. J., & Lee, S. M. (2010). Protective effects of baicalin against ischemia/reperfusion injury in rat liver. *Journal of Natural Products, 73*(12), 2003–2008.
109. Wu, Y. L., Lian, L. H., Wan, Y., & Nan, J. X. (2010). Baicalein inhibits nuclear factor-kappaB and apoptosis via c-FLIP and MAPK in D-GalN/LPS induced acute liver failure in murine models. *Chemico-Biological Interactions, 188*(3), 526–534.
110. Zhao, Y., Li, H., Gao, Z., & Xu, H. (2005). Effects of dietary baicalin supplementation on iron overload-induced mouse liver oxidative injury. *European Journal of Pharmacology, 509*(2–3), 195–200.
111. Freitag, A. F., Cardia, G. F., da Rocha, B. A., Aguiar, R. P., Silva-Comar, F. M., Spironello, R. A., Grespan, R., Caparroz-Assef, S. M., Bersani-Amado, C. A., & Cuman, R. K. (2015). Hepatoprotective effect of silymarin (Silybum marianum) on hepatotoxicity induced by acetaminophen in spontaneously hypertensive rats. *Evidence-based Complementary and Alternative Medicine, 2015*, 538317.
112. Vargas-Mendoza, N., Madrigal-Santillan, E., Morales-Gonzalez, A., Esquivel-Soto, J., Esquivel-Chirino, C., Garcia-Luna, Y. G.-R. M., Gayosso-de-Lucio, J. A., & Morales-Gonzalez, J. A. (2014). Hepatoprotective effect of silymarin. *World Journal of Hepatology, 6*(3), 144–149.
113. Salam, O. M., Sleem, A. A., Omara, E. A., & Hassan, N. S. (2009). Hepatoprotective effects of misoprostol and silymarin on carbon tetrachloride-induced hepatic damage in rats. *Fundamental & Clinical Pharmacology, 23*(2), 179–188.
114. Kim, S. H., Cheon, H. J., Yun, N., Oh, S. T., Shin, E., Shim, K. S., & Lee, S. M. (2009). Protective effect of a mixture of aloe vera and Silybum marianum against carbon tetrachloride-induced acute hepatotoxicity and liver fibrosis. *Journal of Pharmacological Sciences, 109*(1), 119–127.
115. Chen, I. S., Chen, Y. C., Chou, C. H., Chuang, R. F., Sheen, L. Y., & Chiu, C. H. (2012). Hepatoprotection of silymarin against thioacetamide-induced chronic liver fibrosis. *Journal of the Science of Food and Agriculture, 92*(7), 1441–1447.
116. Stanca, E., Serviddio, G., Bellanti, F., Vendemiale, G., Siculella, L., & Giudetti, A. M. (2013). Down-regulation of LPCAT expression increases platelet-activating factor level in cirrhotic rat liver: Potential anti-inflammatory effect of silybin. *Biochimica et Biophysica Acta, 1832*(12), 2019–2026.
117. Li, Y. G., Song, L., Liu, M., Hu, Z. B., & Wang, Z. T. (2009). Advancement in analysis of Salviae miltiorrhizae Radix et Rhizoma (Danshen). *Journal of Chromatography. A, 1216*(11), 1941–1953.
118. Lee, T. Y., Mai, L. M., Wang, G. J., Chiu, J. H., Lin, Y. L., & Lin, H. C. (2003). Protective mechanism of salvia miltiorrhiza on carbon tetrachloride-induced acute hepatotoxicity in rats. *Journal of Pharmacological Sciences, 91*(3), 202–210.
119. Lin, Y. L., Wu, C. H., Luo, M. H., Huang, Y. J., Wang, C. N., Shiao, M. S., & Huang, Y. T. (2006). In vitro protective effects of salvianolic acid B on primary hepatocytes and hepatic stellate cells. *Journal of Ethnopharmacology, 105*(1–2), 215–222.

120. Wu, Z. M., Wen, T., Tan, Y. F., Liu, Y., Ren, F., & Wu, H. (2007). Effects of salvianolic acid A on oxidative stress and liver injury induced by carbon tetrachloride in rats. *Basic & Clinical Pharmacology & Toxicology, 100*(2), 115–120.
121. Lee, C. Y., Sher, H. F., Chen, H. W., Liu, C. C., Chen, C. H., Lin, C. S., Yang, P. C., Tsay, H. S., & Chen, J. J. (2008). Anticancer effects of tanshinone I in human non-small cell lung cancer. *Molecular Cancer Therapeutics, 7*(11), 3527–3538.
122. Liu, J., Shen, H. M., & Ong, C. N. (2001). Role of intracellular thiol depletion, mitochondrial dysfunction and reactive oxygen species in Salvia miltiorrhiza-induced apoptosis in human hepatoma HepG2 cells. *Life Sciences, 69*(16), 1833–1850.
123. Yue, S., Hu, B., Wang, Z., Yue, Z., Wang, F., Zhao, Y., Yang, Z., & Shen, M. (2014). Salvia miltiorrhiza compounds protect the liver from acute injury by regulation of p38 and NFkappaB signaling in Kupffer cells. *Pharmaceutical Biology, 52*(10), 1278–1285.
124. Zhang, Y., Zhang, Y., Xie, Y., Gao, Y., Ma, J., Yuan, J., Li, J., Wang, J., Li, L., Zhang, J., & Chu, L. (2013). Multitargeted inhibition of hepatic fibrosis in chronic iron-overloaded mice by Salvia miltiorrhiza. *Journal of Ethnopharmacology, 148*(2), 671–681.
125. Jin, Q., Jiang, S., Wu, Y. L., Bai, T., Yang, Y., Jin, X., Lian, L. H., & Nan, J. X. (2014). Hepatoprotective effect of cryptotanshinone from Salvia miltiorrhiza in D-galactosamine/ lipopolysaccharide-induced fulminant hepatic failure. *Phytomedicine, 21*(2), 141–147.
126. Yadav, M., Jain, S., Bhardwaj, A., Nagpal, R., Puniya, M., Tomar, R., Singh, V., Parkash, O., Prasad, G. B., Marotta, F., & Yadav, H. (2009). Biological and medicinal properties of grapes and their bioactive constituents: An update. *Journal of Medicinal Food, 12*(3), 473–484.
127. Smoliga, J. M., Baur, J. A., & Hausenblas, H. A. (2011). Resveratrol and health--a comprehensive review of human clinical trials. *Molecular Nutrition & Food Research, 55*(8), 1129–1141.
128. Feng, L. L., Liu, B. X., Zhong, J. Y., Sun, L. B., & Yu, H. S. (2014). Effect of grape procyanidins on tumor angiogenesis in liver cancer xenograft models. *Asian Pacific Journal of Cancer Prevention, 15*(2), 737–741.
129. Scola, G., Laurino, C. C. F. C., Menin, E., & Salvador, M. (2013). Suppression of oncoprotein Her-2 and DNA damage after treatment with flavan-3-ol Vitis labrusca extract. *Anti-Cancer Agents in Medicinal Chemistry, 13*(7), 1088–1095.
130. Tunali-Akbay, T., Sehirli, O., Ercan, F., & Sener, G. (2010). Resveratrol protects against methotrexate-induced hepatic injury in rats. *Journal of Pharmacy & Pharmaceutical Sciences, 13*(2), 303–310.
131. Lee, E. S., Shin, M. O., Yoon, S., & Moon, J. O. (2010). Resveratrol inhibits dimethylnitrosamine-induced hepatic fibrosis in rats. *Archives of Pharmacal Research, 33*(6), 925–932.
132. Roy, S., Sannigrahi, S., Majumdar, S., Ghosh, B., & Sarkar, B. (2011). Resveratrol regulates antioxidant status, inhibits cytokine expression and restricts apoptosis in carbon tetrachloride induced rat hepatic injury. *Oxidative Medicine and Cellular Longevity, 2011*, 703676.
133. Rajasekaran, D., Elavarasan, J., Sivalingam, M., Ganapathy, E., Kumar, A., Kalpana, K., & Sakthisekaran, D. (2011). Resveratrol interferes with N-nitrosodiethylamine-induced hepatocellular carcinoma at early and advanced stages in male Wistar rats. *Molecular Medicine Reports, 4*(6), 1211–1217.
134. Tiwary, M., Naik, S. N., Tewary, D. K., Mittal, P. K., & Yadav, S. (2007). Chemical composition and larvicidal activities of the essential oil of Zanthoxylum armatum DC (Rutaceae) against three mosquito vectors. *Journal of Vector Borne Diseases, 44*(3), 198–204.
135. Kalia, N. K., Singh, B., & Sood, R. P. (1999). A new amide from Zanthoxylum armatum. *Journal of Natural Products, 62*(2), 311–312.
136. Ranawat, L., Bhatt, J., & Patel, J. (2010). Hepatoprotective activity of ethanolic extracts of bark of Zanthoxylum armatum DC in CCl4 induced hepatic damage in rats. *Journal of Ethnopharmacology, 127*(3), 777–780.
137. Lete, I., & Allue, J. (2016). The effectiveness of ginger in the prevention of nausea and vomiting during pregnancy and chemotherapy. *Integrative Medicine Insights, 11*, 11–17.

138. Rahmani, A. H., Shabrmi, F. M., & Aly, S. M. (2014). Active ingredients of ginger as potential candidates in the prevention and treatment of diseases via modulation of biological activities. *International Journal of Physiology, Pathophysiology and Pharmacology, 6*(2), 125–136.
139. Rahnama, P., Montazeri, A., Huseini, H. F., Kianbakht, S., & Naseri, M. (2012). Effect of Zingiber officinale R. rhizomes (ginger) on pain relief in primary dysmenorrhea: A placebo randomized trial. *BMC Complementary and Alternative Medicine, 12*, 92.
140. Grzanna, R., Lindmark, L., & Frondoza, C. G. (2005). Ginger--an herbal medicinal product with broad anti-inflammatory actions. *Journal of Medicinal Food, 8*(2), 125–132.
141. Liu, C. T., Raghu, R., Lin, S. H., Wang, S. Y., Kuo, C. H., Tseng, Y. J., & Sheen, L. Y. (2013). Metabolomics of ginger essential oil against alcoholic fatty liver in mice. *Journal of Agricultural and Food Chemistry, 61*(46), 11231–11240.
142. Lai, Y. S., Lee, W. C., Lin, Y. E., Ho, C. T., Lu, K. H., Lin, S. H., Panyod, S., Chu, Y. L., & Sheen, L. Y. (2016). Ginger essential oil ameliorates hepatic injury and lipid accumulation in high fat diet-induced nonalcoholic fatty liver disease. *Journal of Agricultural and Food Chemistry, 64*(10), 2062–2071.
143. Badawi, M. S. (2019). Histological study of the protective role of ginger on piroxicam-induced liver toxicity in mice. *Journal of the Chinese Medical Association, 82*(1), 11–18.
144. Fahmi, A., Hassanen, N., Abdur-Rahman, M., & Shams-Eldin, E. (2019). Phytochemicals, antioxidant activity and hepatoprotective effect of ginger (Zingiber officinale) on diethylnitrosamine toxicity in rats. *Biomarkers, 24*(5), 436–447.

[illegible]

Chapter 13
Emerging Roles of Phytochemicals in Hepatocellular Carcinoma

Hammad Zafar, Mamoon Ur Rashid, Deepika Sarvepalli, Muzammil Muhammad Khan, Bayarmaa Mandzhieva, Akriti Gupta Jain, Rima Shobar, Anum Jalil, and Sarfraz Ahmad

Abstract Hepatocellular cancer is the most common liver cancer and is the second most common cause of cancer mortality worldwide. Cirrhosis, secondary to viral hepatitis, remains the most common underlying cause worldwide. Surgical resection or liver transplantation is the mainstay of treatment. Various other treatment options include chemoembolization, radiofrequency ablation, and tyrosine kinase inhibitors including sorafenib. More than 30 genetic mutations have been described in peer-reviewed literature affecting multiple signaling pathways. Multiple in vitro and in vivo studies have been reported in the peer-reviewed literature demonstrating the benefit of phytochemicals in the treatment and prevention of hepatocellular cancer. In this chapter, we summarize the role of different phytochemicals including ginger, garlic, turmeric, cinnamon, saffron, coffee, and cruciferous vegetables that have been implicated in playing significant roles in the preventions and management of hepatocellular cancer. We also summarize the theorized pathways affected by these agents. This can lay a groundwork for further studies and randomized clinical trials to address the unmet needs of the topic.

Keywords Hepatocellular cancer · Pathobiology · Molecular pathways · Phytochemicals · Ginger · Turmeric · Cinnamon · Garlic · Saffron · Coffee · Clinical outcomes

---

H. Zafar (✉) · M. U. Rashid · D. Sarvepalli · B. Mandzhieva · A. G. Jain · R. Shobar · A. Jalil
Department of Internal Medicine, AdventHealth, Orlando, FL, USA
e-mail: hammad1190@hotmail.com; mamoon.rashid.MD@adventhealth.com; bayarmaa.mandzhieva.MD@adventhealth.com; akriti.jain.MD@adventhealth.com; rima.shobar.MD@adventhealth.com; anum.jalil.MD@adventhealth.com

M. M. Khan
Khyber Teaching Hospital, Peshawar, Khyber Pakhtunkhwa, Pakistan

S. Ahmad
AdventHealth Cancer Institute and FSU and UCF Colleges of Medicine, Orlando, FL, USA
e-mail: sarfraz.ahmad@adventhealth.com

G. P. Nagaraju (ed.), *Phytochemicals Targeting Tumor Microenvironment in Gastrointestinal Cancers*, https://doi.org/10.1007/978-3-030-48405-7_13

Abbreviations

AC	Antrodia cinnamomea
ARID	AT-rich interactive domain
AX1N1	Ataxin-1
BCL	B-cell lymphoma
BMI	Body mass index
CCND	Cyclin D2
Cdk	Cyclin-dependent kinase
CI	Confidence interval
COX	Cyclo-oxygenase
CT	Computerized tomography
CTNNB1	Catenin B1
DAD	Diallyl disulfide
DAS	Diallyl sulfide
DAT	Diallyl trisulfide
DR5	Death receptor 5
EACG	Ethanolic extracts of AC
EGCG	Epigallocatechin-3-gallate
EGF	Epidermal growth factor
FAS	Apoptosis-stimulating fragment
5-FU	5-Fluorouracil
FGF	Fibroblast growth factor
GP	Ginger polysaccharides
HAT	Histone acetyltransferase
HBV	Hepatitis B virus
HCC	Hepatocellular carcinoma
HCCDB	Human hepatocellular cancer database
HCV	Hepatitis C virus
HGF	Hepatocyte growth factor
IARC	International Agency for Research on Cancer
IGF	Insulin-like growth factor
JAK/STAT	Janus kinase/signal transducer and activator of transcription
MAPK	Mitogen-activated protein kinase
2-MCA	2-Methoxycinnamaldehyde
mTOR	Mammalian target of rapamycin
NAD	Nicotinamide adenine dinucleotide
NAD(P)H	Nicotinamide adenine dinucleotide phosphate
NF-kb	Nuclear factor kappa B
NRF2	Nuclear factor erythroid 2-related factor 2
PDGF	Platelet-derived growth factor
PTEN	Phosphatase and tensin homolog
RAF	Serine/threonine protein kinase
RAS	Retrovirus-associated DNA sequence

SAC	S-allyl cysteine
SAMC	S-allylmercaptocysteine
STAT3	Signal transducer and activator of transcription 3
T2DM	Type 2 diabetes mellitus
TERT	Telomerase reverse transcriptase
TIMP	Tissue inhibitor of matrix metalloproteinase
TGF-β	Transforming growth factor-β
TRAIL	Tumor necrosis factor-related apoptosis-inducing ligand
VEGF	Vascular endothelial growth factor
WCRF	World Cancer Research Fund
WNT	Wingless/integrated

1 Introduction

Hepatocellular cancer constitutes up to 90% of primary liver cancer, which is the sixth most common cancer overall. In men, liver cancer is the fifth most common and in women it is the ninth most common malignancy [1]. Hepatocellular carcinoma (HCC) ranks second most common cause of cancer mortality worldwide. Malignancy is often preceded by cirrhosis, which is the main indication for screening and surveillance [2].

East Asia and Africa are the main hubs of HCC; but its incidence and mortality are on the rise in the Western world also. Overall, viral hepatitis remains the most common cause of HCC. Worldwide implementation of hepatitis vaccination and invention of very effective treatment for hepatitis C are shifting the epidemiology away from disease prevailed by viral hepatitis. Nonalcoholic steatohepatitis is emerging as a significant underlying disease-causing HCC. Biannual surveillance using imaging (e.g., ultrasound/CT), with/without serum α-fetoprotein, has been associated with early diagnosis and relatively improved overall survival (OS) outcomes [3].

Solitary tumor is treated with resection. Poor surgical candidates can qualify for liver transplantation if they meet the Milan Criteria (i.e., single tumor less ≤ 5 cm or up to three tumors ≤ 3 cm). Chemoembolization is the most frequently used therapeutic strategy in patients with multifocal disease without vascular invasion and/or distant metastasis. Radiofrequency ablation and trans-arterial chemoembolization are often used as bridging therapy while waiting for liver transplantation. Additionally, patients who are not eligible for liver-directed therapy and have good performance status, systemic therapy with tyrosine kinase inhibitors (i.e., sorafenib, lenvatinib, and regorafenib) is the standard of treatment with improvement in survival outcomes [4].

Multiple genetic mutations are involved in the development of hepatocellular cancer. More than 30 mutations have been described in peer-reviewed literature; but three most common signaling pathways affected are PTEN, Wnt/B-catenin pathway, and P53 tumor-suppressor gene. Additionally, multiple immunotherapeutic treatment options are also under investigation with potential effects on these pathways which may potentially change/improve the management of HCC. Also, extensive ex vivo and in vivo studies have demonstrated significant role(s) of phytochemicals in the prevention and treatment of hepatocellular cancer. Phytochemicals play their role(s) by modulating these signaling pathways to favor clinical outcomes. This chapter primarily reviews the antineoplastic role(s) of different phytochemicals in the prevention and management of hepatocellular cancer.

2 Pathobiology of Hepatocellular Cancer

Multiple factors are responsible for causing the acute and chronic liver inflammation including viral hepatitis (hepatitis B and C), alcohol, nonalcoholic steatohepatitis, and aflatoxin. HCC is mostly preceded by chronic liver inflammation and fibrosis that results in a disrupted liver architecture, which is the characteristic feature of cirrhosis. Cirrhosis precedes HCC in the majority of cases. Cirrhotic liver has small areas of abnormal, premature cells, and these dysplastic foci (<1 mm) arising in the setting of cirrhosis are considered as precancerous lesions or dysplastic nodules. These dysplastic nodules are further divided into low or high grade on the basis of morphological appearance and cellular atypia. Both types of nodules can be evolved into HCC; but the high-grade nodules have much higher risk [5]. HCC carcinogenesis involves changes in the proliferation markers of cells, tumor-suppressor genes, oncogenes and their receptors, genes involved in such processes as angiogenesis, apoptosis-related factors, and immune response [6].

3 Oncogenes and Their Receptors

Proto-oncogenes inscribe a large variety of proteins, which play a role in such processes as cellular proliferation and differentiation, growth factors and their receptors, transcription factors, and part of signal transduction pathways. Abnormalities in a large variety of oncogenes have been observed in HCC. Epidermal growth factor (EGF) and epidermal growth factor receptor (EGFR) are involved in cell proliferation and differentiation, which are being linked with the late-stage disease, marker of metastasis, and recurrence of HCC (Fig. 13.1).

Hepatoma-derived growth factor (HDGF) is involved in the induction of cell growth, and is considered as a marker of rate of multiplication in tumor (a poor prognostic marker). Transforming growth factor-β1 (TGF-β1) is a strong inhibitor of growth in most epithelial cells and is involved in such processes as cellular proliferation, differentiation, and migration. Notably, the TGF-β1 levels are significantly high in cirrhosis and patients with HCC [7].

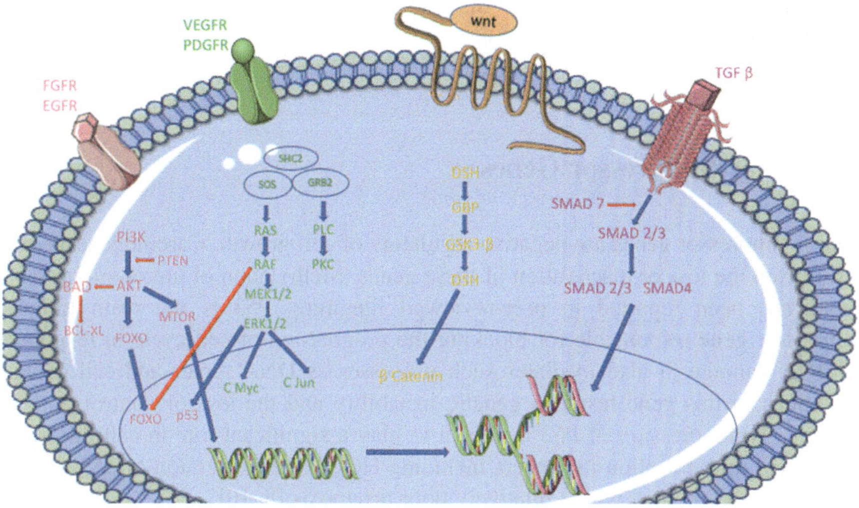

Fig. 13.1 Schematic representation of the major signaling pathways involved in HCC. One of the most important pathways as shown in this figure is receptor tyrosine kinase (RTK) pathway. Various receptors are involved in this pathway including EGF, FGF, HGF, c-MET, PDGF, VEGF, and stem cell growth factor receptor c-KIT. These receptors in turn lead to activation of various downstream signals [15]. VEGF receptor in various studies has been shown to be associated with worse prognosis, recurrence, vascular invasion, and high tumor grade and is now being targeted therapeutically. EGFR is activated by binding of the ligand EGF, which plays complex and imperative role(s) in tumor proliferation and angiogenesis. This is accomplished by the activation of RAF/MEK/ERK and PI3K/AKT/mTOR pathways as shown in this figure. The RAF/MEK/ERK pathway activation leads to tumor development, progression, and metastasis. In HCC, the two main mechanisms that lead to the initiation of this pathway are either oncogenic mutation in RAS gene leading to constitutive CRAF stimulation or a disarray in the overexpression of growth factors and their receptors leading to the same. The PI3K/AKT/mTOR achieves cancer progression and survival. IGF and EGF activate PI3K, which in turn produces PIP3b that leads to the initiation of AKT. This regulates various transcription factors and cytoplasmic proteins comprising BAD and mTOR, which in turn regulate translation and cell cycle. The Wnt/β-catenin pathway is another important pathway which is usually aberrantly activated in HCC by a mutation in β-catenin. Some of the pathways not shown in this figure that might also play role(s) in HCC include but are not limited to RAS and JAK/STAT pathways, Hedgehog signaling pathway, and ubiquitin-proteasome pathway. TGF-β signaling in HCC is important in the activation and trans-differentiation of silent hepatic stellate cells to myofibroblasts [16]. Activation of TGF-β receptor leads to phosphorylation of receptor associated with SMADs (R-SMADs) [15, 17, 18]

4 Epigenetic Pathway Alterations

Persistent viral infection, chronic inflammation, and even normal aging process can result in changes in the epigenetic pathways. These pathways are characterized by three main processes: DNA *hypo*-methylation, DNA *hyper*-methylation, and histone modification, which result in such processes as gene inactivation, gene instability, and changes in chromatin conformation, respectively. DNA methylation can also occur at different stages of liver disease and is the most frequent epigenetic alteration [8].

5 Tumor-Suppressor Genes

Tumor-suppressor genes are negative regulators of cell growth. Carcinogenesis can result from the loss or inactivation of these genes. Methylation of tumor-suppressor genes has been reported in peer-reviewed literature. P53 is the main tumor-suppressor gene responsible for blocking the progression of cell cycle in response to DNA damage. It also mediates such processes as DNA repair and cell death. Mutations in this gene result in genetic instability and the loss of control of cell growth. Overexpression of P53 is shown to play a significant role in cell differentiation and multiplication in cancers including HCC. Overexpression of p53 is also shown to be correlated with a relatively poor prognosis [8–10].

6 Cell Cycle Regulators

Cellular multiplication has multiple checkpoints like between G1 and S phases and another between G2 and M phases. Disruption of these checkpoints can lead to uncontrolled cellular replication and cancer. Overexpression of cyclin proteins has been shown to correlate with the relapse of HCC. Overexpression of cyclin D1 is particularly shown to play a role in progression of HCC. It is also shown to be associated with aggressive form of cancer. In vitro study has demonstrated increased levels and activities of multiple cyclin proteins and cyclin-dependent kinases in proportion with the development of HCC [11, 12]. P27 protein is also involved in cell cycle progression and is a member of cyclin/cyclin-dependent kinase inhibitors. Reduced expression is associated with decreased survival and relatively poor prognosis [13].

7 Angiogenesis

Pathological angiogenesis in hepatocellular cancer has significant role(s) in tumor growth, invasion, and metastasis. Differential expressions of vascular endothelial growth factor (VEGF), platelet-derived growth factor (PDGF), basic fibroblast growth factor (bFGF), angiopoietin-1 and -2, and matrix metalloproteinases (MMPs) and its inhibitors [e.g., tissue inhibitor of matrix metalloproteinase (TIMP)] are related to HCC carcinogenesis and prognosis [6, 14].

8 Signaling Pathways

Multiple signaling pathways are involved in the pathobiology of hepatocellular carcinoma [Fig. 13.1]. Three most common mutations involved are TERT (telomerase reverse transcriptase), CTNNB1 (catenin B1), and TP53. At least 30 other genetic mutations are also identified in the pathogenesis of HCC and some of the most common mutations are summarized in Table 13.1.

9 Role of Phytochemicals in the Prevention of Hepatocellular Carcinoma

Foods rich in fruits, vegetables, and herbs have the potential to decrease the risk of different cancers. This reduction has been attributed to phytochemicals present in them. Phytochemicals are beneficial for health and they impart this benefit by modifying various cellular processes including inflammation, catabolism, growth, and cell death. Multiple studies are ongoing to explain the mechanism of action of different phytochemicals as their therapeutic benefit in different human diseases is increasing. Below we summarize some of the major phytochemicals that are implicated in the prevention and management of HCC.

9.1 Ginger

Globally, ginger is a very commonly used dietary supplement in almost every household. Active ingredients in ginger, i.e., ginger oleoresin, 6-shogaol, zingerone, and 6-gingerol, have been extensively studied for their chemo-protective, antioxidant, and anticancer properties [19], (Table 13.2).

Table 13.1 A summary of the signaling pathways involved with key gene mutations in the pathogenesis of hepatocellular carcinoma

Signaling pathway	Genetic mutation	Frequency of mutation in hepatocellular carcinoma
Wnt	CTNNB1 AXIN1	11–41% 5–19%
P53	TP53	13–48%
Chromatin remodeling	ARID1A ARID2	4–17% 5–7%
Cell cycle	CDKN2A CCND1, FGF3, FGF4, FGF19	8% 5–7%
Growth factors	PTEN	53%

Table 13.2 Summary of some of the key ginger products and their biochemical functions in hepatocellular carcinoma

Active ingredient(s)	Trial results	Mechanism(s) of action
Ginger essential oil (zingiberene, e-citral, z-citral, camphene, ocimene)	Decreases the severity of diethylnitrosamine-induced cytotoxicity suggesting a potent antioxidant activity [20]	Cytoprotective and anticancer potential against HepG2 cells [20]
6-Shogaol	• Enhances the apoptotic activity of TRAIL-induced apoptosis of cancer cells [19, 21] • Anti-metastasis effect [19]	• 6-Shogaol can induce reactive oxygen species (ROS) production, upregulate p53 gene expression, and alter membrane potential of mitochondria • Causes cell cycle arrest in G2/M phase [19, 21] • Anti-metastasis effect through regulation of matrix metalloproteinase-9 and tissue inhibitor of matrix metalloproteinase-1 [19]
Ginger polysaccharides (GP) [d-galactose, 1-rhamnose, d-mannose, d-arabinose, and d-glucose]	Promote cell death by increasing apoptosis [22]	• GP causes cell cycle arrest in G0–G1 phase and promotes apoptosis • Increased expression of FAS, FASL, Bax, caspase-3, and p-21 and decreased expression of Bcl-2 [22]
Zerumbone	• Inhibits proliferation and survival of cancer cells in a dose-dependent manner • Inhibits metastasis of HCC in immunocompromised mice [23]	• Cell cycle arrest at G2/M phase inducing apoptosis • Inhibition of PI3K/AKT/mTOR and STAT3 signaling pathways. It inhibits shunting of glucose-6-phosphate through hexose monophosphate shunt, thereby forcing cancer cells to undergo apoptosis [23]
Zingerone and its derivative (ZD2)	Inhibit metastasis of hepatocellular cancer [24]	Inhibits TGF-β, which results in increased expression of epithelial marker E-cadherin and decreased expression of mesenchymal marker N-cadherin, hence preventing epithelial-mesenchymal transition which is a key step in metastasis [24]

Ginger also works synergistically with many other medicines. Many medicinal fungal species like *Antrodia cinnamomea* (AC) have been used in some Asian countries for the treatment of multiple medical conditions, including cancer. In vitro analysis of Hul-7 and HepG2 cells has shown that co-cultivation of ginger with Antrodia EACG (ethanolic extracts of AC co-cultivated with ginger) is significantly more effective then ethanolic extracts of AC alone in targeting these cell lines. EACG modified cyclin protein expression and many signaling pathways including mitogen-activated protein kinase (MAPK) in favor of cancer cell apoptosis. It also works by promoting cell cycle arrest at G2/M phase in Huh-7 and HepG2 cells [25].

9.2 Turmeric

Bioactive chemical in turmeric is curcumin, which has been reported to have antineoplastic activity against multiple cancers, including hepatocellular cancer. It has anti-inflammatory properties, promotes apoptosis, reduces angiogenesis and tumor invasion, and reverses chemotherapy resistance [26]. In a study done in rats, curcumin improved the survival and decreased serum aspartate aminotransferase activity and fetoprotein concentrations. It also induced autophagy and reduced oxidative stress in liver. In vitro, curcumin decreased the concentration of SQSTM1 in HepG2 cells, which is a marker for viability [27].

Curcumin affects multiple signaling proteins including cytokine signaling receptors, growth factors, protein kinases, and adhesion molecules. It also causes time-dependent activation of pro-apoptotic proteins, i.e., caspase-9 and caspase 3, and reduction in anti-apoptotic protein Bcl-2, hence promoting cell death in hepatocellular cancer cells. It has also been shown to work synergistically with doxorubicin and cisplatin. Increased level of cisplatin has been observed with simultaneous administration with curcumin. Curcumin-loaded nanostructured lipid carrier (Cur-NLC) is found to be superior in inducing apoptosis of HepG2 cells and inhibiting proliferation when compared to the native curcumin. Cur-NLC notably increases the expression of death receptor 5 (DR5), caspase-3, and caspase-8, which translates into increased apoptosis [28].

The Human Hepatocellular Cancer Database (HCCDB) has shown that HCC with poor prognosis and primitive features is more likely to improve from nuclear factor (NF)-kB inhibition. Curcumin has been shown to increase cell death in cancer stem cells, which correlates with the degree of NF-kB inhibition. Hence, it can be a potential treatment option for hepatocellular cancer with improved progenitor features. In contrast, some cancer stem cells in hepatocellular cancer can show paradoxical response to curcumin by increased proliferation [29].

Curcumin has also a good chemo-sensitizing effect and can be used as an adjunct with chemotherapy to overcome potential chemoresistance. Lin28B is associated with and is a potential marker for HCC resistance to paclitaxel chemotherapy in Hep3B and HepG2 cell lines. Curcumin is shown to decrease Lin28B expression in hepatocellular cancer and exhibit paclitaxel-sensitizing effect [26]. In rats, curcumin is shown to protect hepatocytes against diethylnitrosamine-induced hepatocarcinogenesis [19].

A decade of preclinical research on cell cultures and in animals has shown that curcumin from saffron can increase sensitization of tumor to different chemotherapy agents including 5-fluorouracil (5-FU), oxaliplatin, vincristine, paclitaxel, doxorubicin, melphalan, cisplatin, gemcitabine, butyrate, vinorelbine, etoposide, and bortezomib. It also sensitizes many tumors to gamma radiation therapy. Mechanism involves downregulation of various growth regulatory pathways including multidrug resistance proteins, growth factor receptors, anti-apoptotic proteins, Akt, COX2, NF-kB, and STAT3. On the other hand, it protects normal organs like kidney, oral mucosa, heart, and liver from chemo- and radiotherapy-induced toxicity. This effect is thought to be mediated through the activation of NRF2 (nuclear factor erythroid 2-related factor 2) and increased expression of antioxidant enzymes (for example, glutathione peroxidase, modulatory subunit of γ-glutamyl-cysteine ligase, hemeoxygenase-1, and NAD(P)H:quinone oxidoreductase 1), increasing glutathione, inhibiting the activity of p300 histone acetyltransferase (HAT), and directly quenching free radicals [30].

9.3 Garlic

Garlic (*Allium sativum*) is commonly used as a flavoring agent in cooking and as medicinal food for its anticancer, antibacterial, and immunomodulatory properties. It is most commonly used as herbal remedy [31]. Multiple organosulfur compounds are present in garlic, which include diallyl trisulfide (DAT), diallyl disulfide (DAD), allicin, and diallyl sulfide (DAS), which are lipid soluble. S-allyl cysteine (SAC) and S-allylmercaptocysteine (SAMC) are water soluble [32]. Aged garlic is a good source of SAMC, which has strong hepatoprotective properties. A recent study has shown that SAMC affects the interface between MAPK pathway and TGF-β and induces apoptosis of HepG2 cells [33]. In another study, SAMC promoted apoptosis of hepatic cancer cells without influencing the normal liver cells via direct interaction with Wnt-pathway co-receptor LRP6 on the cell membrane [34]. Allicin induces cell death by apoptosis in hepatocyte cancer cells HepG2 (p53 (wild type)) cells.

Another trial demonstrated caspase-dependent and -independent apoptosis in Hep3B cells by allicin through the overproduction of reactive oxygen species (ROS) [35, 36]. Multiple studies have demonstrated antitumor properties of SAC against different human malignancies including hepatocellular cancer. It inhibits the proliferation of hepatocellular cells, induces apoptosis, causes cell cycle arrest of HCC cells in S phase, and inhibits migration and invasion of HCC cells [32]. Diallyl trisulfides were shown to have significant antitumor activity against orthotopic transplantation model through the induction of apoptosis and the inhibition of proliferation of liver cancer cells [37].

As noted earlier, garlic also has chemopreventive properties which include scavenging ROS and electrophiles, decreasing inflammation, enhancing DNA repair, inhibiting proliferation, inhibiting angiogenesis, and enhancing immunity [31].

9.4 Cinnamon

Cinnamon is obtained from the bark of *Cinnamomum verum* and is traditionally used all across the world for its flavor. It has been used for multiple medical conditions including cancer. Its antineoplastic activity is attributed to two bioactive compounds: (1) 2-methoxycinnamaldehyde (2-MCA) and (2) cuminaldehyde. 2-MCA is shown to have antiproliferative effect on human HCC SK-Hep-1 cells in both the in vitro and in vivo studies. Tumor-suppressive effect is due to apoptosis downregulation of proliferative controls of cell, inhibition of DNA-binding activity of NF-kB, and decreased level of COX-2 and prostaglandin E2 [38]. Cuminaldehyde has been reported to induce apoptosis and inhibit growth of HCC by depleting mitochondrial membrane potential and activation of caspase-9 and caspase-3 [19].

9.5 Saffron

Saffron is a spice acquired from the flower of *Crocus sativus* [39]. Biologically active ingredients include carotene, crocin, anthocyanin, and lycopene. Saffron treatment has been shown to inhibit the growth of QGY-7703 cancer cells by decreasing telomerase activity, increasing Bax/Bcl-2 ratio, and enhancing expression of P21, hence promoting apoptosis. The number of senescent cells increases markedly [40]. Saffron carotenoids inhibit STAT3 (signal transducer and activator of transcription 3), a protein involved in survival, growth, new blood vessel formation, invasion, and metastasis in Hep3B and HepG2 hepatocellular cells. Carotenoids also inhibited STAT3-regulated anti-apoptotic (Bcl-2, survivin), invasive (CXCR4), angiogenic (VEGF), and proliferative (cyclin) proteins [41]. Crocin has pro-apoptotic and antiproliferative properties which are shown in the induced HCC models. Crocin inhibits NF-kB and imparts anti-inflammatory and antineoplastic activity. In vitro studies have demonstrated that crocin arrests the cell cycle at S and G2/M phases and induces cell death in HepG2 cells. Further analysis confirmed the role of NF-kB as a potential regulator of this action. Hence, crocin prevents early dysplasia in liver cells [42]. Crocin is shown to decrease the expression of catalytic subunit of telomerase enzyme in HepG2 cells, hence imparting antiproliferative activity [43].

9.6 Coffee

Coffee is a very common beverage all over the world and billions of cups are consumed daily. Bioactive molecules in coffee include caffeine, diterpenes, and chlorogenic acid. Coffee has been studied in multiple studies for several medical conditions for its anti-fibrotic, antineoplastic, anti-inflammatory, and antioxidant properties [19]. Reports by the International Agency for Research on Cancer (IARC) [44] and the World Cancer Research Fund (WCRF) have shown coffee to be helpful in preventing against HCC [45]. A meta-analysis on the benefit of coffee has reported that the relative risk of HCC for one additional cup of coffee every day was 0.75 [95% confidence interval (CI) 0.65–0.83] [46]. In another meta-analysis involving more than two million participants, 35% risk reduction in HCC was seen by increasing the coffee consumption by two cups per day. This reduction in risk was not dependent on the etiology of HCC: HBV/HCV, T2DM, high BMI, and high alcohol intake [45].

As per data from few studies in which both caffeinated and decaffeinated coffee were evaluated, risk reduction for decaffeinated coffee was 14% for two additional cups per day. As this protective effect is not dependent on the etiology of HCC, coffee is believed to affect a common pathway in the development of HCC. As noted earlier, 90% of HCC develops on the background of cirrhosis and many studies have shown a protective effect of coffee against cirrhosis—this can be a major factor responsible for the antineoplastic effect of coffee. Caffeine is also believed to have antitumor effect, which can explain the lesser benefit obtained from the decaffeinated drinks. Caffeine has also been demonstrated to reduce the proliferation of HCC cancer cells [45].

There are some regional differences between the protective effects of coffee on HCC. Preventive effect of coffee consumption on hepatocellular cancer is somewhat smaller in Japan as compared to Europe. This is believed to be due to the differences in the original composition of coffee such as kahweol, chlorogenic acid, and cafestol [47]. One study showed that the quantity of kahweol and cafestol in instant coffee is much lower than in the French press or boiled coffee. Instant coffee or drip filtered is the main drink in Japan [48]. However, in another prospective cohort study with 7.5-year follow-up, instant and ground coffee were found to be similar in the protective effects against hepatocellular cancer (hazard ratio 0.51 vs. 0.47) [49]. The preventive effect was found to be dose dependent. A prospective cohort study with 16-year follow-up showed adjusted hazard ratio for liver cancer of 0.65 for less than one cup of coffee per day, 0.63 for one cup per day, and 0.40 for two or more cups per day compared with the nondrinkers [50].

Coffee ($\geq$3 cups per day) is also found to have a preventive role against recurrence of HCC after orthotopic liver transplant for HCC. The hazard ratio was 0.29 (CI 0.12–0.17). Postoperative coffee intake was also found to result in an improved overall survival. This effect is shown to be mediated by antagonistic effect of caffeine on adenosine A2AR-mediated growth enhancing the effects on HCC cells [51]. Data from green and black tea is however conflicting with some studies reporting no benefit [50]. A principal catechin of green tea, epigallocatechin-3-gallate (EGCG), is shown to have antioxidant and antineoplastic activity. Many in vitro experiments and some in vivo analyses in animals have shown that EGCG induces cell death and inhibits progression of HCC by acting on different molecular pathways. More studies are obviously desirable in this domain to have more conclusive outcomes [52].

10 Cruciferous Vegetables

Multiple studies have reported that daily use of cruciferous vegetables is helpful in preventing cancer. Glucosinolates are important bioactive chemicals present in cruciferous vegetables and their metabolites, i.e., isothiocyanates, are found to have chemoprotective properties. Other chemicals have shown to inhibit NF-kB and have beneficial anticancer properties [53]. Other bioactive molecules in cruciferous vegetables like iberin and alyssin are shown to increase intracellular reactive oxygen species (ROS) and depolymerization of tubulin in cell cultures of HepG2 [54].

11 Conclusions and Future Perspectives

Hepatocellular carcinoma is the most common primary liver cancer and is the most common cause of cancer-related morbidity and mortality in chronic liver disease. Despite significant advances in translational oncologic research, mortality remains very high. Allopathic medicine does not have many options for patients who do not qualify for the surgical interventions. Phytochemicals have emerging role(s) in the prevention and treatment of multiple malignancies including hepatocellular carcinoma. Evidence is mainly based on preclinical (in vitro) studies conducted on cells. Few in vivo studies are also available which are mainly observational. Promising results are seen with ginger, garlic, coffee, cruciferous vegetables, and saffron. Biologically active ingredients in these phytochemicals seem to play important role(s) in the prevention and management of hepatocellular carcinoma. Some agents are also shown to augment the role of chemo- and radiotherapy, which is the cornerstone for the treatment for metastatic disease. Very few, if any, adverse effects of phytochemicals are reported and these spices are commonly used in almost every household globally. Good-quality randomized controlled trials are needed to further evaluate their role(s) and quantify the benefits. Also, it is unknown yet if the combination of these phytochemicals would have synergistic or augmentative benefits. Furthermore, nanotechnology can enhance bioavailability of these active ingredients into bloodstream which can theoretically enhance the antineoplastic activity. Multiple other food items also contain many phytochemicals and their role(s) in hepatocellular cancer needs further research and implementation.

Acknowledgements *Author Contributions*: Dr. Hammad Zafar conceived the idea and subsequently all the authors have diligently contributed to the development and preparation of this research manuscript (book chapter), including the literature search, concept organization, data interpretation, and writings. All the authors have read and approved the final draft for publication.

Conflict of Interest: The authors declare that they have no conflicts of interest associated with this book chapter.

Financial Disclosures: None to disclose.

References

1. Pocha, C., & Xie, C. (2019). Hepatocellular carcinoma in alcoholic and non-alcoholic fatty liver disease-one of a kind or two different enemies? *Translational Gastroenterology and Hepatology, 4*, 72.
2. Hartke, J., Johnson, M., & Ghabril, M. (2017). The diagnosis and treatment of hepatocellular carcinoma. *Seminars in Diagnostic Pathology, 34*(2), 153–159.
3. Singal, A. G., Lampertico, P., & Nahon, P. (2020). Epidemiology and surveillance for hepatocellular carcinoma: New trends. *Journal of Hepatology, 72*(2), 250–261.
4. Forner, A., Reig, M., & Bruix, J. (2018). Hepatocellular carcinoma. *Lancet, 391*(10127), 1301–1314.
5. International Consensus Group for Hepatocellular Neoplasia The International Consensus Group for Hepatocellular Neoplasia. (2009). Pathologic diagnosis of early hepatocellular carcinoma: A report of the international consensus group for hepatocellular neoplasia. *Hepatology, 49*(2), 658–664.
6. Braicu, C., Burz, C., Berindan-Neagoe, I., et al. (2009). Hepatocellular carcinoma: Tumorigenesis and prediction markers. *Gastroenterology Research, 2*(4), 191–199.
7. Gomaa, A. I., Khan, S. A., Leen, E. L., Waked, I., & Taylor-Robinson, S. D. (2009). Diagnosis of hepatocellular carcinoma. *World Journal of Gastroenterology, 15*(11), 1301–1314.
8. Lim, S. O., Gu, J. M., Kim, M. S., et al. (2008). Epigenetic changes induced by reactive oxygen species in hepatocellular carcinoma: Methylation of the E-cadherin promoter. *Gastroenterology, 135*(6), 2128–2140, 2140.e2121-2128.
9. Itoh, T., Shiro, T., Seki, T., et al. (2000). Relationship between p53 overexpression and the proliferative activity in hepatocellular carcinoma. *International Journal of Molecular Medicine, 6*(2), 137–142.
10. Zhou, L., Liu, J., & Luo, F. (2006). Serum tumor markers for detection of hepatocellular carcinoma. *World Journal of Gastroenterology, 12*(8), 1175–1181.
11. Baek, H. J., Lim, S. C., Kitisin, K., et al. (2008). Hepatocellular cancer arises from loss of transforming growth factor beta signaling adaptor protein embryonic liver fodrin through abnormal angiogenesis. *Hepatology, 48*(4), 1128–1137.
12. Masaki, T., Shiratori, Y., Rengifo, W., et al. (2000). Hepatocellular carcinoma cell cycle: Study of Long-Evans cinnamon rats. *Hepatology, 32*(4 Pt 1), 711–720.
13. Lévy, L., Renard, C. A., Wei, Y., & Buendia, M. A. (2002). Genetic alterations and oncogenic pathways in hepatocellular carcinoma. *Annals of the New York Academy of Sciences, 963*, 21–36.
14. Zhu, A. X., & Raymond, E. (2009). Early development of sunitinib in hepatocellular carcinoma. *Expert Review of Anticancer Therapy, 9*(1), 143–150.
15. Dimri, M., & Satyanarayana, A. (2020). Molecular signaling pathways and therapeutic targets in hepatocellular carcinoma. *Cancers (Basel), 12*(2), 491. https://doi.org/10.3390/cancers12020491.
16. Fabregat, I., & Caballero-Díaz, D. (2018). Transforming growth factor-β-induced cell plasticity in liver fibrosis and hepatocarcinogenesis. *Frontiers in Oncology, 8*, 357.
17. Elsonbaty, S. M., Zahran, W. E., & Moawed, F. S. (2017). Gamma-irradiated β-glucan modulates signaling molecular targets of hepatocellular carcinoma in rats. *Tumour Biology, 39*(8), 1010428317708703.
18. Goyal, L., Muzumdar, M. D., & Zhu, A. X. (2013). Targeting the HGF/c-MET pathway in hepatocellular carcinoma. *Clinical Cancer Research, 19*(9), 2310–2318.
19. Rawat, D., Shrivastava, S., Naik, R. A., Chhonker, S. K., Mehrotra, A., & Koiri, R. K. (2018). An overview of natural plant products in the treatment of hepatocellular carcinoma. *Anti-Cancer Agents in Medicinal Chemistry, 18*(13), 1838–1859.
20. Fahmi, A., Hassanen, N., Abdur-Rahman, M., & Shams-Eldin, E. (2019). Phytochemicals, antioxidant activity and hepatoprotective effect of ginger. *Biomarkers, 24*(5), 436–447.

21. Akhtar, T., & Sheikh, N. (2016). Chemopreventive prospective of dietary spices against hepatocellular carcinoma. *Current Science, 110*(4), 579–583.
22. Wang, Y., Wang, S., Song, R., et al. (2019). Ginger polysaccharides induced cell cycle arrest and apoptosis in human hepatocellular carcinoma HepG2 cells. *International Journal of Biological Macromolecules, 123*, 81–90.
23. Wani, N. A., Zhang, B., Teng, K. Y., et al. (2018). Reprograming of glucose metabolism by zerumbone suppresses hepatocarcinogenesis. *Molecular Cancer Research, 16*(2), 256–268.
24. Kim, Y. J., Jeon, Y., Kim, T., et al. (2017). Combined treatment with zingerone and its novel derivative synergistically inhibits TGF-β1 induced epithelial-mesenchymal transition, migration and invasion of human hepatocellular carcinoma cells. *Bioorganic & Medicinal Chemistry Letters, 27*(4), 1081–1088.
25. Chen, S. Y., Lee, Y. R., Hsieh, M. C., et al. (2018). Enhancing the anticancer activity of Antrodia cinnamomea in hepatocellular carcinoma cells via cocultivation with ginger: The impact on cancer cell survival pathways. *Frontiers in Pharmacology, 9*, 780.
26. Tian, N., Shangguan, W., Zhou, Z., Yao, Y., Fan, C., & Cai, L. (2019). Lin28b is involved in curcumin-reversed paclitaxel chemoresistance and associated with poor prognosis in hepatocellular carcinoma. *Journal of Cancer, 10*(24), 6074–6087.
27. Elmansi, A. M., El-Karef, A. A., Shishtawy, M. M. E., & Eissa, L. A. (2017). Hepatoprotective effect of curcumin on hepatocellular carcinoma through autophagic and apoptotic pathways. *Annals of Hepatology, 16*(4), 607–618.
28. Wang, F., Ye, X., Zhai, D., et al. (2020). Curcumin-loaded nanostructured lipid carrier induced apoptosis in human HepG2 cells through activation of the DR5/caspase-mediated extrinsic apoptosis pathway. *Acta Pharmaceutica, 70*(2), 227–237.
29. Marquardt, J. U., Gomez-Quiroz, L., Arreguin Camacho, L. O., et al. (2015). Curcumin effectively inhibits oncogenic NF-κB signaling and restrains stemness features in liver cancer. *Journal of Hepatology, 63*(3), 661–669.
30. Goel, A., & Aggarwal, B. B. (2010). Curcumin, the golden spice from Indian saffron, is a chemosensitizer and radiosensitizer for tumors and chemoprotector and radioprotector for normal organs. *Nutrition and Cancer, 62*(7), 919–930.
31. Aly, S. M., Fetaih, H. A., Hassanin, A. A. I., Abomughaid, M. M., & Ismail, A. A. (2019). Protective effects of garlic and cinnamon oils on hepatocellular carcinoma in albino rats. *Analytical Cellular Pathology (Amsterdam), 2019*, 9895485.
32. Ng, K. T., Guo, D. Y., Cheng, Q., et al. (2012). A garlic derivative, S-allyl cysteine (SAC), suppresses proliferation and metastasis of hepatocellular carcinoma. *PLoS One, 7*(2), e31655.
33. Tong, D., Qu, H., Meng, X., et al. (2014). S-allylmercaptocysteine promotes MAPK inhibitor-induced apoptosis by activating the TGF-β signaling pathway in cancer cells. *Oncology Reports, 32*(3), 1124–1132.
34. Xiao, J., Xing, F., Liu, Y., et al. (2018). Garlic-derived compound. *Acta Pharmaceutica Sinica B, 8*(4), 575–586.
35. Chu, Y. L., Ho, C. T., Chung, J. G., Raghu, R., Lo, Y. C., & Sheen, L. Y. (2013). Allicin induces anti-human liver cancer cells through the p53 gene modulating apoptosis and autophagy. *Journal of Agricultural and Food Chemistry, 61*(41), 9839–9848.
36. Kim, H. J., Han, M. H., Kim, G. Y., Choi, Y. W., & Choi, Y. H. (2012). Hexane extracts of garlic cloves induce apoptosis through the generation of reactive oxygen species in Hep3B human hepatocarcinoma cells. *Oncology Reports, 28*(5), 1757–1763.
37. Belloir, C., Singh, V., Daurat, C., Siess, M. H., & Le Bon, A. M. (2006). Protective effects of garlic sulfur compounds against DNA damage induced by direct- and indirect-acting genotoxic agents in HepG2 cells. *Food and Chemical Toxicology, 44*(6), 827–834.
38. Perng, D. S., Tsai, Y. H., Cherng, J., et al. (2016). Discovery of a novel anticancer agent with both anti-topoisomerase I and II activities in hepatocellular carcinoma SK-Hep-1 cells in vitro and in vivo: Cinnamomum verum Component 2-methoxycinnamaldehyde. *Drug Design, Development and Therapy, 10*, 141–153.

39. Bolhassani, A., Khavari, A., & Bathaie, S. Z. (2014). Saffron and natural carotenoids: Biochemical activities and anti-tumor effects. *Biochimica et Biophysica Acta, 1845*(1), 20–30.
40. Liu, T., Tian, L., Fu, X., Wei, L., Li, J., & Wang, T. (2019). Saffron inhibits the proliferation of hepatocellular carcinoma via inducing cell apoptosis. *Panminerva Medica*. https://doi.org/10.23736/S0031-0808.18.03561-9.
41. Kim, B., & Park, B. (2018). Saffron carotenoids inhibit STAT3 activation and promote apoptotic progression in IL-6-stimulated liver cancer cells. *Oncology Reports, 39*(4), 1883–1891.
42. Amin, A., Hamza, A. A., Daoud, S., et al. (2016). Saffron-based crocin prevents early lesions of liver cancer: In vivo, in vitro and network analyses. *Recent Patents on Anti-Cancer Drug Discovery, 11*(1), 121–133.
43. Noureini, S. K., & Wink, M. (2012). Anti-proliferative effects of crocin in HepG2 cells by telomerase inhibition and hTERT down-regulation. *Asian Pacific Journal of Cancer Prevention, 13*(5), 2305–2309.
44. Humans IWGotEoCRt. Drinking coffee, mate, and very hot beverages. 2018.
45. Kennedy, O. J., Roderick, P., Buchanan, R., Fallowfield, J. A., Hayes, P. C., & Parkes, J. (2017). Coffee, including caffeinated and decaffeinated coffee, and the risk of hepatocellular carcinoma: A systematic review and dose-response meta-analysis. *BMJ Open, 7*(5), e013739.
46. Bravi, F., Tavani, A., Bosetti, C., Boffetta, P., & La Vecchia, C. (2017). Coffee and the risk of hepatocellular carcinoma and chronic liver disease: A systematic review and meta-analysis of prospective studies. *European Journal of Cancer Prevention, 26*(5), 368–377.
47. Bøhn, S. K., Blomhoff, R., & Paur, I. (2014). Coffee and cancer risk, epidemiological evidence, and molecular mechanisms. *Molecular Nutrition & Food Research, 58*(5), 915–930.
48. Tamura, T., Hishida, A., & Wakai, K. (2019). Coffee consumption and liver cancer risk in Japan: A meta-analysis of six prospective cohort studies. *Nagoya Journal of Medical Science, 81*(1), 143–150.
49. Tran, K. T., Coleman, H. G., McMenamin, Ú., & Cardwell, C. R. (2019). Coffee consumption by type and risk of digestive cancer: A large prospective cohort study. *British Journal of Cancer, 120*(11), 1059–1066.
50. Tamura, T., Wada, K., Konishi, K., et al. (2018). Coffee, green tea, and caffeine intake and liver cancer risk: A prospective cohort study. *Nutrition and Cancer, 70*(8), 1210–1216.
51. Wiltberger, G., Wu, Y., Lange, U., et al. (2019). Protective effects of coffee consumption following liver transplantation for hepatocellular carcinoma in cirrhosis. *Alimentary Pharmacology & Therapeutics, 49*(6), 779–788.
52. Bimonte, S., Albino, V., Piccirillo, M., et al. (2019). Epigallocatechin-3-gallate in the prevention and treatment of hepatocellular carcinoma: Experimental findings and translational perspectives. *Drug Design, Development and Therapy, 13*, 611–621.
53. Soundararajan, P., & Kim, J. S. (2018). Anti-carcinogenic glucosinolates in cruciferous vegetables and their antagonistic effects on prevention of cancers. *Molecules, 23*(11), E2983. https://doi.org/10.3390/molecules23112983.
54. Pocasap, P., Weerapreeyakul, N., & Thumanu, K. (2019). Alyssin and iberin in cruciferous vegetables exert anticancer activity in HepG2 by increasing intracellular reactive oxygen species and tubulin depolymerization. *Biomolecules & Therapeutics (Seoul)., 27*(6), 540–552.

Chapter 14
Phytochemicals: Current Understandings of the Modern Therapeutic Approaches for Hepatocellular Carcinoma

Austin Cook and Shadab A. Siddiqi

Abstract The growing occurrence of hepatocellular carcinoma (HCC) worldwide poses major concerns because of high mortality rate and poor prognosis. A lack of explicit diagnostics makes early detection of HCC implausible accentuating the demand of novel therapeutic approaches. In this chapter we discuss briefly major risk factors that contribute to the development of HCC and progress made in the identification of new molecular biomarkers and their significance in the detection of HCC. Here, our main focus is on recent advances made in the development of phytochemicals as novel prophylactics and therapeutic agents. First, we discuss a number of phytochemicals that are used to prevent or treat a variety of cancers. Subsequently, our emphasis is shifted on phytochemicals that are specifically significant in the treatment or prevention of HCC. A number of phytochemicals are emerging as plausible therapeutic agents for the treatment of HCC and are discussed in this chapter.

Keywords Hepatocellular carcinoma (HCC) · Phytochemicals · Hepatic steatosis · Nonalcoholic fatty liver disease (NAFLD) · Cancer stem cells (CSCs) · Hepatitis B virus (HBV) · Hepatitis C virus (HCV)

Abbreviations

ABCG2	Adenosine triphosphate (ATP)-binding cassette subfamily G member 2
ACVR1	Activin A receptor type I
AFLD	Alcoholic fatty liver disease
AFP	Alpha fetoprotein
ALD	Alcohol-related liver disease
ALT	Alanine transaminase

A. Cook · S. A. Siddiqi (✉)
Burnett School of Biomedical Sciences, College of Medicine, University of Central Florida, Orlando, FL, USA
e-mail: shadab.siddiqi@ucf.edu

G. P. Nagaraju (ed.), *Phytochemicals Targeting Tumor Microenvironment in Gastrointestinal Cancers*, https://doi.org/10.1007/978-3-030-48405-7_14

AST	Aspartate transaminase
Bcl-2	B-cell lymphoma 2
BMP	Bone morphogenetic protein
$CD8^+$ T cell	Cluster of differentiation 8 T cell
COX-2	Cyclooxygenase-2
CRAE	*C. rhizome* aqueous extract
CSC	Cancer stem cell
CT	Computed tomography
CTL-4	Cytotoxic T-lymphocyte-associated protein 4
CXCL1	Chemokine (C-X-C motif) ligand 1
CXCR4	C-X-C motif chemokine receptor 4
DIHS	Drug-induced hepatic steatosis
DLK-1	Delta-like 1/fetal antigen-1
DNA	Deoxyribonucleic acid
EGCG	Epigallocatechin-3-gallate
EMT	Epithelial-mesenchymal transition
EpCAM	Epithelial cell adhesion molecule
GLB1	Galactosidase beta 1
GSTM1	Glutathione S-transferase mu 1
GSTT1	Glutathione S-transferase theta 1
GTP	Guanosine-5′-triphosphate
HA	Hyaluronic acid
HAV	Hepatitis A virus
HBeAg	Hepatitis B e-antigen
HBV	Hepatitis B virus
HBx	HBV-encoded X antigen
HCC	Hepatocellular carcinoma
hCSC	Human CSC
HCT-15	Human colorectal adenocarcinoma
HCV	Hepatitis C virus
HLA	Human leukocyte antigen
HPC	HCC progenitor cell
Hsp	Heat-shock protein
IBD	Inflammatory bowel disease
IGF	Insulin-like growth factor 1
IKK	IκB kinase
IL	Interleukin
iNOS	Inducible nitric oxide synthase
JAK2	Janus kinase 2
JNK	c-Jun N-terminal kinase
LGR5	Leucine-rich repeat-containing G-protein-coupled receptor 5
MAPK	Microtubule-associated protein kinase
MCF-7	Michigan Cancer Foundation-7
MDM2	Mouse double minute 2 homolog

miRNA	microRNA
MKK7	Mitogen-activated protein kinase kinase 7
MRA	Magnetic resonance angiogram
MRI	Magnetic resonance imaging
mTOR	Mammalian target of rapamycin
NAFLD	Nonalcoholic fatty liver disease
NASH	Nonalcoholic steatohepatitis
NF-kB	Nuclear factor kappa-light-chain-enhancer of activated B cells
OCT4	Octamer-binding transcription factor 4
PAE	Prostate artery embolization
PARP	Poly-ADP-ribose polymerase
PD-1	Programmed cell death protein 1
PDGF-BB	Platelet-derived growth factor subunit BB
PDL-1	Programmed death ligand-1
PI3K	Phosphoinositide 3-kinase
PKB	Protein kinase B
PKC	Protein kinase C
PPAR	Peroxisome proliferator-activated receptor
PTEN	Phosphatase and tensin homolog
RNA	Ribonucleic acid
ROCK	Rho-associated protein kinase
ROS	Reactive oxygen species
SMAD7	Mothers against Dpp homolog 8
SNP	Single-nucleotide polymorphism
STAT3	Signal transducer and activator of transcription 3
STRAP	Serine/threonine kinase receptor-associated protein
T2DM	Type 2 diabetes
TACE	Transarterial chemoembolization
TAE	Transarterial embolization
TCTP	Translationally controlled tumor protein
TERT	Telomerase reverse transcriptase
TGF-β1	Transforming growth factor-beta 1
TGP	Total glucosides of peony
TIPRL	TOR signaling pathway regulator
TNFα	Tumor necrosis factor alpha
TRAIL	TNF-related apoptosis-inducing ligand
VEGF	Vascular endothelial growth factor
XRCC3	X-ray repair cross complementing 3

1 Background

Hepatocellular carcinoma (HCC) is recognized as one of the largest contributors to cancer mortalities with the incidence rate increasing globally. In the USA alone, over 42,000 new cases arose in 2019 and nearly 32,000 deaths occurred as a result of this disease [1]. Not to mention, the prognosis is poor with an average 5-year survival rate of less than 10% [2]. Some causes of hepatic cancer are known, which include hepatitis C virus (HCV), hepatitis B virus (HBV), and alcohol-induced cirrhosis. Other links to hepatic cancer have been speculated in recent years. Such links include genetics, obesity, type 2 diabetes, alcohol-related liver disease (ALD), nonalcoholic steatohepatitis, and nonalcoholic fatty liver disease (NAFLD) [3–7]. The amplified attention to genetic studies in the recent years revealed numerous genetic correlations in hepatic cancer [8]. HCC development and metastasis can also be due to dysregulation of factors related to epigenetics, such as DNA methylation, modifications of histones, noncoding miRNAs, and other related modulations [8, 9]. Diagnostic methods are currently insufficient to achieve early detection of the disease, and patients remain largely asymptomatic until the later stages of development. Current therapeutic strategies involve surgical resection, transplantation, radiofrequency ablation, chemotherapy, etc. and have yet to prove efficient in treating these patients. Moreover, the extensive variability of subtypes of cell populations in HCC further complexes successful treatment [10]. Cancer stem cells (CSCs) have recently been deemed a main contributor to the development, progression, and recurrence of cancer, since it is thought that this characteristic provides the cell with proliferative and invasive traits [9, 11, 12]. Due to these predicaments, we bring our focus to phytochemicals as potential candidates in the optimal treatment of hepatic cancer. Specialties of phytochemicals include lack of side effects and their unique targeting of hepatic CSCs, which happens to be a trait that most current treatments lack.

1.1 Causes and Pathogenesis of HCC

Two classifications exist for hepatic cancer: primary and metastatic. HCC and hepatic angiosarcoma are two primary hepatic cancers with HCC accounting for nearly all cases. As depicted in Fig. 14.1, various risk factors of HCC have been identified, including HBV, HCV, obesity, type 2 diabetes, alcohol-related liver disease (ALD), nonalcoholic steatohepatitis (NASH), and NAFLD [3–7, 9, 13, 14]. Obesity and diabetes are known to be connected to NASH, consequently leading to HCC [3, 4, 7, 9]. Incidence due to viral and alcohol-related causes is declining, while new cases due to NASH and NAFLD are taking their place [4, 5, 13]. Of course, the genome-wide association studies have revealed the large role of genetics in relation to several diseases, including HCC. For instance,

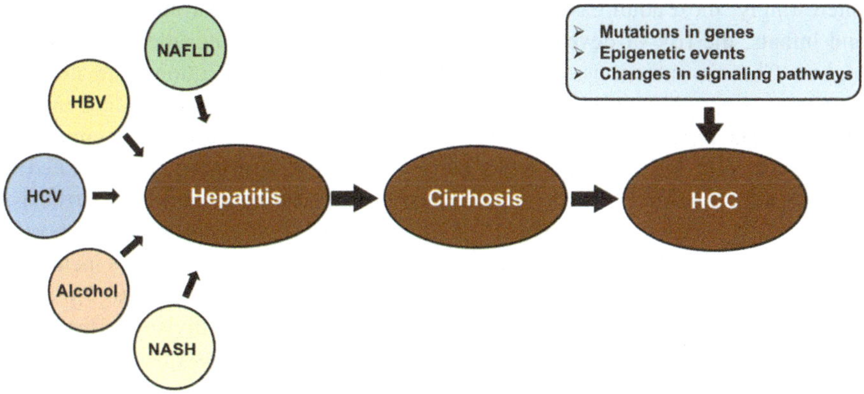

Fig. 14.1 Major risk factors that contribute to the development of hepatocellular carcinoma (HCC)

single-nucleotide polymorphisms (SNPs) have been found in GTSM1, GSTT1, MDM2, XRCC3, HLA, CTL-4, GLB1, TGF-β1, and many more [10].

Furthermore, hepatitis is an infection of the liver, and there are three types: hepatitis A virus (HAV), HBV, and HCV. We will focus on HBV and HCV, as they are the two main contributors to HCC. Although viral causes of HCC are decreasing, compared to metabolic causes, they are currently the largest contributors. Upon chronic infection, individuals are susceptible to liver cirrhosis, which could lead to liver cancer [10]. Natural killer cells and $CD8^+$ T cells specific to HBV and HCV were recently described as possible drivers of liver damage. More postulations included macrophages and neutrophils releasing DNA-damaging ROS and nitrogen compounds during inflammation, as well as epigenetic changes, mitochondrial disfunction, senescence, and alterations of chromosomes [9, 10]. A few studies focused on the roles of PPARα/γ in relation to HCC. Intriguingly, they mentioned that several studies have found connections between PPARα/γ and the onset of not only HCC, but also NAFLD, HBV, and HCV. Therefore, there might be a relation between the regulation of PPARα/γ during NAFLD, HBV infection, and HCV infection and the development of HCC. miRNA regulation has been postulated as the relation [10, 15, 16]. The inflammatory cytokine IL-8 was concluded as a contributor to inflammation leading to HCC by promoting cancer growth, progression, and metastasis [6, 11]. IL-8 plays a role in upregulating neurotensin, CXCL1, and MAPK pathway to accomplish tumorigenic characteristics [11].

Over 250 million people have chronic HBV infection with an associated death rate of nearly 900,000 per year [17]. Some reports claim HBV as Eastern Asia's and sub-Saharan Africa's major cause of HCC, accounting for 70% of cases [9]. Because of its high incidence and mortality, HBV is clearly dangerous and accounts for its importance in the prevention of HCC. Sexual contact and contact with blood of an infected individual are the methods of transmission for HBV. Contact with blood can occur in several ways, such as sharing needles, coming into contact with sores, or exposure to an infected mother during birth. HBV can be acute or chronic.

Interestingly, most adult cases of acute HBV do not become chronic. For toddlers and infants, the risk of developing chronic HBV from an acute infection is much higher. Chronic infections, typically defined as lifelong infections, are notably important, since they pose the risk of hepatic cancer onset. Chronic infection and inflammation result in liver cirrhosis [18]. Subsequently, the chronic infections typically cause HCC, due to the development of liver cirrhosis [6, 10, 17, 19, 20]. Notably, however, HBV can initiate HCC without the development of cirrhosis. This is thought to be due to HBV's ability to transfer its genome into its host's genome. Disruption to chromosomes was observed to affect several genes including those related to the immune system, cell cycle, and DNA processing [6, 10]. Notably, integration into host DNA is conserved through replication and division. Therefore, upregulation of hepatocyte proliferation caused by the virus consequently promotes the rapid increase of damage [10].

The prevalence of HCV was estimated to be nearly 140 million globally, with an associated death rate of greater than 350,000 [19]. HCV is stated to be responsible for 50–70% of HCC cases in North American and European countries [9]. Transmission of this viral infection is known to occur from contact with blood of infected individuals. However, unlike with HBV sexual contact and mother-to-child transmission are less likely to result in infection. Similar to HBV, HCV may begin as acute and have the potential to develop into a chronic infection. The majority of individuals with acute infection are susceptible to chronic infection, although slightly less likely than those with HBV infection [17, 20–24]. As previously discussed, chronic infection and inflammation pose as risk factors for HCC, due to the development of cirrhosis. Interestingly, only a small amount of liver cirrhosis cases due to HCV develop into HCC, complicating the elucidation of the responsible mechanisms. A few ideas are thought to indirectly lead to HCC development: promotion of hepatocyte proliferation and fatty liver, genetic mutations and disruptions causing inflammation and oxidative stress, stimulation of reactive oxygen species and mitochondrial damage, and finally immune responses triggered from the host [6, 7, 10, 18].

NAFLD and AFLD (alcoholic fatty liver disease) are the main diseases related to hepatic steatosis. The most prevalent form, NAFLD, is found in nearly 30% of all people, and is also the most prevalent cause of pediatric hepatic steatosis [3]. The connection between NAFLD and hepatocellular carcinoma lies behind its progression into NASH. Nearly half of all NASH-related deaths are observed due to HCC [5, 25, 26]. NASH occasionally develops into liver cirrhosis, which we previously determined to be a main risk factor for HCC. Oxidative stress and inflammation from excess lipid deposition cause the progression into NASH and liver cirrhosis, and also previously determined mechanisms responsible for HCC [3]. Here, inflammation is thought to be caused by TNFα and IL-6 via their activation of IKK, JNK, and STAT3 [5, 27–32]. NAFLD is known to correlate with diabetes and obesity, which were also previously mentioned as risk factors for HCC, as well [3]. As commonly known, obesity has become extremely prevalent worldwide. Over 90% of obese individuals present with NAFLD and 25% with NASH, 50% on average for T2DM. These same individuals have four and a half times higher risk of hepatic cancer

[5]. Leptin, known to be increased in obesity, was observed as a contributor to carcinogenesis and NAFLD advancement. This hormone can stimulate JAK2/STAT3 and PI3K/Akt pathways. The inverse effects of adiponectin were simultaneously observed to be downregulated, since adiponectin is decreased in obesity [27–32]. Several studies evaluated the relationship of diabetes to NAFLD and HCC. Diabetes was concluded to increase the risk of HCC and to be found more often among HCC patients compared to those without HCC [5]. Obesity is a main promoter of AFLD, as well. Alcoholic steatohepatitis, as a result of alcohol abuse, potentially accounts for around 20% of HCC cases in North America and Europe [9]. Found in nearly all alcoholic patients, AFLD can likely result in liver cirrhosis [3, 33–37]. As commonly known, obesity has become extremely prevalent worldwide. Hepatic steatosis is caused by metabolic, viral, and drug-induced routes. Metabolic determinants can be separated by inborn errors and acquired metabolic disfunction. Galactosemia, hereditary fructose intolerance, tyrosinemia, glycogen storage disease, Refsum syndrome, Shwachman syndrome, and Wilson disease are among the many inborn errors. Acquired metabolic disorders include IBD, Kwashiorkor, and starvation. On average, 60% of HCV-infected individuals develop hepatic steatosis, and is thought to be due to the insulin resistance and steatogenic nature of HCV. HBV, on the other hand, likely leads to hepatic steatosis indirectly, as a result of metabolic disruptions caused by HBV. Drug-induced hepatic steatosis (DIHS) has been associated with several medications used for neurological disorders, cardiovascular disorders, and infections, as well as chemotherapy medications [3, 27–37].

1.2 Heterogeneity and the Role of Cancer Stem Cells in Development of HCC

Heterogeneity exists between separate hepatic tumors, as well as within each tumor. They are referred to as intertumoral heterogeneity and intratumoral heterogeneity, respectively. Hundreds of genes responsible for encoding drug catabolism, inflammatory responses, and cell proliferation are found, through RNAseq screening, to be transcriptionally dysregulated. Cancer-associated genes, kinases, and cell cycle pathways comprise most of the variably expressed genes in HCC, as well as telomerase reverse transcriptase (TERT) and chromatin modifiers. These contribute to the difficulties of diagnosis, treatment, and recurrence of tumors. However, studying heterogeneity of tumors can also provide insight into the development of successful interventional strategies. Of particular importance, cancer stem cells are thought to be key promoters of heterogeneity among HCC cells [8, 9, 11, 12, 38–40]. Cancer stem cells (CSCs) are being recognized as a core component behind the mechanisms of cancer development and recurrence [11, 12, 39, 40]. This subpopulation of cells owe to the self-renewal, differentiating, and tumorigenic properties that promote malignancy. CSCs are heavily responsible for the difficulties of treatment and recurrence, as a result of their unique properties and the variety of CSCs coexisting within hepatic cancers. Several signaling pathways, epigenetic modulators, miRNAs, and metabolic enzymes collectively contribute to the maintenance and characteristics of hCSCs. Among the many mechanisms, some are shared by cells expressing certain markers, and others are unique to groups of cells. Notably, cellular markers are not specific only to CSCs. They are expressed among other cells of the body, and this should be taken into account when identifying CSCs. Furthermore, HCC cells expressing markers, such as CD133, CD44, CXCR4, OCT4, and NANOG, show increased initiation of cloning. CD133 HCC cells are even shown to persist when hypoxic and nutrient deprived by utilizing autophagy. Furthermore, it was shown that H-Ras and SV40LT promote the development of hepatic CSCs from three different lineages: differentiated adult hepatocytes, hepatic progenitor cells (HPCs), and lineage-committed hepatoblasts. HPCs are the most susceptible to alteration, although the overall understanding of formation has not been completely elucidated. CD47 hCSCs are one group that have portrayed traits of tumorigenesis, metastasis, and self-renewal. This group of cells is associated with upregulation of cathepsin S, protease-activated receptor 2, IL-8, and IL-6, which stimulate NF-kB, MAPK, and LIN28. CSCs are also capable of promoting each other through IL-6 mechanisms. Tumor-associated macrophages of CD14 cells can secrete IL-6, as well as TGF-β1, that induces STAT3-mediated cancer progression of CD44 hCSCs. TGF-β1 also causes hepatic cancer cells to undergo epithelial-mesenchymal transition. EMT is a core element of cancer progression and malignancy. One group demonstrated upregulating of Ras/Raf/MAPK and PI3K/Akt/mTOR pathways to be associated with hCSC-expressing markers CITED1, DLK1, CD133, LGR5, SOX9, SOX4, and AFP. Another group observed Akt- and miRNA-216a-mediated PTEN pathways, in conjunction with TGF-β, to be dysregulated in hCSCs with CD133, CD90, and EpCAM. CD133 hCSCs are enhanced from miRNA-130b inhibiting tumor protein 53-induced nuclear protein 1. These cells specifically complicate treatment strategies by employing Akt/PKB, Bcl-2, and MAPK/PI3K pathways. STAT3 and NANOG have large roles in CD24 hCSCs, along with Twist2. Twist2 is a transcription factor that exerts control over EMT by binding to a promoter region and providing self-renewal traits through STAT3/NANOG. Nanog is a transcription factor related to pluripotency with the ability to stimulate IGF. hCSCs' characteristics are also regulated by zinc finger protein-X linked. This transcription factor, known to have a large presence in embryonic and hematopoietic stem cells, exhibits control in hCSCs by binding to NANOG and SOX2 promoters. CD133, CD49, and CD45 HCC cells demonstrated CSC traits following knockout of *Mat1a*. This gene encodes methionine adenosyltransferase, which is necessary for the synthesis of S-adenosylmethionine; SAM is important in the body's management of liver injury and HCC. Histone deacetylase 3 and DNA methyltransferase 1 are two epigenetic modulators in the tumorgenicity, pluripotency, and self-renewal traits of hCSCs. MicroRNAs 148a, 142-3p, 216a, and 217 are found to be related to the CSC nature of some HCC cells. miRNA 148a interacts with BMP receptor ACVR1, whereas the latter two act through PTEN and SMAD7, initiating EMT [11, 41–50].

1.3 Current Diagnostic Approaches for HCC

Patients diagnosed with hepatic cancer typically do not present with symptoms until the end stages of the disease, at which point medical treatment is finally sought. In conjunction with its chronic onset, this hinderance in patient presentation complicates the early diagnosis of hepatic cancer. Upon presentation, if suspicion of hepatic dysfunction is raised during physical examination and patient history, then blood tests are suggested. Blood samples are examined for liver function and serum tumor markers, such as alpha-fetoprotein (AFP). Due to the difficulty of sufficiently diagnosing hepatic cancer, imaging exams are also recommended to confirm suspicions. Imaging exams used in the detection of hepatic cancer include CT, MRI, MRA, and ultrasound. The first three involve a technique referred to as triple phase, in which three success images are captured following injection of dye. More invasive approaches are sometimes necessary, such as biopsies. Biopsy is accomplished by a few methods: fine aspiration, core needle, or laparoscopy. The invasiveness of each procedure increases, respectively, although all of them are minimally invasive [51].

Further studies are warranted to determine more successful detection of early-onset hepatic cancer. Knowledge of cellular/chemical markers is emerging, as well as more clear understandings about the progression of diseases that are risk factors for hepatic cancer. Their implications could significantly improve interventional and preventive guideline [52]. For instance, if hepatic steatosis can be identified and treated at earlier stages, then its progression to HCC is potentially preventable [3]. However, hurdles present themselves, such as fibrosis [53]. The progression of fibrosis is not uniform, making it difficult to unravel and use in prognosis. HBV progression and potential development into HCC can possibly be determined from the expression of HBeAg/HBV-DNA levels [10]. Primary tumor cytokine mRNA levels were tested for prognostic capabilities. IL-8 expression was found to be heavily correlated with HCC development [6]. Accordingly, identification and examination of early-stage hepatic cancer tissue would be more achievable.

Molecular profiles of hepatocytes are potential predictors of survival and tumor recurrence. Observed through genome-wide and proteome-wide studies, they were found to be unique to various grades of hepatocyte maturation. Knowledge of specific molecular profiles also assists in diagnoses and provides insight towards therapeutic strategies. Many molecular markers of CSCs identified so far include CD90, EpCAM, CD133, CD24, CD13, CD34, SOX9, ABCG2, and DLK-1 [9, 11, 39, 41–50]. ABCG2 expression was observed in side-population cells, while the rest were all found to be expressed as CSC surface markers. EpCAM, CD24, and CD90 expressions were also found to be associated with sphere formation. However, the most frequently utilized molecular markers for identifying populations of hepatic CSCs are CD133, CD90, EpCAM, CD24, CD44, calcium channel $\alpha 2\delta$ 1 isoform 5, CD47, OV6, and CD13 [9, 11, 12]. Specific molecular markers for virally induced HCC have been elucidated, as well. HBV-encoded X antigen (HBx) is upregulated in HCC caused by HBV. This protein component stimulates activation of oncogenic and proliferative genes in the promotion of tumor and stem cell characteristics. This is supported by the observation that HCC progenitor cells (HPCs) are more tumorigenic when EpCAM and HBx are expressed, as compared to expression of EpCAM alone [11]. A separate group demonstrated a similar relationship between aflatoxin B1 and HBx; they are more tumorigenic together, as opposed to the single expression of either one [11, 40]. In a report from 2018, numerous epigenetic modulators were described in association to HCC. Such components included DNA methyltransferases, microRNAs, histone deacetylases, and more [8].

1.4 Current Treatment Modalities for HCC

Depending on the stage of the disease at the time of diagnosis and the overall health of the individual diagnosed, various treatment strategies are available. Specifically, patients are diagnosed on the basis of a few stages: 0, A, B, C, and D. A team of oncology and transplant surgeons, radiologists, and pathologists will assist in the advisement of treatments pending their agreed-upon diagnosis. In any case, if the patient's status is severe enough or unfit for standard treatments, then clinical trials are discussed as options. As appropriate for the patient and their stage of disease, strategies range from periodical surveillance to ablation therapy for stages 0, A, and B. Patients with lesions observed with only small lesions are suggested for surveillance, in which they are reevaluated every 3 months. As the severity increases, patients are recommended for surgeries including partial hepatectomy or total hepatectomy coupled with transplantation. The determined surgery is based on the ratio of effected tissue to healthy tissue. When a substantial amount of healthy tissue is intact, partial hepatectomy is performed. The effected tissue, as well as some healthy tissue in the surrounding environment, is excised. In some cases, tissue regeneration occurs, and the liver replaces the removed portion. In the event a total hepatectomy is necessary, only some individuals will qualify. Even those who qualify will only receive transplantation if a healthy liver donation is available. Many patients require alternative treatment in these cases, and as the second option results in poorer outcomes. Not to mention, surgical excision is usually not entirely successful with a recurrence rate of 70% [6]. Radiofrequency ablation, microwave therapy, percutaneous ethanol injection, and cryoablation are methods employed for tumor ablation. Radiofrequency is the application of high-energy radio waves to a tumor. The radio waves are transmitted to the tip of a needle that is inserted through the abdomen, in order to kill cancer cells. Microwave therapy utilizes the high-temperature nature of microwaves to kill cancer cells. This strategy has the added benefit of making the cancer cells more susceptible to further chemotherapy. Percutaneous ethanol injection is characterized by multiple ethanol injections into a tumor. Cryoablation, sometimes assisted by ultrasound, is a method of killing cancer cells by freezing them. Clinical trials for patients in stages 0, A, and B include electroporation therapy. An electrode implanted in a tumor aims to kill cancer cells by administering direct electrical impulses. Patients in stages C and D require advanced treatments, ranging from embolization therapy to radiation therapy. An embolism is defined as a blockage of an artery. As you might infer, embolization therapy is characterized by the blockage of arteries connecting to a tumor, in order to deprive the tumor of oxygen and nutrients. For tumors of the liver, this is accomplished through the hepatic artery, allowing the hepatic portal vein to continue supplying healthy liver tissue. Two embolization therapies are currently used: transarterial embolization (TAE) and transarterial chemoembolization (TACE). TAE is the administration of an agent into the hepatic artery that will cease blood supply. The agent is transmitted through a catheter typically inserted through the inner thigh and pushed superiorly until it reaches the hepatic artery. TACE is a similar method, but a chemotherapeutic drug is also administered. Embolizing the artery not only prevents blood supply, but also hinders the drug from escaping the tumor environment. Tyrosine kinase inhibitors are an available drug used in the therapy referred to as targeted therapy. Here, the goal is to block growth, division, and angiogenic factors of specific cancer cells while sparing healthy cells from harm. Currently used tyrosine kinase inhibitors include sorafenib, lenvatinib, and regorafenib. Sorafenib and regorafenib have been the drugs of choice, although their benefit only slightly exceeds that of other choices, an average increase in survival of about 3 months. Nivolumab is a drug in immunotherapy. The goal of immunotherapy is to enhance the body's immune responses to cancer. Drugs like nivolumab achieve this by acting as an immune checkpoint inhibitor, in which PD-1 (T-cell surface protein) is exploited. The normal physiological responsibility of PD-1 involves recognition and attachment to PDL-1 on cancer cells. Doing so prevents the T cells from killing the cancer cells. PD-1 inhibitors block this action by binding to PDL-1. Finally, there are two types of radiation therapy. This type of therapy kills cancer cells and inhibits progression by applying radiation, such as high-energy X-rays. First, external radiation involves targeted radiation using three various methods from outside the body. Conformal radiation therapy is achieved through a computer-generated 3-D conformation of a tumor and radiation administered in that conformation. Stereotactic body radiation therapy is performed by applying radiation through a radiation machine, directly towards the overlying region of the tumor. This is performed numerous times with one treatment per day. Proton beam radiation therapy is another method affording less damage to surrounding healthy cells. As the name implies, protons are beamed at tumors to destroy cancer cells. Internal radiation is accomplished with the use of needles, catheters, wires, and seeds. The goal is to internally deposit a radioactive agent in the tumor environment [54].

These currently utilized approaches have not proven to be efficient in treating patients [8, 11, 12, 23, 24, 39–42, 52, 53, 55]. This is mostly due in part to the heterogeneity of HCC cell lines and insufficient early diagnosis of the disease [8, 11, 12, 23, 24, 39–42, 52, 53, 55]. However, they are the best options available, thus suggesting the necessity for alternative strategies. For this reason, phytochemicals are receiving increasing attention as therapeutic agents against cancer. Their unique ability to target cancer stem cells partially accounts for their success in reducing recurrence and further tumor formation. A combination of medicinal agents might be the optimal route towards complete treatment.

1.5 Phytochemicals as Therapeutic Agents for Cancer

Phytochemicals are active compounds naturally derived from plants. Their medicinal properties are used around the world and have been for a long time. It was not until the past century or so that these active compounds started gaining increased attention. By identifying the specific components of plants that were found to have therapeutic qualities, phytochemicals emerged as a new group of candidates for cancer treatment. Our interest is focused on phytochemical effects in relation to hepatic cancer. Intriguingly though, these therapeutic compounds are successful in treating many types of cancer, including pancreatic, cervical, renal, lung, skin, ovarian, breast, and colon cancer. Conditions involving the skin, lungs, inflammation, infection, gastrointestinal dysfunction, urogenital dysfunction, obesity, and diabetes are all known to be treated with the use of phytochemicals and associated plants. Even cough, insomnia, asthma, and headaches have been treated with these compounds. Polyphenols are a prominent group of phytochemicals that display use of several mechanisms. Flavonoids, the most common subgroup of polyphenols, inhibit autoimmunity, control metabolic processes, disrupt gene expression, and interfere with signaling pathways. Each of these is an example of mechanisms most commonly employed by anticancer phytochemicals. When considering the use of phytochemicals in the treatment of hepatic cancer, particular attention should be given to the ones with unique mechanisms. For instance, some phytochemicals coordinate the expression of DNA in exclusive patterns. Alternatively, some can target CSCs, while others do not express this trait. Fortunately, their wide range of actions can be used together. Therefore, they should be considered in combination to achieve complete effectiveness.

1.6 Mode of Action and Therapeutic Targets of Phytochemicals

Here, we perform an overview of the most commonly utilized and thoroughly examined phytochemicals along with associated plants. Following with discussion of various mechanisms, we provide a clear, inclusive picture of phytochemicals' potential in hepatic cancer treatment. Several phytochemicals have been observed as especially effective against hepatic cancer, and they will be reviewed with emphasis. As phytochemicals are being studied for unique benefits against hepatic cancer, we find that many of them share mechanisms of action and effectiveness against additional types of cancer. For this reason, we will begin by describing the many phytochemicals and plants associated with effectiveness against the spectrum of cancers (Fig. 14.2).

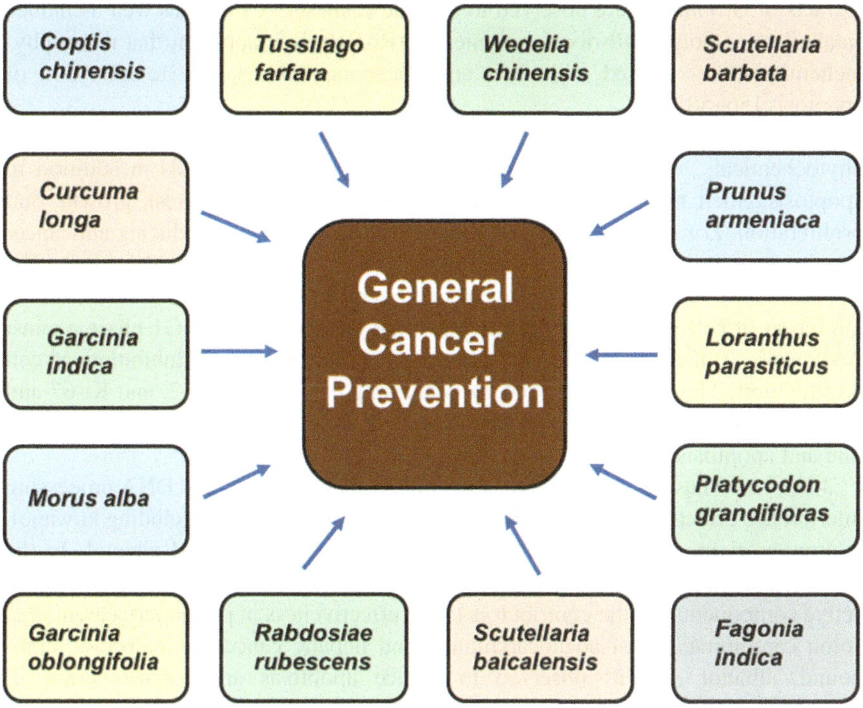

Fig. 14.2 Phytochemicals that are being used in the prevention or treatment of various types of cancers

1.7 Phytochemicals: General Overview

Compounds in *Coptis chinensis* accomplish anticancer behavior through apoptosis. Specifically, berberine alkaloids cause downregulation of nucleophosmin/B23 and telomerases, leading to the induction of apoptosis in HL-60 human leukemia cells. Curcumin is responsible for the active properties of *Curcuma longa*, which act through apoptosis. Comparatively, curcumin achieves this by preventing mRNA and protein expression of COX-2 in colon cancer cells. After performing cell viability and cytotoxicity tests on human breast cancer cells, curcumin was found to induce apoptosis, as well as upregulate activity of caspase 3/9. Also observed was the stimulation of signaling pathways, PTEN/Akt, in order to downregulate miR-21. Apoptotic activity of *Garcinia oblongifolia* is due to the metabolites oblongifolin A-G and oblongizanthones A-C, as well as other components. Specifically, oblongifolins F and G, xanthone, nigrolineaxanthone T, and garcicowin B showed the most effectiveness in inducing apoptosis in HeLa cervical cancer cells. Garcinol, found in *Garcinia indica*, exhibits anticancer effects in colon cancer cells. Another study demonstrated that this effectiveness was accomplished by substantially inhibiting cell invasion activities. In preventing leukemia in human HL-60 cells, extracts of *G. indica* were observed to activate caspase-3/CPP32, as well as induce catabolism of poly-ADP-ribose polymerase (PARP). It is apparent that many phytochemicals are credited with their anticancer capabilities, due to induction of apoptosis [56–58].

As we further discuss the mechanisms generating the therapeutic actions of phytochemicals, we will see that many of them employ methods in addition to apoptosis. Such methods include interference with cell cycle arrest, growth, and proliferation. *Loranthus parasiticus* is proved to be effective in inducing anticancer activity in ovarian cancer cells, such as SKOV3, CAOV3, and OVCAR-3. The flavonoids extracted from *L. parasiticus* exhibited pro-apoptotic behavior, as well as inhibition of cell proliferation and arrest of the cell cycle in G0–G1 phase against AML cells. When applied to sarcoma in mice, extract caused inhibition of cell proliferation. This is accomplished by decreasing cyclin D1, Bcl-2, and Ki-67 and increasing Bax protein, consequently inhibiting the progression of the cancer cell line and apoptosis [56–58].

Morus alba has antiproliferative, apoptotic, cell cycle arrest, and DNA processing interference effects. Many phytochemicals are found in *M. alba*, including kuwanol, hydroxymoricin, moranoline, morusin, calystegin, albafuran, and albanol. In the leaves, quercetin, rutin, apigenin, and 1-deoxynojirimycin can be found. These active components are the contributors to the effectiveness in pulmonary carcinoma, colon carcinoma, breast adenocarcinoma, and hepatic cancer. One specific compound, albanol A, was observed to induce apoptosis and topoisomerase II, downregulate pro-caspase-3/8/9, and upregulate Bax/Bcl-2. Phenolic compounds are also specific contributors. Through regulation of $p27^{Kip1}$, increased activity of caspases, and prevention of topoisomerase IIa, the phenolic compounds portray effects of preventing proliferation, arresting cell cycle at G2/M phase, and inducing apoptosis. *M. alba* also contains lectin, which was observed to inhibit proliferation, arrest cell cycle, and induce apoptosis via caspase-3 in MCF-7 and HCT-15 cell lines. Interestingly, extracts of *M. alba* were also shown to downregulate the expression of NF-kB, and two new anticancer compounds have been extracted, soroceal B and sanggenol Q. *Platycodon grandiflorus* consists of saponins, flavonoids, anthocyanins, phenolics, and polysaccharides that are responsible for its activity, which includes immune, anti-inflammatory, hepatoprotective, and antitumor capabilities. Cell death in HT-80 cells is induced by decreasing the enhancement of MmP-9 and MmP-2 matric metallopeptidases from PKC. Platycodin D is an active component that induces apoptosis and hinders cell viability and cell proliferation when applied to MCF-7 cells. This activity is accomplished through the regulation of particular cellular components. Specifically, caspase-8/9 and Bid are stimulated, Bax and Bcl-2 are increased, and PARP is cleaved. Platycodin D applied to human leukemia cells decreased transcription and post-translation of human telomerase reverse transcriptase (hTERT), in order to prevent telomerase activity. Upregulation of *Egr-1* increases reactive oxygen species, which causes dysfunction in mitochondrial membrane potential, leading to stimulation of caspase-3 and cleavage of PARP, finally inducing apoptosis. Through similar mechanisms extract is also successful against ovarian cancer cells, such as SKOV3 [56–58].

Metabolites such as β-carotene, flavonoids, organic acids, thiamine, minerals, and oils, as well as cyanogenic glycosides and phenolic compounds, are present in *Prunus armeniaca*. One particular glycoside, amygdalin, is effective against prostate cancer. Extract from *P. armeniaca* proves to be effective against colon, breast, and hepatic cancer cells, especially hepatic [56–58].

The many active components in *Rabdosia rubescens* include monoterpenes, sesquiterpene, diterpene, and terpenoids. Among this composition, oridonin is the notably effective component. It was observed to express pro-apoptotic and growth inhibitory behavior in hepatocellular carcinoma, as well as skin, gastric, breast, pancreatic, colorectal, and gallbladder cancers. When applied to HepG2 cells, oridonin caused growth inhibition, cell cycle arrest at G2, and induction of apoptosis. These mechanisms are also characterized through regulation of cellular components. Cell cycle arrest and apoptosis are achieved by increasing the expression of STRAP, Hsp70.1, Stil1, TCTP, and PPase while simultaneously decreasing hnRNP-E1. Growth inhibition is caused by tyrosine kinase and telomerase through the increase of HP1 beta and GlyRS. By decreasing Bcl-2:Bax, NF-kB, caspase-8, phosphor-mTOR, IKKβ, and IKKα while upregulating PPARγ, PARP, and Fas cleaving, oridonin causes growth inhibition from cell cycle arrest and induction of apoptosis. Also, oridonin can inhibit cell invasion and migration by regulating the integrin β1/FAK pathway and matrix metallopeptidases [56–58].

Therapeutic properties of *Scutellaria baicalensis* can be attributed to flavone extracts, particularly baicalein, and prove useful against brain cancer, prostate cancer, and HNSCC (head-and-neck squamous cell carcinoma). Through regulation of p27, Bcl, and c-myc, extract can hinder cell growth in lymphoma and myeloma. Baicalin is especially pro-apoptotic, upregulates caspases-3 and -9, prevents cell proliferation, and downregulates angiogenic genes. *Scutellaria barbata* has an interesting anticancer effect of decreasing the synthesis of ATP, in order to inhibit cancer cell growth. This is caused from the buildup of superoxide and peroxide in mitochondria and inhibiting glycolysis. The phytochemical components comprising *S. barbata*, such as apigenin, luteolin, scutellarein, scutebarbatine A, and other alkaloid, flavone, steroid, and polysaccharide metabolites, are responsible for the anticancer mechanisms. Finally, they are particularly effective against colon cancer, lung cancer, hepatic cancer, and skin cancer [56–58].

Tussilago farfara was shown to be effective against human colon cancer cells through pro-apoptotic and cytotoxic behavior. Antimutagenic activity and favorable activity against genotoxicity were also observed. Anticancer effects in human hepatocellular carcinoma cells were portrayed by *T. farfara* as inhibiting mTOR signaling pathway regulator-like protein, MKK7-TIPRL, and MKK7/JNK activation, causing apoptosis through TRAIL (TNF-related apoptosis-inducing ligand). The active contents of *T. farfara* are comprised of quercetin glycosides, phenolic compounds, flavonoids, and trace elements, such as Zn, Mg, and Se and are attributable to the anticancer effects [56–58].

Carvacrol and trans-caryophyllene, along with metabolites such as phenol, flavonoids, and tannin, are components of *Wedelia chinensis* effective against melanoma cells and lung cancer. Catalase, superoxide dismutase, and glutathione peroxidase are antioxidant enzymes found upregulated along with glutathione caused by these components [56–58].

1.8 Phytochemicals Specific to HCC

Considerable advances have recently been made in the development of phytochemicals as prophylactics or therapeutic agents specifically for HCC as shown in Fig. 14.3. *Fagonia indica* is another plant with compounds capable of inducing apoptosis in HCC cells, as well as breast cancer and colon cancer cells. Observation of pan-caspase inhibitor Z-VAD-fmk activity, caspase cleavage, and DNA ladder assays supported this mechanism. The phytochemicals contained by *F. indica* accomplishing these effects are amino acids, proteins, saponins, terpenoid, alkaloids, and flavonoids. Recently, cell lysis of breast cancer cells by a steroidal saponin glycoside was achieved through necrosis [56, 59–61].

Methyl anthraquinone is a main active component in *Hedyotis diffusa* and activates the caspase-4/Ca^{2+}/calpain pathway, as well as S-phase arrest of the cell

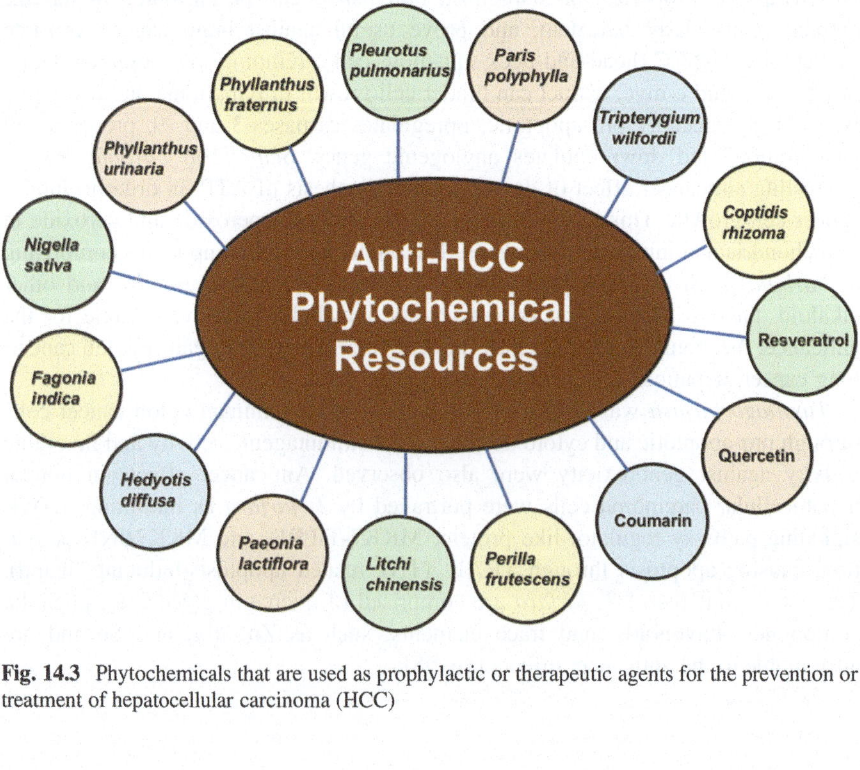

Fig. 14.3 Phytochemicals that are used as prophylactic or therapeutic agents for the prevention or treatment of hepatocellular carcinoma (HCC)

cycle in breast cancer cells. These attribute to the apoptotic and inhibitory capabilities of this compound. Another demonstration showed the prevention of proliferation and induction of apoptosis when applied to Hela cells [56, 59, 60, 62].

Paris polyphylla is effective against hepatic cancer, colon cancer, and esophageal cancer through the activity of metabolite extracts. Such metabolites include polyphyllin D, formosanin C, β-ecdysterone, dioscin, daucosterol heptasaccharide, oligosaccharides, octasaccharide, protogracillin, trigofoenoside A, yunnanosides G-J, padelaoside B, pinnatasterone, and other saponins. Extracts proved to be effective in preventing cell proliferation and inducing apoptosis by upregulating connexin 26 and *Bad* genes while downregulating Bcl-2 [56, 59, 60, 63].

Triptolide, characterized by a five-membered unsaturated lactone ring, is the notable component of *Tripterygium wilfordii*. Effective against hepatic cancer breast cancer cells, neuroblastoma, melanoma, bladder cancer, and gastric cancer, triptolide utilizes various signaling pathways to induce apoptosis. Inhibition of proliferation, induction of apoptosis, and antiangiogenic properties of triptolide were observed. Antiangiogenic properties were observed as decreased Tie2 and VEGFR-2. *T. wilfordii* also contains the anticancer component, celastrol, which interferes with IkB kinase and NF-kB activation by TAK1 [56, 59, 60, 64].

Astragalus membranaceus contains flavonoid, polysaccharide, saponin, and amino acid phytochemicals that contribute to its anticancer effects. Such effects include inhibiting growth and angiogenesis, as well as inducing apoptosis [56, 65]. Among these compounds, their polysaccharides (AMP) have the most noticeable effects against hepatic cancer. AMP from *A. membranaceus* seem to exhibit anticancer activity via upregulation of host immune responses. At various doses, AMP inhibited tumor growth at rates ranging from ~50% to ~70%, as a measure of tumor weight. An increase of cytokines IL-2, IL-12, and TNF-α was observed following doses of AMP, which are known as immune responses for attacking tumors. Interestingly, IL-10 was found to be lower. The phagocytic activity of macrophages was also found to be much higher in AMP-treated HCC. Macrophages are key components of the immune system, and their phagocytic activity is important for inhibiting cancer progression [56, 66, 67]. Kiani et al. described AMP effects on Treg cells of HCC. They prevent the progression of CD4/CD25 Treg cells and do so through immune functions, as well. Specifically, they stabilize cytokine expression and decrease mRNA expression of FOXp3 [56, 67]. CASE, Astragalus and Salvia Compound, showed major activity against HCC. CASE acts through TGF-β/SMAD signaling and DEN. Fibrosis and PAI-1 mRNA transcription were prevented by CASE inhibition of DEN [56, 67]. Altogether, these traits attribute to the anticancer effects found in *A. membranaceus*.

Coptidis rhizoma portrays anticancer properties with pro-apoptotic, tumor proliferation inhibiting, and angiogenic traits, as well as prevention of migration and invasion. MicroRNA arrays, qRT-PCR, and cluster analysis of miRNA expression in CRAE (*C. rhizome* aqueous extract, includes berberine) treated HCC revealed upregulated activity of miRNA 23a, thought to mediate various signaling pathways. A 48-h treatment of CRAE showed to cause major cell death in HCC while exhibiting the increase of miR-23a. Upregulation of miR-21 was also found and thought to be a large contributor. However, qRT-PCR only revealed the expression of miR-23a gene targets, NEK6 and SLC [56, 68, 69]. In analyzing the preventive capabilities of CRAE in migration, Rho/ROCK signaling pathway is considered. This pathway promotes HCC cell migration. When administered with a Rho-ROCK inhibitor, doses of CRAE enhanced the blocking of this pathway, supporting its claim as a migration inhibitor. This is further proven via its suppression of ROCK-1 and Rho GTPase. Finally, small doses of CRAE, below its IC_{50} value, disrupt the cytoskeleton of HCC cells by interfering with polymerization of F-actin [56, 69].

Litchi chinensis is known for its anti-inflammatory, anticancer, and antioxidant nature. The phytochemicals accounting for the activity of *L. chinensis* include flavonoids, sterols, triterpenes, polyphenols, and more. Polyphenol extract inhibited hepatic cancer progression through apoptosis. Pumilaside A, funingensin A, kaempferol-7-O-neohesperidosid, and litchioside D are a few more compounds with anticancer activity, here, observed to be highly cytotoxic in HepG2 cells. Moreover, several oxygen radical scavengers are found among these. Specifically, litchi polysaccharide fraction, LFP3, portrayed a significantly strong effect on superoxide and hydroxyl radicals. Epicatechin and procyanidin from *L. chinensis* showed similar effects. Cinnamtannin B1, PFLP, and PDLP tested against HepG2 cells caused cell cycle arrest and apoptosis to reduce growth and proliferation. Interestingly, anti-obesity effects are found with litchi extracts. This is seen as the decreased expression of adipogenesis genes and lipase activity. Since obesity is a main risk factor of NAFLD and HCC, phytochemicals from *L. chinensis* exhibit preventive benefits, too [56, 70, 71].

Paeonia lactiflora contains paeoniflorin, albiflorin, benzoylpaeoniflorin, oxypaeoniflorin, and paeonin, referred to as total glucosides of peony (TGP). One group already tested TGP against human hepatoma cells and proved its ability to prevent proliferation in these cells. It is widely understood that combination treatments are typically more effective than treating with agents individually. Subsequently, the group previously mentioned performed a treatment of *P. lactiflora/A. membranaceus* combination extract (PAE) on HCC cells, demonstrating inhibition of proliferation, migration, and invasion, as well as utilization of apoptosis. Their findings were obtained following treatments of 48-h durations. Immunocytochemistry and western blotting showed that PAE is capable of inducing apoptosis by means of Bcl-2, Bax, and caspase-3. Finally, migration and invasion of HCC are inhibited by PAE, as demonstrated by wound healing assays and transwell invasion assays [56, 65]. Another group focused on the preventive benefits of PAE by testing it against liver fibrosis, a known risk factor leading to hepatic cancer. Alanine transaminase (ALT) and aspartate transaminase (AST), two liver enzymes elevated during liver damage, were decreased by PAE. Hydroxyproline, hyaluronic acid (HA), and type III pre-collagen (PC III) are known indicators of liver fibrosis and fibrogenesis. Both levels were found to be decreased after PAE treatment. Proliferation of hepatic cancer cells is stimulated through the alterations from platelet-derived growth factor subunit BB (PDGF-BB). This glycoprotein regulates the uptake of [^{3}H]-thymidine, which is markedly decreased when exposed to certain concentrations of PAE [56, 72].

Perilla frutescens has significant effectiveness against hepatic cancer through preventing proliferation and inducing apoptosis by upregulating genes involved in the process. Isoegomaketone is a specific component acquired from extraction of this plant. By cleaving caspases-3/8/9, cell growth is inhibited. Isoegomaketone is also capable of inducing apoptosis by triggering cleavage of PARP and Bid protein, translocating Bax protein, and causing release of cytochrome *c* from mitochondria. *Perilla frutescens* exhibits abilities to treat HCC from the antiproliferative and proapoptotic traits discovered when analyzing its extract. Active phytochemicals present in *P. frutescens* extract (PLE) include luteolin, caffeic acid, triterpene acid, and rosmarinic acid. MTT assays, used in the evaluation of metabolic activity, apoptosis assays, and cDNA microarrays, were applied in the investigation of antiproliferative and apoptotic activity of PLE on HCC cells. Upon determining an IC_{50} value for growth inhibition, they analyzed the effects of this dose in apoptosis assays. Results showed an increase in apoptotic cells after periodic measurements. cDNA microarray analysis demonstrates the increased expression of genes over time after exposure to PLE with an increase of some genes being time dependent. Importantly, the genes increased are those related to apoptosis, including caspase-8, NFkBIA, TNFSF9, Jun, Jun-8, Fos-B, and Bax. Bcl-2, an important apoptotic factor, was observed to decrease [56, 73]. Wang et al. proposed that the antiproliferative properties of isoegomaketone were achieved through additional methods. Results following isolation of IK and administration to HCC cells revealed an interference with the PI3K/Akt signaling pathway. Evidence of lowered phosphorylated-Akt levels and unperturbed levels of Akt supported this claim [56, 74].

Pleurotus pulmonarius is a potent antioxidant that prevents growth and proliferation of hepatic cancer. This edible mushroom also causes downregulation of PI3K/Akt pathways in HCC cells. Its extracts, containing polysaccharides, triterpenoids, polyphenols, nucleotides, sterols, and steroids, are responsible for the antiproliferation and anti-invasion traits. Additionally, they reduce drug resistance of hepatic cancer cells. PP is a specific polysaccharide/protein complex contained in extracts. Western blot analysis shows HCC cells exposed to PP results in lowered p-Akt and iNOS, with a higher amount of cleaved caspase-3. Ki-67, elevated during proliferation, is downregulated in HCC cells exposed to the extract [56, 75]. One group provided similar findings, except that they described a VEGF-mediated PI3K/Akt disruption. Their western blots showed lowered p-Akt and VEGF. Since VEGF can activate PI3K/Akt, their combined decrease in HCC when exposed to PP suggests a relationship. Addition of recombinant human VEGF to the same HCC causes reactivation of proliferative characteristics [56, 76].

Milk thistle and members of the Phyllanthus family together exhibit strong hepatoprotective benefits [56, 77, 78]. Although both are effective against steatohepatitis, milk thistle alone is recognized as one of the leading plants for treating NASH and ALD. Blood glucose and cholesterol levels can be stabilized phytochemicals in milk thistle, thereby reducing the risk of obesity and diabetes-related hepatic cancer. Silymarin is the main compound of milk thistle. The active component of silymarin, silibinin, enhances treatment of ALD and acute/chronic hepatitis. Silibinin and isosilibinin A and B, silicristin, and silidianin specifically make up silymarin. Flavonoids, taxifolin, and quercetol can be found, too [56, 79–81]. Regulation of reactive oxygen species, cytochrome P459, and high-mobility group box 1 (HMGB1) are a few ways through which the Phyllanthus family exhibits anticancer effects. Fraternus, urinaria, polyphyllus, and *Glycyrrhizin glabra* are each members of this family. *Phyllanthus fraternus* controls ROS and cytochrome P459 via phyllanthin. *Phyllanthus urinaria* assists in preventing lipid accumulation to treat steatohepatitis [56, 82–84]. *Glycyrrhizin glabra* mainly portrays preventive effects through treating viral hepatitis. Its active compounds are called glycyrrhizin, a triterpene, and glycyrrhetinic acid. Together, these two phytochemicals induce apoptosis and necrosis, alter cell membrane permeability, and decrease HMGB1, an inflammatory component [56, 77, 85–91].

Quercetin and resveratrol are both detected in red wine, grapes, and berries. Quercetin is also found in apples, onions, and licorice root, and several cellular molecules and processes. By exhibiting control over cyclin D1, a cell cycle component, quercetin can impede proliferation of hepatic cancer cells. Studies have also observed this phytochemical to stimulate p53 and p21 tumor suppressors, apoptosis, and tumor necrosis while downregulating tyrosine kinase and angiogenesis [56, 77]. Resveratrol, on the other hand, takes advantage of COX-2, p53, and some other cell cycle regulators. The combined manipulation of COX-2 and cell cycle regulators accounts for the antiangiogenic, antiproliferative, anti-metastasis, and pro-apoptotic traits of this phytochemical [77].

Other noteworthy phytochemicals recognized for targeting hepatic cancer are coumarin, berberine, and nigella. Coumarin, identified in numerous plants, is unique in preventing the onset of hepatic cancer by delaying the progression of hepatitis B and C. Its preventive qualities are owed to coumarin's strong influence over immune responses. Immune system responses include upregulation of T cells, NK cells, and cytokines while decreasing immune-suppressing factors, such as TGF-β. Coumarin also stabilizes Th1:Th2, boosts cytotoxic white blood cells, and decreases cytochrome P450 activity. More so, HBV- and HCV-infected patients who do not respond to interferon treatments are found to benefit from coumarin [56, 92]. Berberine is an alkaloid widely present as a phytochemical. Barberry is known to contain berberine and vitamin C. Previously mentioned, diabetes, dyslipidemia, hepatitis, and cirrhosis are main causes of hepatic cancer. Berberine is especially effective at treating each of those disorders. Although it was recognized as toxic in the past, studies since then have revealed ideal tolerance in human subjects. Blood glucose levels in type 2 diabetic patients and damage from liver disorders are restored with the application of berberine [56, 93]. *Nigella sativa* has been used for its medicinal qualities for over 3000 years being reported in the Bible and by people of ancient Greece. Hundreds of studies exist at this point, heavily supporting its credibility as a therapeutic agent for hepatic cancer. Besides its benefits against hepatic cancer, nigella oil is known for treating renal disorders, hypertension, diabetes, and inflammatory disorders. The oil contains thymoquinone, nigellone, melanthin, nigellinine, tannin, linoleic acid, and many other fatty acids. Vitamins, minerals, and some proteins are also active components [56].

The importance of cancer stem cells in the onset, progression, and treatment of cancer warrants discussion on the phytochemicals that can target this subpopulation. The revelation of CSCs' role in cancer is relatively new to the research world. For this reason, only a few phytochemicals have been reported for their targeting capabilities. Rottlerin, retinoic acid, paclitaxel, and camptothecin are some active compounds effective against CSCs of various cancers [94]. Epigallocatechin-3-gallate (EGCG) and curcumin are two polyphenol phytochemicals widely reported as beneficial treatments for hepatic disorders. They are also the two phytochemicals best studied for targeting hepatic CSCs. Many people around the world use green tea for health benefits and have been using it for a long time. Green tea happens to contain EGCG in its extract, owing to the potency of green tea compared to other teas. This phytochemical regulates reactive oxygen species and iron buildup in the liver to reduce oxidative stress. EGCG is proapoptotic, anti-inflammatory, antiproliferative, and antioxidative. It accomplishes these features by interfering with signaling pathways and other cellular processes. For instance, proliferation of cancer cells is inhibited by EGCG through downregulation of DNA methylation via DNA methyltransferase. It enhances this effect with the stimulation of tumor-suppressor genes [56, 92]. Turmeric is the plant best known for curcumin. This curcuminoid polyphenol is an anti-inflammatory and antioxidant. It has long been used for treating liver disorders, especially those with bile secretion dysfunction. Interestingly, curcumin exhibits a hepatoprotective effect of neutralizing the liver toxicity caused by other medications. Anticancer effects are achieved through apoptosis and cell cycle arrest. This compound can regulate NF-kB signaling and cell cycle genes to reduce invasion and angiogenesis [56, 93]. Furthermore, Wnt/β-catenin and Notch signaling pathways are two important factors of tumorigenesis via CSCs. EGCG and curcumin are special for their interference with these pathways. EGCG is thought to target hCSCs by downregulating their Wnt/β-catenin pathways. Curcumin utilizes inhibition of both pathways in targeting hCSCs [95–102]. Together with future studies, these phytochemicals, and many more, can prove to be successful tools in the prevention and treatment of hepatic cancer.

2 Conclusions

Hepatocellular carcinoma with poor prognosis and high mortality rate demands the development of novel therapeutic approaches to improve health span and life span of HCC patients. The use of phytochemicals provides promising effects to limit the progression of hepatitis infection or liver cirrhosis to HCC. Despite the promising effects that we now understand about phytochemicals, there are negative effects that should be acknowledged and controlled. These are mainly from the plants containing phytochemicals. Accordingly, with proper knowledge of the active components in anticancer plants, isolation and purification could potentially alleviate most effects. Generally, the medicinal use of phytochemicals and related plants is safe, especially compared to current treatment strategies. Some are even great additions to current treatments. Combination treatment of various phytochemicals and standard therapies might be the ideal suggestion. Of course, this raises the concern of drug-drug interactions. Fortunately, these do not display unwanted interactions. As attributed to the heterogeneity of hepatic cancer and the mechanisms unique to various phytochemicals, a combination of these compounds is necessary to provide a well-rounded treatment strategy. There are some minor barriers, however. Curcumin expresses resistance when administered. Because administration is currently an oral route, absorption issues arise as the hinderance. Many methods were studied in recent years, so there has been an increase in success rate. Further research is warranted, though. Treatment with this phytochemical, and several others, has great potential if their therapeutic traits can be properly exploited.

Acknowledgement This work was supported by NIH's R01-DK81413 (to SAS) from the National Institute of Diabetes and Digestive and Kidney Diseases and by the UCF Reach for the Stars Award (to SAS). The content is solely the responsibility of the authors and does not necessarily represent the official views of the National Institute of Diabetes and Digestive and Kidney Diseases or the National Institutes of Health.

References

1. Siegel, R. L., Miller, K. D., & Jemal, A. (2019). Cancer statistics, 2019. *CA: a Cancer Journal for Clinicians, 69*, 7–34.
2. Liver cancer survival rates. American Cancer Society. Accessed January 8, 2020 from https://www.cancer.org/cancer/liver-cancer/detection-diagnosis-staging/survival-rates.html.
3. Idilman, I. S., Ozdeniz, I., & Karcaaltincaba, M. (2016). Hepatic steatosis: Etiology, patterns, and quantification. *Seminars in Ultrasound, CT, and MRI, 37*(6), 501–510.
4. Moore, J. B. (2019). From sugar to liver fat and public health: Systems biology driven studies in understanding non-alcoholic fatty liver disease pathogenesis. *The Proceedings of the Nutrition Society, 78*, 290–304.
5. Marengo, A., Rosso, C., & Bugianesi, E. (2016). Liver cancer: Connections with obesity, fatty liver, and cirrhosis. *Annual Review of Medicine, 67*, 103–117.
6. Peng, S., Chen, Y., Gong, Y., Li, Z., Xie, R., Lin, Y., et al. (2019). Predictive value of intratumour inflammatory cytokine mRNA levels of hepatocellular carcinoma patients and activation of two distinct pathways govern IL-8 induced epithelial-mesenchymal transition in human hepatic cancer cell lines. *Cytokine, 119*, 81–89.
7. Jena, P., Sheng, L., Liu, H. X., Kalanetra, K. M., Mirsoian, A., Murphy, W., et al. (2017). Western diet-induced dysbiosis in farnesoid X receptor knockout mice causes persistent hepatic inflammation after antibiotic treatment. *The American Journal of Pathology, 187*(8), 1800–1813.
8. Mani, S. K. K., & Andrisani, O. (2018). Hepatitis B virus-associated hepatocellular carcinoma and hepatic cancer stem cells. *Genes, 9*(3), 137.
9. Sukowati, C. H. C. (2019). Heterogeneity of hepatic cancer stem cells. *Advances in Experimental Medicine and Biology, 1139*, 59–81.
10. Ringelhan, M., Mckeating, J. A., & Protzer, U. (2017). Viral hepatitis and liver cancer. *Philosophical Transactions of the Royal Society B: Biological Sciences*, 372(1732).
11. Chan, L. H., Luk, S. T., & Ma, S. (2015). Turning hepatic cancer stem cells inside out – A deeper understanding through multiple perspectives. *Molecules and Cells, 38*(3), 202–209.

12. Oh, J., Hlatky, L., Jeong, Y. S., & Kim, D. (2016). Therapeutic effectiveness of anticancer phytochemicals on cancer stem cells. *Toxins, 8*, 199.
13. Yamashita, T., & Kaneko, S. (2016). Liver cancer. *Rinsho Byori, 64*, 787–796.
14. Pocha, C., & Xie, C. (2019). Hepatocellular carcinoma in alcoholic and non-alcoholic fatty liver disease – One of a kind or two different enemies? *Translational Gastroenterology and Hepatology, 4*, 72–84.
15. Portius, D., Sobolewski, C., & Foti, M. (2017). *MicroRNAs-dependent regulation of PPARs in metabolic diseases and cancers*. PPAR Research.
16. Wu, L., Guo, C., & Wu, J. (2020). Therapeutic potential of PPARgamma natural agonists in liver diseases. *Journal of Cellular and Molecular Medicine*.
17. Hepatitis B: key facts. World Health Organization. Accessed July 18, 2019 from https://www.who.int/news-room/fact-sheets/detail/hepatitis-b.
18. Hoshida, Y., Nijman, S. M. B., Kobayashi, M., Chan, J. A., Brunet, J.-P., Chiang, D. Y., et al. (2009). Integrative transcriptome analysis reveals common molecular subclasses of human hepatocellular carcinoma. *Cancer Research, 69*, 7385–7392.
19. Hepatitis C questions and answers for the public. CDC. Accessed January 13, 2020 from https://www.cdc.gov/hepatitis/hcv/cfaq.htm.
20. Hepatitis B questions and answers for the public. CDC. Accessed January 13, 2020 from https://www.cdc.gov/hepatitis/hbv/bfaq.htm.
21. Ferlay, J., Soerjomataram, I., Dikshit, R., Eser, S., Mathers, C., Rebelo, M., Parkin, D. M., Forman, D., & Bray, F. (2015). Cancer incidence and mortality worldwide: Sources, methods and major patterns. *GLOBOCAN. International Journal of Cancer, 136*, 359–386.
22. El-Serag, H. B. (2012). Epidemiology of viral hepatitis and hepatocellular carcinoma. *Gastroenterology, 142*, 1264.
23. Llovet, J. M., Bru, C., & Bruix, J. (1999). Prognosis of hepatocellular carcinoma: The BCLC staging classification. *Seminars in Liver Disease, 19*, 329–338.
24. Bruix, J., & Sherman, M. (2011). Management of hepatocellular carcinoma: An update. *Hepatology, 53*, 1020–1022.
25. Yatsuji, S., Hashimoto, E., & Tobari, M. (2009). Clinical features and outcomes of cirrhosis due to nonalcoholic steatohepatitis compared with cirrhosis caused by chronic hepatitis C. *Journal of Gastroenterology and Hepatology, 24*, 248–254.
26. Sanyal, A. J., Banas, C., & Sargeant, C. (2006). Similarities and differences in outcomes of cirrhosis due to nonalcoholic steatohepatitis and hepatitis C. *Hepatology, 43*, 682–689.
27. Shoelson, S. E., Herrero, L., & Naaz, A. (2007). Obesity, inflammation and insulin resistance. *Gastroenterology, 132*, 2169–2180.
28. Hirosumi, J., Tuncman, G., Chang, L., et al. (2002). A central role for JNK in obesity and insulin resistance. *Nature, 420*, 333–336.
29. Hodge, D. R., Hurt, E. M., & Farrar, W. L. (2005). The role of IL-6 and STAT3 in inflammation and cancer. *European Journal of Cancer, 41*, 2502–2512.
30. Jiang, N., Sun, R., & Sun, Q. (2014). Leptin signaling molecular actions and drug target in hepatocellular carcinoma. *Drug Design, Development and Therapy, 8*, 2295–2302.
31. Villanueva, A., Chiang, D. Y., Newell, P., et al. (2008). Pivotal role of mTOR signaling in hepatocellular carcinoma. *Gastroenterology, 135*, 1972–1983.
32. Sharma, D., Wang, J., Fu, P. P., et al. (2010). Adiponectin antagonizes the oncogenic actions of leptin in hepatocellular carcinogenesis. *Hepatology, 52*, 1713–1722.
33. Angulo, P. (2007). Obesity and nonalcoholic fatty liver disease. *Nutrition Reviews, 65*, 57–63.
34. Teli, M. R., Day, C. P., Burt, A. D., et al. (1995). Determinants of progression to cirrhosis or fibrosis in pure alcoholic fatty liver. *Lancet, 346*, 987–990.
35. Mandayam, S., Jamal, M. M., & Morgan, T. R. (2004). Epidemiology of alcoholic liver disease. *Seminars in Liver Disease, 24*, 217–232.
36. González-Reimers, E., Quintero-Platt, G., Rodríguez-Gaspar, M., et al. (2015). Liver steatosis in hepatitis C patients. *World Journal of Hepatology, 7*, 1337–1346.

37. Amacher, D. E., & Chalasani, N. (2014). Drug-induced hepatic steatosis. *Seminars in Liver Disease, 34*(2), 205–214.
38. Martins-Filho, S. N., Paiva, C., Azevedo, R. S., & Alves, V. A. F. (2017). Histological grading of hepatocellular carcinoma-a systematic review of literature. *Frontiers in Medicine, 4*, 193.
39. DePeralta, D. K., Wei, L., Ghoshal, S., Schmidt, D., Lauwers, G., Lanuti, M., et al. (2016). Metformin prevents hepatocellular carcinoma development by suppressing hepatic progenitor cell activation in a rat model of cirrhosis. *Cancer, 122*(8), 1216–1227.
40. Li, S., Yang, F., & Ren, X. (2015). Immunotherapy for hepatocellular carcinoma. *Drug Discoveries & Therapeutics, 9*, 363–371.
41. Haraguchi, N., Ishii, H., Mimori, K., Tanaka, F., Ohkuma, M., Kim, H. M., et al. (2010). CD13 is a therapeutic target in human liver cancer stem cells. *The Journal of Clinical Investigation, 120*, 3326–3339.
42. Ma, S., Chan, K. W., Hu, L., Lee, T. K., Wo, J. Y., Ng, I. O., et al. (2007). Identification and characterization of tumorigenic liver cancer stem/progenitor cells. *Gastroenterology, 132*, 2542–2556.
43. Yamashita, T., Ji, J., Budhu, A., Forgues, M., Yang, W., Wang, H. Y., et al. (2009). EpCAM positive hepatocellular carcinoma cells are tumor-initiating cells with stem/progenitor cell features. *Gastroenterology, 136*.
44. Yang, Z. F., Ho, D. W., Ng, M. N., Lau, C. K., Yu, W. C., Ngai, P., et al. (2008). Significance of CD90+ cancer stem cells in human liver cancer. *Cancer Cell, 13*, 153–166.
45. Tang, K. H., Ma, S., Lee, T. K., Chan, Y. P., Kwan, P. S., Tong, C. M., et al. (2012). CD133(+) liver tumor-initiating cells promote tumor angiogenesis, growth, and self-renewal through neurotensin/interleukin-8/CXCL1 signaling. *Hepatology, 55*, 807–820.
46. Schrader, J., Gordon-Walker, T. T., Aucott, R. L., van Deemter, M., Quaas, A., Walsh, S., et al. (2011). Matrix stiffness modulates proliferation, chemotherapeutic response, and dormancy in hepatocellular carcinoma cells. *Hepatology, 53*, 1192–1205.
47. He, G., Dhar, D., Nakagawa, H., Font-Burgada, J., Ogata, H., Jiang, Y., et al. (2013). Identification of liver cancer progenitors whose malignant progression depends on autocrine IL-6 signaling. *Cell, 155*.
48. Fan, Q. M., Jing, Y. Y., Yu, G. F., Kou, X. R., Ye, F., Gao, L., et al. (2014). Tumor-associated macrophages promote cancer stem cell-like properties via transforming growth factor-beta1-induced epithelial-mesenchymal transition in hepatocellular carcinoma. *Cancer Letters, 352*, 160–168.
49. Chen, H., Luo, Z., Dong, L., Tan, Y., Yang, J., Feng, G., et al. (2013). CD133/prominin-1-mediated autophagy and glucose uptake beneficial for hepatoma cell survival. *PLoS One, 8*.
50. Chen, H., Luo, Z., Sun, W., Zhang, C., Sun, H., Zhao, N., et al. (2013). Low glucose promotes CD133 mAb-elicited cell death via inhibition of autophagy in hepatocarcinoma cells. *Cancer Letters, 336*, 204–212.
51. Wang, X., Hassan, W., Zhao, J., Bakht, S., Nie, Y., Wang, Y., et al. (2019). The impact of hepatocyte nuclear factor-1alpha on liver malignancies and cell stemness with metabolic consequences. *Stem Cell Research & Therapy, 10*, 315.
52. Haznadar, M., Diehl, C. M., Parker, A. L., Krausz, K. W., Bowman, E. D., Rabibhadana, S., et al. (2019). Urinary metabolites diagnostic and prognostic of intrahepatic cholangiocarcinoma. *Cancer Epidemiology, Biomarkers & Prevention, 28*, 1704–1711.
53. Kubo, N., Araki, K., Kuwano, H., & Shirabe, K. (2016). Cancer-associated fibroblasts in hepatocellular carcinoma. *World Journal of Gastroenterology, 22*, 6841–6850.
54. Adult primary liver cancer treatment (PDQ®)–patient version. National Cancer Institute. Accessed July 2, 2019 from https://www.cancer.gov/types/liver/patient/adult-liver-treatment-pdq#_44.
55. McDonald, G. B., Freston, J. W., Boyer, J. L., & DeLeve, L. D. (2019). Liver complications following treatment of hematologic malignancy with anti-CD22-calicheamicin (Inotuzumab Ozogamicin). *Hepatology, 69*, 831–844.
56. Calkic, L. (2019). Phytotherapy and liver disease. *Liver Cirrhosis – Debates and Challenges*.

57. Madrigal-Santillán, E., MadrigalBujaidar, E., Álvarez-González, I., Sumaya-Martínez, M. T., GutiérrezSalinas, J., et al. (2014). Review of natural products with hepatoprotective effects. *World Journal of Gastroenterology, 20*(40), 14787–14804.
58. Pratheeshkumar, P., Son, Y. O., Korangath, P., Manu, K. A., & Siveen, K. S. (2015). Phytochemicals in cancer prevention and therapy. *BioMed Research International, 2015*, 324021.
59. Khan, T., Ali, M., Khan, A., Nisar, P., Jan, S., Afridi, S., et al. (2020). Anticancer plants: A review of the active phytochemicals, applications in animal models, and regulatory aspects. *Biomolecules, 10*(1), 47.
60. Mohammad, A., Anuradha, M., Afreen, U., & Parwez, A. (2017). Dietary agents and phytochemicals in the prevention and treatment of hepatocellular carcinoma: Review article. *Med Phoenix, 2*(1), 56–62.
61. Azam, F., Sheikh, N., Ali, G., & Tayyeb, A. (2018). Fagonia indica repairs hepatic damage through expression regulation of toll-like receptors in a liver injury model. *Journal of Immunology Research, 2018*, 7967135.
62. Chen, X. Z., Cao, Z. Y., Chen, T. S., Zhang, Y. Q., Liu, Z. Z., Su, Y. T., et al. (2012). Water extract of Hedyotis diffusa Willd suppresses proliferation of human HepG2 cells and potentiates the anticancer efficacy of low-dose 5-fluorouracil by inhibiting the CDK2-E2F1 pathway. *Oncology Reports, 28*, 742–748.
63. Liu, J., Man, S., Li, J., Zhang, Y., Meng, X., & Gao, W. (2016). Inhibition of diethylnitrosamine-induced liver cancer in rats by Rhizoma paridis saponin. *Environmental Toxicology and Pharmacology, 46*, 103–109.
64. Chen, S. R., Dai, Y., Zhao, J., Lin, L., Wang, Y., & Wang, Y. (2018). A mechanistic overview of triptolide and celastrol, natural products from Tripterygium wilfordii Hook F. *Frontiers in Pharmacology, 9*, 104.
65. Wu, J. J., Sun, W. Y., Hu, S. S., Zhang, S., & Wei, W. (2013). A standardized extract from Paeonia lactiflora and Astragalus membranaceus induces apoptosis and inhibits the proliferation, migration and invasion of human hepatoma cell lines. *International Journal of Oncology, 43*, 1643–1651.
66. Yang, B., Xiao, B., & Sun, T. (2013). Antitumor and immunomodulatory activity of *Astragalus membranaceus* polysaccharides in H22 tumor-bearing mice. *International Journal of Biological Macromolecules, 62*, 287–290.
67. Miraj, S., & Kiani, S. (2016). *Astragalus membranaceus*: A review study of its anti-carcinoma activities. *Der Pharmacia Lettre, 8*(6), 59–65.
68. Zhu, M., Wang, N., Tsao, S., Yuen, M. F., Feng, Y., Wan, T., et al. (2011). Up-regulation of microRNAs, miR21 and miR23a in human liver cancer cells treated with *Coptidis rhizoma* aqueous extract. *Experimental and Therapeutic Medicine, 2*, 27–32.
69. Wang, N., Feng, Y., Lau, E., Tsang, C., Ching, Y., Man, K., et al. (2010). F-actin reorganization and inactivation of Rho signaling pathway involved in the inhibitory effect of Coptidis rhizoma on hepatoma cell migration. *Integrative Cancer Therapies, 9*(4), 354–364.
70. Ibrahim, S. R., & Mohamed, G. A. (2015). Litchi chinensis: Medicinal uses, phytochemistry, and pharmacology. *Journal of Ethnopharmacology, 174*, 492–513.
71. Bhoopat, L., Srichairatanakool, S., Kanjanapothi, D., Taesotikul, T., Thananchai, H., & Bhoopat, T. (2011). Hepatoprotective effects of lychee (Litchi chinensis Sonn.): A combination of antioxidant and anti-apoptotic activities. *Journal of Ethnopharmacology, 136*, 55–66.
72. Sun, W. Y., Wang, L., Liu, H., Li, X., & Wei, W. (2012). A standardized extract from Paeonia lactiflora and Astragalus membranaceus attenuates liver fibrosis induced by porcine serum in rats. *International Journal of Molecular Medicine, 29*, 491–498.
73. Lin, C. S., Kuo, C. L., Wang, J. P., Cheng, J. S., Huang, Z. W., & Chen, C. F. (2007). Growth inhibitory and apoptosis inducing effect of Perilla frutescens extract on human hepatoma HepG2 cells. *Journal of Ethnopharmacology, 112*, 557–567.

74. Wanga, Y., Huangb, X., Hanc, J., Zhenga, W., & Maa, W. (2013). Extract of *Perilla frutescens* inhibits tumor proliferation of HCC via PI3K/AKT signal pathway. *African Journal of Traditional, Complementary and Alternative Medicines., 10.*
75. Xu, W. W., Li, B., Lai, E. T., Chen, L., Huang, J. J., Cheung, A. L., et al. (2014). Water extract from Pleurotus pulmonarius with antioxidant activity exerts in vivo chemoprophylaxis and chemosensitization for liver cancer. *Nutrition and Cancer, 66*, 989–998.
76. Xu, W., Huang, J. J., & Cheung, P. C. (2012). Extract of Pleurotus pulmonarius suppresses liver cancer development and progression through inhibition of VEGF-induced PI3K/AKT signaling pathway. *PLoS One, 7.*
77. Jacobs, E. C. (2018). Potential therapeutic effects of phytochemicals and medicinal herbs for cancer prevention and treatment. *Archives of General Internal Medicine., 02.*
78. Nishino, H. (2009). Phytochemicals in hepatocellular cancer prevention. *Nutrition and Cancer, 61*, 789–791.
79. Ahmed-Belkacem, A., Ahnou, N., Barbotte, L., Wychowski, C., Pallier, C., Brillet, R., et al. (2010). Silibinin and related compounds are direct inhibitors of hepatitis C virus RNA-dependent RNA polymerase. *Gastroenterology, 138*, 1112–1122.
80. Ferenci, P., Scherzer, T. M., Kerschner, H., Rutter, K., Beinhardt, S., Hofer, H., et al. (2008). Silibinin is a potent antiviral agent in patients with chronic hepatitis C not responding to pegylated interferon/ribavirin therapy. *Gastroenterology, 135*, 1561–1567.
81. Falasca, K., Ucciferri, C., Mancino, P., Vitacolonna, E., De Tullio, D., Pizzigallo, E., et al. (2008). Treatment with silybin-vitamin E-phospholipid complex in patients with hepatitis C infection. *Journal of Medical Virology, 80*, 1900–1906.
82. Gopi, S., & Setty, O. H. (2010). Protective effect of Phyllanthus fraternus against bromobenzene induced mitochondrial dysfunction in rat liver mitochondria. *Food and Chemical Toxicology, 48*, 2170–2175.
83. Chirdchupunseree, H., & Pramyothin, P. (2010). Protective activity of phyllanthin in ethanol-treated primary culture of rat hepatocytes. *Journal of Ethnopharmacology, 128*, 172–176.
84. Shen, B., Yu, J., Wang, S., Chu, E. S., Wong, V. W., Zhou, X., et al. (2008). Phyllanthus urinaria ameliorates the severity of nutritional steatohepatitis both in vitro and in vivo. *Hepatology, 47*, 473–483.
85. Koike, K. (2011). Expression of junB is markedly stimulated by glycyrrhizin in a human hepatoma cell line. *Oncology Reports, 25*, 609–617.
86. Ashfaq, U. A., Masoud, M. S., Nawaz, Z., & Riazuddin, S. (2011). Glycyrrhizin as antiviral agent against hepatitis C virus. *Journal of Translational Medicine, 9*, 112.
87. Nakamura, T., Fujii, T., & Ichihara, A. (1985). Enzyme leakage due to change of membrane permeability of primary cultured rat hepatocytes treated with various hepatotoxins and its prevention by glycyrrhizin. *Cell Biology and Toxicology, 1*, 285–295.
88. Lin, G., Nnane, I. P., & Cheng, T. V. (1999). The effects of pretreatment with glycyrrhizin and glycyrrhetinic acid on the retrorsine-induced hepatotoxicity in rats. *Toxicon, 37*, 1259–1270.
89. Gumpricht, E., Dahl, R., Devereaux, M. W., & Sokol, R. J. (2005). Licorice compounds glycyrrhizin and 18β-glycyrrhetinic acid are potent modulators of bile acid-induced cytotoxicity in rat hepatocytes. *The Journal of Biological Chemistry, 280*, 10556–10563.
90. Ogiku, M., Kono, H., Hara, M., Tsuchiya, M., & Fujii, H. (2011). Glycyrrhizin prevents liver injury by inhibition of high-mobility group box 1 production by Kupffer cells after ischemia-reperfusion in rats. *The Journal of Pharmacology and Experimental Therapeutics, 339*(1), 93–98.
91. Korenaga, M., Hidaka, I., Nishina, S., Sakai, A., Shinozaki, A., Gondo, T., et al. (2011). A glycyrrhizin-containing preparation reduces hepatic steatosis induced by hepatitis C virus protein and iron in mice. *Liver International, 31*, 552–560.
92. Saewong, T., Ounjaijean, S., Mundee, Y., Pattanapanyasat, K., Fucharoen, S., Porter, J. B., et al. (2010). Effects of green tea on iron accumulation and oxidative stress in livers of iron-challenged thalassemic mice. *Medicinal Chemistry, 6*, 57–64.

93. Kim, H. J., Yoo, H. S., Kim, J. C., Park, C. S., Choi, M. S., Kim, M., et al. (2009). Antiviral effect of Curcuma longa Linn extract against hepatitis B virus replication. *Journal of Ethnopharmacology, 124*, 189–196.
94. Tuorkey, M. J. (2015). Cancer therapy with phytochemicals: Present and future perspectives. *Biomedical and Environmental Sciences, 28*, 808–819.
95. Lee, S. H., Nam, H. J., Kang, H. J., Kwon, H. W., & Lim, Y. C. (2013). Epigallocatechin-3-gallate attenuates head and neck cancer stem cell traits through suppression of Notch pathway. *European Journal of Cancer, 49*, 3210–3218.
96. Mineva, N. D., Paulson, K. E., Naber, S. P., Yee, A. S., & Sonenshein, G. E. (2013). Epigallocatechin-3-gallate inhibits stem-like inflammatory breast cancer cells. *PLoS One, 8*.
97. Lin, C. H., Shen, Y. A., Hung, P. H., Yu, Y. B., & Chen, Y. J. (2012). Epigallocatechin gallate, polyphenol present in green tea, inhibits stem-like characteristics and epithelial-mesenchymal transition in nasopharyngeal cancer cell lines. *BMC Complementary and Alternative Medicine, 12*.
98. Clarke, N., Germain, P., Altucci, L., & Gronemeyer, H. (2004). Retinoids: Potential in cancer prevention and therapy. *Expert Reviews in Molecular Medicine, 6*, 1–23.
99. Ying, M., Wang, S., Sang, Y., Sun, P., Lal, B., Goodwin, C. R., et al. (2011). Regulation of glioblastoma stem cells by retinoic acid: Role for Notch pathway inhibition. *Oncogene, 30*, 3454–3467.
100. Palmer, H. G., Gonzalez-Sancho, J. M., Espada, J., Berciano, M. T., Puig, I., Baulida, J., et al. (2001). Vitamin D3 promotes the differentiation of colon carcinoma cells by the induction of E-cadherin and the inhibition of beta-catenin signaling. *The Journal of Cell Biology, 154*, 369–387.
101. Garcia, J. J., Lopez-Pingarron, L., Almeida-Souza, P., Tres, A., Escudero, P., & Garcia-Gil, F. A. (2014). Protective effects of melatonin in reducing oxidative stress and in preserving the fluidity of biological membranes: A review. *Journal of Pineal Research, 56*, 225–237.
102. Kakarala, M., Brenner, D. E., Korkaya, H., Cheng, C., Tazi, K., & Ginestier, C. (2010). Targeting breast stem cells with the cancer preventive compounds curcumin and piperine. *Breast Cancer Research and Treatment, 122*, 777–785.

Index

G. P. Nagaraju (ed.), *Phytochemicals Targeting Tumor Microenvironment in Gastrointestinal Cancers*, https://doi.org/10.1007/978-3-030-48405-7

The manufacturer's authorised representative in the EU is Springer Nature Customer Service Centre GmbH, Europaplatz 3, 69115 Heidelberg, Germany. If you have any concerns regarding our products, please contact ProductSafety@springernature.com

Printed and bound by CPI Group (UK) Ltd, Croydon, CR0 4YY
30/07/2026
02181727-0004